Trauma and Recovery

nova
Medicine & Health
New York

Trauma and Recovery

Adversity after the Crash: The Physical, Psychological and Social Burden of Motor Vehicle Crashes
Ashley Craig, Ph.D. and Rebecca Guest, Ph.D. (Editors)
2019. ISBN: 978-1-53614-563-2 (Hardcover)
2018. ISBN: 978-1-53614-564-9 (eBook)

More information about this series can be found at
https://novapublishers.com/product-category/series/trauma-and-recovery/

**VD Sinha, Amit Chakraborty, Jitin Bajaj,
Gaurav Jain and Amit Agrawal**
Editors

Rehabilitation in Neurotrauma

Current Concepts, Practices and Recommendations

nova
Medicine & Health
New York

https://doi.org/10.52305/FLNG2422

NOTICE TO THE READER

Library of Congress Cataloging-in-Publication Data

ISBN: 978-1-68507-787-7

Published by Nova Science Publishers, Inc. † New York

There is a scarcity of books on the topic of rehabilitation following neurotrauma in the existing neurosurgical literature, yet neurotrauma occurs so frequently, and is the condition that neurosurgeons, especially those in the LMIC countries in the Asian-Australian region and in the rest of the world, encounter the most.

As neurosurgeons, whilst we may not be directly involved in the rehabilitation of these patients (although we would have operated on many of them immediately following the neurotrauma), knowing and understanding what management and further care they will need following our neurosurgical interventions is an important part of the care continuum.

I applaud and highly commend Prof. Virenda D Sinha and the authors of this book for their tremendous effort to give us a book that will help and update us in managing patients who suffer the aftermath of neurotrauma. It is what most of us need in the continual care of our patients. I am sure the readers will appreciate the efforts that have gone into the publication of this book, and I am thankful to Prof. Sinha and his team for this book.

Dr. Seow Wan Tew
President,
Asian Australasian Society of Neurological Surgeons (AASNS)

Contents

Preface

Neurorehabilitation is an upcoming area and has become a vital aspect in the management of every neurologic disorder. Neurorehabilitation is a vital aspect in the holistic management of neurological diseases, which includes but is not limited to stroke, trauma, epilepsy, tumors, spine injuries, movement disorders, etc. The book is divided into sections for easy readability. It encompasses all aspects of this modality from basic research to advanced technology and is written by eminent authors working in these fields. The problem-solving approach is a key feature of this book. A special emphasis is given on evaluation and techniques helpful for resource-limited settings. Tables, figures, schemas, and videos are embedded at suitable places for better understanding. Case studies are also included at relevant places. Separate chapters on neurologic problems like cognition, vision, audition, etc. are made for quick and easy grasp. The book is intended for broad academia including neurologists, neurosurgeons, physical therapists, ophthalmologists, otolaryngologists, general practitioners, medical students, paramedical staff, and researchers working in this field. The spectrum includes, but is not limited to, rehabilitation before and after stroke, trauma, tumors, epilepsy, spine injuries, movement disorders, etc. The spectrum is enlarging due to an aging population. Newer advances like robot and automation-assisted rehabilitation, exoskeletons, brain-computer interface, and transcranial magnetic stimulation have added to the armamentarium of this modality. This book is dedicated to basic and advanced aspects of neurorehabilitation. It is intended for a broad academic level including neurologists, neurosurgeons, physical therapists, ophthalmologists, otolaryngologists, general practitioners, paramedical staff, and researchers working in this field. We believe that the book shall benefit neurologists, neurosurgeons, physical therapists, ophthalmologists, otolaryngologists, general practitioners, medical students, paramedical staff, and researchers working in the field of neurorehabilitation.

VD Sinha
Amit Chakraborty
Jitin Bajaj
Gaurav Jain
Amit Agrawal

Chapter 1

Basic Research on TBI Rehabilitation

Narges Ali Kadhem[1,*] and Manar Ahmed Kamal[2]
[1]College of Medicine, Thi-Qar University, Thi-Qar, Iraq
[2]Faculty of Medicine, Benha University, Benha, Egypt

Abstract

Traumatic brain injury (TBI) is related to the brain, skull, and scalp. TBI occurs when sudden, external, or forced injuries damage the brain. TBI is significantly associated with seizures, disorders, handicaps, morbidity, mortality, and death. Brain injury rehabilitation helps patients heal their injuries by preventing, detecting, managing, regular, and advanced medical follow-up. Many brain injury rehabilitation methods are surgical, medical, nutritional, and supplementary interventions. Surgical interventions include craniectomy to extract the injured bone, and hematoma evacuation, whereas medical interventional drugs include sedation and analgesia. Vitamin and mineral supplementation has been shown to improve outcomes for preclinical models in TBI management. This chapter concludes that patients with moderate and severe brain injuries usually require neuroimaging and should be transferred to tertiary centers for intensive neurological monitoring.

Keywords: traumatic brain injury, rehabilitation, basic research, medical interventions, surgical interventions

---

* Corresponding Author's Email: nargesali309@gmail.com.

In: Rehabilitation in Neurotrauma
Editors: VD Sinha, Amit Chakraborty, Jitin Bajaj et al.
ISBN: 978-1-68507-787-7

Introduction

Traumatic brain injury (TBI) occurs when sudden, external, or forced injuries damage the brain. This damage changes brain function and increases the incidence of the signs of brain pathology. TBI is a widespread type of injury significantly associated with seizures, disorders, handicaps, morbidity, mortality, and death worldwide (Al et al., 2014).

Moreover, it has a substantial impact on the standard of living, with a global annual incidence of 106 per 100,000 people (Hyder et al., 2007). -Brain damage changes are characteristic of the following symptoms: consciousness and mental disturbance or impairment, memory loss for previous events or immediately after the mishap, confusion, slow thinking, disorientation, and neurological deficits, including weakness, loss of balance, and distorted vision (Maas et al. 2010). Brain injury rehabilitation helps people heal by preventing, detecting, and managing injuries with regular, advanced medical follow-ups. However, treatment, physiotherapy, speech and language therapy, and other medicines, including neuropsychology, facilitate neuroplasticity, restore body function, and provide compensatory rehabilitation interventions. For example, independent mobility can be achieved using a wheelchair (Turner-Stokes et al., 2015). However, there are still many areas where the evidence is inadequate for comprehensive recovery preparation for each patient (Jolliffe et al., 2018). This book chapter discusses TBI rehabilitation.

Epidemiology

TBI has been dubbed a "silent disease" because of its high incidence and prevalence, but insufficient public awareness (Tandelilin 2010). The epidemiology of TBI has been changing. The majority of TBI among the elderly in high-income countries is increasing owing primarily to drop; traffic-related incidents are more common in developing countries, mainly responsible for the rise in TBI prevalence (Huijben et al. 2020). Individually, however, the total number of TBI-related deaths has decreased in recent years, partly because of increased awareness. Increased knowledge, management, and guidance are structured and significant technological advances in today's world care regimens (Canty et al. 2014). Patients with mild TBI seldom seek medical attention or are treated by general practitioners. As a result, the actual incidence and prevalence of mild TBI are likely to be underreported (Prince and Bruhns, 2017). TBI has been described at 811–979 per 100,000 people per year [16–18]. Thus, the incidence rates for TBI are significantly higher than those in research focused on annual hospital discharge rates (475–6435 per 100,000 people) (Fu et al., 2016).

Medical Intervention

Elevating the Head

Raising an individual's head with TBI usually has immediate consequences. The displacement of intracranial pressure (ICP) lowers this pressure. The promotion of cerebrospinal fluid (CSF) from the intracranial compartment venous outflow describes the blood flow through the veins (Greenberg 2006). Even though the mean carotid pressure is decreased when the bed's head is elevated, the cerebral blood flow (CBF) is unchanged (Feldman et al. 1992).

Prophylaxis for Seizures

To help avoid early seizures, TBI in progress recommendations declare that one week of preventative medicine anti-epileptics is appropriate. However, since there is no evidence that anti epileptics help avoid seizures after a TBI that lasts for a long time, they are usually stopped after seven days (Torbic et al., 2013).

Hyperventilation

It induces cerebral vasoconstriction, which reduces ICP and blood supply to the brain. A lower blood volume is needed for patients with a low level of enforcement to significantly improve ICP (Stocchetti, et al. 1993). As vasoconstriction reduces CBF, prophylactic hyperventilation is not commonly recommended. Additionally, focal areas of ischemia may develop in sites where autoregulation is maintained (Darby et al., 1988). 19 In extreme TBI, hyperventilation is usually only used for a short time during acute neurological deterioration (Greenberg 2006).

ICP Monitoring

The importance of ICP regulation in patients with TBI is reflected in current treatment guidelines (Greenberg 2006). Management of serious traumatic brain injury, 4th Edition (Greenberg 2006). The following are the reasons for ICP monitoring of severe TBI: To reduce mortality in the hospital and for the first two weeks after an accident, it is suggested that severe TBI patients be managed using information from ICP monitoring. Owing to the scarcity of high-quality data to agree with the suggestion, the recommendations no longer specify which patients should be selected for observation. Clinicians should use their clinical judgment and perform intracranial monitoring in patients at high risk of intracranial hypertension and clinical decline (Srinivasan et al., 2014). If the ICP is not carefully controlled, severe consequences may occur. Other thresholds, such as oxygen tension in the brain, can also be monitored, providing physicians with another tool to use brain injury (Bratton et al., 2007). The cornerstone of ICP surveillance is the external ventricular drain, which can drain blood from the heart. Accessed with a catheter, it is still in use. This device18 has both diagnostic and therapeutic applications. Another choice to be implanted if the patient's ventricles are too small is a diagnostic fiber-optic ICP monitor to support a ventricular drain. Because there is evidence that this parameter decreases in cases of severe TBI, new models are now being used to calculate brain oxygen stress more frequently (Chesnut et al., 2012). These modalities assist neurosurgeons in determining which patients are eligible for secure treatment, and patients may need neurosurgical intervention if medical management alone is ineffective in the future (Keddie and Rohman 2012).

Sedation and Analgesia

It is widely agreed that reducing sedation in intensive care unit (ICU) patients improves their results, especially by shortening the time on the ventilator, reducing the duration of hospital stay, and the amount of time spent on the ventilator, facilitating mobilization and lowering the occurrence of delirium (Srinivasan et al. 2014). Sedatives have neuroprotective effects on the brain rather than exacerbating neurochemical cascades that contribute to excitotoxicity and secondary injury. For neurological evaluation, any agent used for this purpose should be short-acting, not increase ICP, and not decrease cerebral perfusion (Baharoglu et al., 2016). Propofol and opioids are the most used sedatives in TBI, followed by benzodiazepines being a less ideal option. However, TBI patients are essential when using large doses of propofol; sufficient intravascular volume should be maintained to prevent the unusual complication of propofol infusion syndrome (Mangat et al., 2015); this is distinguished by renal failure, cardiovascular collapse, rhabdomyolysis, and metabolic (Greenberg 2006) acidosis; barbiturate coma can treat difficult-to-control intracranial hypertension, but not as a preventative measure (Cottenceau et al. 2011). Barbiturate therapy often reduces the rate of metabolism of the brain. Patients may be responders or non-responders, and the test doses may be administered before inducing a barbiturate coma. Because of the possibility of morbidity, the desired effect on ICP is ensured. A coma is caused by barbiturate (infection or; hypotension) (Burke et al. 1981). Table 1 shows some of the most widely used sedatives for acute TBI; as well as their risks and benefits.

Table 1. Sedatives and analgesics commonly used after traumatic brain injury

Sedatives	Hazard	Benefits
Propofol	Propofol infusion syndrome and hypotension	Decrease ICP, CMRO2 and suppresses seizures
Midazolam	Increase delirium and the duration of the MV	Decrease ICP, CMRO2, and amnesia
Barbiturates	Immune suppression, hypotension, ileus	Strongly decrease ICP
Fentanyl/remifentanil	Increase ICP, hypotension, and prolonged MV	Analgesia
Dexmedetomidine	Limited effect on ICP, hypotension, and bradycardia	Quick onset and minimal respiratory depression
Morphine	Unpredictably effect on ICP	Low cost
Ketamine	Variable effect on ICP, hallucinations, and dysphoria	Fat onset suppresses seizures and minimal hypotension

Abbreviations: ICP stands for intracranial pressure, and CMRO2 stands for cerebral metabolic rate of oxygen.

Hyperosmolar Therapy

Hyperosmolar therapy is one of the most commonly used treatments for elevated blood pressure. Hyperosmolar agents (mannitol and hypertonic saline) were injected intravenously. ICP is an acronym for integrated control processes (Keddie & Rohman, 2012). There was no difference in mortality between the hypertonic saline group and the other groups (Mangat et al., 2015). Richard and colleagues 21 performed a meta-analysis of 171 patients from six osmotic therapy trials. They found that hypertonic saline and mannitol effectively lowered ICP in patients with TBI, with hypertonic saline having a statistically insignificant benefit. A group of 47 patients with severe TBI was recruited prospectively by a French group: Twenty-two people were administered 7.5% hypertonic saline, and twenty-five people were 20% mannitol. Both agents effectively lowered ICP; however, the hypertonic saline group had a much more robust and longer-lasting effect. However, there was no difference in functional outcomes (Cottenceau et al., 2011). Osmotic diuretic properties were observed for mannitol. After the immediate impact, the ice is thought to be lowered (Burke et al., 1981).

Surgical Intervention

Surgical Administration of Skull Fracture

The parietal bone, the most frequently fractured bone in the skull, is the occipital bone. The temporal, head, and frontal bones are next (Guyot and Michael 2000). Patients with TBI often experience the following symptoms: depressed fractures and fractures at the skull base are less common than linear fractures. Evidence-based and expert-recommended practices (Petroni et al. 2010). Open skull fractures that are depressed more than the cranium's thickness or more than five mm below the adjacent inner table should be raised and washed out. Fractures with an underlying hematoma (expanding) can also require emergency surgery. Elevating fractures in cases of significant bone displacement improves cosmetics. Bone fragments are typically used for reconstruction; if this is not an option, implants may be used as skull cover defects (Bullock et al., 2006). Patients with open skull fractures are usually administered antibiotics; however, existing evidence does not support regular prophylaxis for all skull fractures (Marbacher et al., 2008).

Craniotomy

Craniotomy is a surgical intervention that involves removing part of the skull to access the intracranial space. It helps neurosurgeons remove intracranial hematomas after TBI (Lazaridis and Czosnyka 2012). Intracranial hematomas can result from increased intracranial pressure, a drop in cerebral perfusion pressure (CPP), hypoxia in the blood, and increased brain edema. Removal of hematomas breaks this vicious cycle. However, if a hematoma is sufficiently large, it can cause herniation and death (Wagner et al. 2001). Therefore, surgical alternatives (craniotomy or decompression craniectomy) are often more suitable for extreme TBI (Compagnone et al., 2007). Radiological examinations, papillary responses, age, and other factors play a role. With the seriousness of this condition, the possible advantages of surgical treatment have increased. Mild or moderate TBI with small hematomas, on the other hand, is often treated conservatively (Compagnone et al., 2007). Although the recommendations often reference essential criteria, such as hematoma length, the decision to proceed with surgical management is based on a more comprehensive image that includes the Glasgow Coma Scale (GCS), pupil anomalies, and details derived from advanced cerebral testing, if applicable (Compagnone et al. 2007).

Epidural Hematomas

Extramural hematomas often occur because of a direct hit to the head, and hematoma typically occurs ipsilateral to the blow. Because significant parenchymal damage is uncommon in isolated extramural hematomas, craniotomy is the preferred surgical procedure in cases of extradural hematomas (Hutchinson and Kolias 2010). Regardless of GCS ranking, existing guidelines suggest epidural hematoma (EDH) evacuation for volumes > 30 ml (Wang et al., 2011). In practice, the patient's neurological condition, age, pre-existing medical conditions, systemic status, hematoma location, and hematoma mass effect are considered when determining whether to perform surgery (Walcott et al., 2011). The skin incision and bone flap are customized to the hematoma size and location; a trauma skin incision and large trauma bone flap are rarely required for EDH. Before the bone flap is removed, the underlying subdural space should be tested for any additional hematuria clots in the subdural space (Polin et al., 1997).

Subdural Hematomas

Torn bridging veins cause acute subdural hematomas (ASDH) during an acceleration-deceleration injury. A plunge down several stairs or a high-speed road traffic collision is the most common mechanism (Paoletti et al., 1983). Compared to EDH, venous bleeding is the most common mechanism of bleeding. Arterial bleeding from small cortical arteries is uncommon, occurring in approximately 20% to 30% of cases (Low et al., 2013). Those with related brain pathologies which are older and have a greater degree of ash have a higher mortality rate (Low et al., 2013). All adult patients with a hematoma thickness of at least one-centimeter Sgt; ten mm or a change in the midline according to existing guidelines and expert consensus, Sgt; five mm should undergo ash surgery (Anthony Marmarou et al. 1996). The two surgical options are craniotomy (replacement of the bone flap at the end of the procedure) and decompression craniectomy (DC) (the bone flap is left out at the end of the process). Since TBI patients with ash may have a significant parenchymal injury and swelling on imaging, they may be affected by ICP increased (Rahme et al. 2010). In 2001, the European Brain Injury Consortium stated that DC was used in approximately one-quarter of all operations for ASH (Honeybul et al., 2018). The RESCUE-aSDH research started in 2014 with the help of the National Institutes of Health (NIH) (NIHR) in the United Kingdom to compare primary DC (bone flap left out) with craniotomy (bone flap replacement) for severe TBI patients undergoing ASDH evacuation (Gladstone, McDermott, and Cooke 1995).

Decompression Craniectomy

A sufficiently large portion of the skull was removed to prevent neurological degradation, allowing for ICP reduction and maintenance of cortical compliance. Prefixing, or removing a part of the skull, has been practiced since the Neolithic times, as evidenced by heads dating from that time (Drosos et al., 2012). The use of DCs in clinical medicine is controversial. ICP reduction and advances in brain tissue oxygen, brain perfusion, and neurochemistry have also been demonstrated (Schuss et al., 2012). However, patient outcomes were less noticeable, prompting randomized trials in the early 2000s (Honeybul & Ho, 2011). DCs is divided into primary and secondary based on when they are performed. First, the bony decompression must be large enough to prevent herniation through the craniectomy window, which would result in compression of the bridging veins, causing a venous infarction and, paradoxically, a worse outcome (Klinger et al. 2014). Several authors recommend a minimum bone flap diameter of 11–12 cm to allow sufficient bony removal and avoid related complications (Klinger et al., 2014). Second, broad durotomy is needed for bony decompression to allow adequate brain expansion. Therefore, a large durotomy is necessary, if not essential, to perform a good DC. The sub-temporal, bifrontal, and front temporoparietal DC methods are the most commonly used (classically considered decompression hemicraniectomy) (Dujovny et al., 1997).

Management of Post-Traumatic Hydrocephalus

Post-traumatic hydrocephalus (PTH) is a well-known complication of TBI. Due to the various diagnostic criteria used, PTH ranges (0.7-29%) (Paoletti, Pezzotta, and Spanu 1983). If VM is used as a diagnostic criterion, the prevalence varies between 30 and 86%. PTH may cause high-pressure headaches and vomiting, deterioration of neurological status, or lack of progress (Anthony Marmarou et al., 1996). There are no specific guidelines for PTH treatment. Adjustable or flow-regulated ventriculoperitoneal shunt appears to be the most frequently defined operation for PTH treatment. Success rates have ranged from 45 to 74% (Low et al., 2013). Shunting has several risks, including infection, shunt failure, occlusion, and overshunting; therefore, patient selection is crucial (Low et al., 2013). PTH has been considered a contraindication to endoscopic third ventriculostomy, although several studies have shown that it can be used safely (Paoletti, Pezzotta, and Spanu 1983). Identifying CSF dynamics and circulation may assist in determining the difference between atrophy and PTH (Anthony Marmarou et al., 1996). It has been suggested that DC could be a risk factor for the onset of PTH. 63, 65 DC performed within 25 mm of the midline were closely linked to hydrocephalus growth. In contrast, others rule out the possibility of a connection between DCs and PTH (Low et al., 2013).

Management of Posttraumatic CSF Leaks

After a closed head injury occurs in 1-3% of all cases, CSF leaks skull base fractures are seen in 10-30% of severe TBI cases. CSF leaks can appear within 48 hours, but they can also appear months later (Paoletti et al., 1983). In an analysis of the treatment of 81 patients with CSF leaks complicating a skull base fracture,

GCS score was found to be a strong predictor of prognosis. A total of 56 CSF leaks were identified (Low et al., 2013). Leaks in the CSF can lead to infection and meningitis in the brain. According to the same report, patient with a GCS score of 8 was significantly more likely to develop meningitis than those with a GCS score of 9 (P = 0.0006) (Anthony Marmarou et al. 1996). It was also discovered that prophylactic antibiotic use for skull base fractures (instead of open fractures) did not affect meningitis rates in either community (Paoletti et al., 1983). As most CSF fistulas, conservative care heals on their own. Lumbar drainage or surgery was the preferredchoicechoices. Even though the transcranial route is still used when there are other indications for transcranial surgery, the latter is more often conducted using an endoscopic transnasal approach (e.g., debridement, depressed fragment, and reconstruction) (Paoletti, Pezzotta, and Spanu 1983). Lumbar drainage helps reduce CSF pressure, which aids in spontaneous resolution and surgery (Rahme et al., 2010).

Therapeutic Studies in Animal Models of TBI

Several TBI animal models have been proposed, all of which have attempted to simulate clinical TBI. TBI animal models, such as control cortical impact injury (CCI), fluid percussion injury (FPI), blast injury model, and weight drop impact acceleration injury (WDIAI), have all been widely utilized in research (Table 2). (Xiong et al., 2013). According to the Federal Publication Institute (FPI), TBI symptoms include cerebral edema, cortical neuronal injury, and intraparenchymal bleeding. A lateral FPI model, which generates localized cortical contusions and transfers traumatic injury to subcortical regions, including the hippocampus and thalamus, was recently added to the FPI model (Thompson et al., 2005). Neuronal failure can develop minutes after a TBI and persist for seven days. However, chemical alterations in subcortical regions such as the septum pellucidum, thalamus, amygdala, and stratum, may take months to complete (Hall et al., 2005). This TBI model features symptoms similar to those in humans and severe neurobehavioral deficits that persist for more than a year after the injury. CCI must be kept in check.

In contrast to the FPI model, the CCI control model displays better injury control, particularly in velocity, force, duration, and depth of damage. This model causes cortical damage, subdural hematoma (SDH), axonal injury, and subcortical injury in the thalamus and hippocampus. The CCI model generates long-term neurobehavioral impairments linked to cortical atrophy and diminished brain perfusion (Goldstein et al., 2012). WDIAI is still expanding. Closed or open head injuries were generated using the WDIAI model. The earliest consequences result in cortical contusion with probable subcortical intracerebral bleeding, which causes a necrotic cavity to form within two weeks after trauma. In this paradigm, the recuperation time ranged from two to three months. In this model, closed head injury results in neurological abnormalities, BBB collapse, neurodegeneration, an inflammatory response with microglial activation, and DAI. The pathophysiology of this model is similar to that of human TBI induced by vehicular accidents or sports injuries (Goldstein et al., 2012). A blast can inflict harm. High-velocity ballistic penetration or the stub of an explosion produces a blast injury model. The path of damage with intraparenchymal bleeding and subsequent cavity development is influenced by blast injury's anatomical and morphological aspects. This model also produces inflammation caused by BBB collapse, cerebral edema, neurodegeneration, tauopathy, and axonal degeneration (Williams and Hartings 2005).

Table 2. TBI animal models that have been commonly used for research

<table>
<tr><th>Focal impact</th><th>Diffuse impact</th><th>Nonimpact</th></tr>
<tr><td>Penetrating and ballistic injury(Ley et al. 2011)</td><td rowspan="3">Impact acceleration (Long et al. 2009)</td><td rowspan="2">Blast injury (Gentner et al. 2009)</td></tr>
<tr><td>Controlled cortical impact (McIntosh, Vink, and Noble n.d.)</td></tr>
<tr><td>Fluid percussion injury</td><td rowspan="2">Rotational TBI (Xiong et al. 2012)</td></tr>
<tr><td>Midline (McIntosh n.d.)</td><td rowspan="3">Diffuse injury (Xia et al. 2017)</td></tr>
<tr><td>Lateral (A Marmarou, Foda, and MA 1994)</td><td rowspan="2">Inertial acceleration (Marklund and Hillered 2011)</td></tr>
<tr><td>Weight drop (Cernak et al. 2004)</td></tr>
</table>

Abbreviations: TBI stands for traumatic brain injury.

Investigation of Therapeutic Strategies in TBI Animal Models

Therapeutic strategies are being investigated in animal models of TBI. This animal model aids in our understanding of the pathological progression of TBI. TBI causes primary and secondary neuron loss, which manifests clinically as varying degrees of neurological impairment depending on the condition and, thus, the magnitude of the neuron loss (Langham et al., 2003). Several studies have been conducted to decrease or avoid TBI-induced neuronal failure. TBI treatment that shows neuroprotective benefits in animal models requires intervention within a few hours after the acute impact (Vergouwen, Vermeulen, and Roos 2006). However, the outcomes of many neuroprotective treatment clinical trials have been inconsistent. Consequently, the neuroprotection therapeutic potential of neuroprotection in TBI studies has been questioned. A few neuroprotective techniques have been investigated in TBI clinical trials and animal models, as listed below (McIntosh n.d.). Calcium channel blockers are a class of medications that prevent calcium from passing through the the body. Calcium accumulation inside the cells may be a significant issue. TBI-induced cellular death can be avoided by neutralizing intracellular calcium using two calcium channel blockers (L-type and N-type) during the cellular damage cascade following TBI (A Marmarou et al., Foda, and MA 1994). The neuroprotective action of nimodipine was identified in 198438, indicating that it might assist in managing brain perfusion and preventing additional neuronal damage. Nimodipine is an L-type calcium channel blocker that has been shown to aid individuals with spontaneous subarachnoid hemorrhage (Cernak et al., 2004). However, a scientific investigation refuted such findings, showing no significant difference in mortality and morbidity in patients with TBI treated with placebo or nimodipine (Long et al., 2009). N-type calcium channel blocker ziconotide (SNX-111). When patients are administered ziconotide41, their mitochondrial activity improves from 15 minutes to six hours after TBI; nonetheless, substantially adverse effects such as hypotension have been noted (Xia et al., 2017). Calcium channel blockers. Increased intracellular calcium may play a critical role in the cellular damage cascade after a TBI. Using two calcium channel blockers (L and N-type) to neutralize intracellular calcium can prevent TBI-induced cell death (Gentner et al., 2009). In 198438, the neuroprotective action was identified, and it was shown to assist in controlling brain circulation and preventing t additional neuronal damage. Nimodipine, an L-type calcium channel blocker, improves patient outcomes with spontaneous subarachnoid hemorrhage (Xiong et al., 2012). However, a scientific investigation refuted such findings, showing no significant difference in mortality and morbidity in patients with TBI treated with placebo or nimodipine (Marklund and Hillered 2011). Ziconotide is a calcium channel blocker that acts on N-type calcium channels (SNX-111). Although ziconotide has been proven to restore mitochondrial activity in individuals 15 minutes to six hours after TBI, significant adverse effects, such as hypotension, have been described. When injected directly into the hippocampal CA2 and CA3, another N-type calcium channel blocker, SNX-185, showed neuroprotective characteristics (Kostron et al. 1984). Hyperosmolar drugs are used to measure ICP in patients with severe TBI. Hyperosmolar saline injections are therapeutic in patients with TBI. Mannitol, hyperosmolar drug, has been shown to reduce ICP in patients with TBI in a dose-dependent manner. Mannitol treatment increases blood perfusion and decreases inflammatory response after TBI (Langham et al., 2003). Amantadine, a dopamine agonist, is used to treat Parkinson's disease. The (NMDA) receptor, which is found in the frontal lobes, is blocked by amantadine. According to one theory, amantadine may protect neurons from glutamate excitotoxicity during the acute phase of TBI (Vergouwen, Vermeulen, and Roos 2006). Amantadine (100–400 mg/d) has been proven to promote arousal and improve cognitive function when administered within 12 weeks of TBI65. The glycoprotein erythropoietin (EPO) has a molecular weight of 30 kD a is secreted. The role of EPO in erythropoiesis regulation was originally recognized in the hematopoietic system (Jelkmann, 1992). EPO and its receptor, EpoR, are extensively expressed in the brain, suggesting that it may have a role in the central nervous system (Hasselblatt, 2006). The brain parenchyma has been found to contain exogenous EPO. Although its relative molecular mass is larger than the molecular threshold of the BBB, it functions in neuroprotection following brain damage (Brines et al., 2000). In various investigations of TBI, EPO was found to have anti-excitotoxic, antioxidant, anti-edematous, and anti-inflammatory characteristics (Cerami et al. 2001). EpoR expression increases following brain damage (Ponce et al., 2013). EPO receptor-deficient mice exhibit fewer neural progenitor cells (NPCs) and a greater incidence of apoptosis (Yu et al., 2002). Neuroprotection is aided by the EPO/EpoR signaling pathway (Ghezzi and Brines 2004). After TBI, EPO receptors in neurons, glia, and endothelial cells. Binding to EpoR activates the JAKNF and PI3K signaling pathways (Ghezzi and Brines 2004). Phosphorylation of AK-2 also activates the PI3K/AKT and Ras/MAPK pathways, as well as STAT-5 homodimerization, all of which have anti-apoptotic and neurotrophic effects (Byts et al., 2008). However, according to a new double-blind, randomized controlled clinical study, EPO does not appear to reduce the number of individuals with severe neurological impairment. The effect of EPO on mortality in patients with moderate or severe TBI is unknown (Digicaylioglu and Lipton, 2001). To corroborate this experimental research findings, more clinical trials must be conducted. Galgano et al. 1123, S100B protein. The BBB was opened following brain injury, and S100B protein was detected in the serum. In neurons, S100B exhibits a dose-dependent dual action. At low doses, S100B acts as a neurotrophic factor for neuroprotection. In large doses, S100B, on the other hand, increases neuroinflammation and decreases neuronal survival (Jia et al., 2014). Hypothermia used refers to decreasing body temperature and becoming cold. In 1945, Fay suggested hypothermia to cure severe brain trauma (Nichol et al., 2015). Since then, many experiments have shown that hypothermia increases TBI outcomes in animal models (Fay, 1943). After a cerebral injury, it is important to keep the brain's temperature under control (MULLAN, RAIMONDI, and SUWANWELA 1961). Deep hypothermia (below 30°C) appears to have little benefit for TBI, whereas mild to moderate hypothermia (32–35°C) appears to have a neuroprotective effect (Hasselblatt et al., 2006). Hypothermia's neuroprotective mechanisms after TBI, on the other hand, remain unclear. Hypothermia has been shown to have various health benefits, including effects on metabolism, excitotoxicity, inflammatory mediators, and autophagy (Lee et al., 2014). Reduction Reduced brain oxygen intake and glucose rate have been related to hypothermia's neuroprotective effect. High-energy phosphate compounds are preserved in the brain, and tissue pH is retained (Fay 1943). Therapeutic hypothermia has been shown to substantially alter genomic transcripts and microRNA responses in rat models of TBI and regulate protein synthesis and translation (Jia et al., 2014). The responses of the genes, miRNAs, and proteins were modified. Hypothermia following TBI may be used to target the delayed responses that regulate secondary brain damage. Although therapeutic cooling has been shown to have strong neuroprotective effects in animal models of TBI, it remains unclear whether hypothermia treatment can provide long-term protection or prolong the injury phase (Byts et al., 2008). The district of Columbia's capital is Washington, DC. DC is a form of neurosurgery in which a swollen brain expands without compression. In brain tumors, strokes, and serious TBI, DCs have been used to lower ICP (Yu et al., 2002). Kocher was the first to mention DC as a treatment for TBI (Cerami et al. 2001). Owing to conflicting clinical and experimental trial findings, most national and international recommendations recommend DC as a third-tier therapy to treat elevated ICP (Ponce et al., 2013).

The role of DCs in the development of brain edema and secondary injury after TBI has been studied in animal models. Using a controlled cortical impact model of TBI, Zweckberger et discovered that early craniectomy prevented secondary brain damage and significantly reduced brain edema in mice (Lee et al., 2014). According to a recent study, DCs can minimize brain edema after TBI by affecting AQP4 expression. On the other hand, Szczygielski and colleagues obtained the opposite results. According to the researchers, surgical decompression exacerbated functional impairments in mice with closed head injuries by fostering brain edema and contusion blossoming (MULLAN, RAIMONDI, and SUWANWELA 1961). Different injury severities from other TBI models may also factor in the performance variations. The severity of the original injury is strongly correlated with the outcome of craniectomy surgery (Nichol et al., 2015). Although the findings of laboratory trials remain controversial, TBI patients' lives are still being saved, and their functional neural conditions are improving owing to DC. Further research is required to determine the types of TBI suitable for DC and the physiological and pathological processes linked to functional outcomes following DC in TBI (Lee et al., 2014).

Nutrition and Supplements

Supplementation and diet can be options for treating the secondary effects of TBI. Nutritional guidelines based on evidence are recommended for TBI patients. Advanced nutritional preparation should begin 24–48 h after TBI, according to a consensus reached in 2011 (Cook, et al., 2009). The survival rates and GCS scores of patients who received enteral nutrition within 48 hof injury were high. A multicenter cohort analysis conducted in 201281 confirmed this. According to other studies, patients should increase their caloric intake and add 1–1.5 g/kg of protein to the diet for the first two weeks after an accident (Wahls et al., 2014). Relevant nutrients can be supplemented based on their function in the mechanisms of brain injury. TBI results in neuronal membrane dysfunction and vascular damage, all of which can lead to ischemia (Girgis et al., 2013). Ischemia can disrupt cellular metabolism and lead to reactive oxygen species (ROS) production, further damaging neuronal membranes (Ten and Starkov 2012). Intracellular Ca^{+2} homeostasis is disrupted when neuronal membranes are weakened, leading to endoplasmic reticulum (ER) stress and possibly apoptosis. Inflammation can be decreased by nutritional targets, development of reactive oxygen species (ROS), neuronal cell death, and complications of TBI. The following are some of the most commonly used dietary supplements for TBI (Maroon et al., 2012).

Vitamins and Minerals

Mineral and vitamin supplementation have been shown to increase outcomes in preclinical models of mild TBI (Cekic et al., 2011). Vitamin D deficiency in rats has been shown to have a worse effect after TBI (Tang et al., 2015). Vitamin D (1 g/kg) and progesterone (16 mg/kg) were found to reduce inflammatory markers and neuronal cell death in a TBI model (Xiao et al., 2008). Progesterone has also been shown to have neuroprotective properties (Conte et al., 2004). Another vitamin to consider in TBI clinical trial therapy is vitamin E. After chronic concussive brain damage in mice, vitamin E supplementation (2 IU/g) significantly enhances memory (Peterson et al., 2015). Vitamin E minimizes oxidative stress and improves learning and memory in a fluid percussion TBI (Maroon et al., 2012). When combined with progesterone, the water-soluble vitamin nicotinamide helps rodents recover faster after mild TBI (Vonder Haar, 2012). After mild TBI in rodents, the most successful neuroprotective neuroprotection effect is a continuous infusion of nicotinamide (150 mg/kg per day) (Cope et al., 2011). This long-term administration method has been associated with better functional recovery (Maes et al. 1994).

On the other hand, folic acid therapy for TBI has been controversial. According to Nail et al., folic acid helps piglets recover more quickly from mild TBI. However, after mild TBI, Wonder Hear and colleagues found that folic acid administration did not affect rodents (Vonder Haar, Emery, and Hoane 2012), indicating that vitamin supplementation has different effects depending on the species (Maroon et al., 2012). Vitamins have yet to be tested in TBI clinical trials. They may be most effective when used as adjuvants to increase the efficacy of promising therapeutics (Sen and Gulati, 2010).

Zinc, a cofactor of superoxide dismutase, has shown promise as a TBI supplement. Zinc has been shown to minimize inflammation, apoptosis, and autophagy in preclinical models of neural injury, in addition to reducing oxidative stress (Cope et al., 2011). In rats after TBI, zinc supplementation (180 ppm) for four weeks was shown to reduce depression and anxiety (Maes et al. 1994). Hypozincemia has been attributed to depression and can be linked to depression following TBI (McClain et al. 1986). Zinc serum levels are lower in patients with moderate TBI, which may be due to hypoalbuminemia, disrupting serum zinc supply after injury (Vonder Haar, Emery, 2012). However, this finding has yet to be verified in cases of mild TBI, necessitating a double-blind clinical trial. Zinc supplementation can help in the preservation of brain tissue and the reduction of neuropsychiatric symptoms in TBI patients. Magnesium aid in recovery after TBI82 in preclinical models (Wahls et al., 2014).

Furthermore, when magnesium was supplemented following mild TBI in humans, Walls et al. colleagues discovered that it is one of the four primary nutrients associated with enhanced somatic scores (Cook et al., 2009). Magnesium depletion is normal after TBI, most likely because of interactions with transient receptor potential metastasis, which results in neuronal cell death. Magnesium reaches the brain readily in rodents after mild TBI, but it has not been shown to increase dramatically in the CNS when supplemented in humans (Wu, Ying, and Gomez-Pinilla 2010). Combined Sen and Multi discovered that taking magnesium with mannitol increases human brain bioavailability. Further research is required to determine whether combining therapy with magnesium supplementation will increase the effectiveness of magnesium supplementation in humans with mild TBI (Haar, Anderson, and Hoane 2011)

Conclusion

TBI is a significant public health problem affecting people worldwide, with a disproportionately high incidence and mortality rate. Although there is currently no successful treatment for TBI, attempts to establish therapeutic methods for TBI recovery have been ongoing for decades. Standard medical and surgical procedures are often essential for the acute management of patients with TBI. A systematic approach is suitable for patients with mild to severe brain injuries. The method identifies high-risk injury pathways, signs, and symptoms that indicate severe head injury. The airway, respiratory physiology, and hemodynamics are all aggressively regulated, with the primary aim of maintaining adequate cerebral perfusion. Following life-threatening situations, a comprehensive head-to-toe examination of the patient was performed for significant injuries. Our book chapter concludes that patients with moderate or severe brain injuries usually require neuroimaging and should be transferred to tertiary centers for intensive neurological monitoring.

References

Al, Wafa, Loganathan Venkatachalam, Somaya Al, and Fatma Al. 2014. "Traumatic Brain Injury Rehabilitation: An Overview." In *Traumatic Brain Injury*, InTech. http://www.intechopen.com/books/traumatic-brain-injury/traumatic-brain-injury-rehabilitation-an-overview.

Baharoglu, M Irem et al. 2016. "Platelet Transfusion versus Standard Care after Acute Stroke Due to Spontaneous Cerebral Haemorrhage Associated with Antiplatelet Therapy (PATCH): A Randomised, Open-Label, Phase 3 Trial." *The Lancet*, 387(10038): 2605–13.

Bratton, S L et al. 2007. "Brain Trauma Foundation; American Association of Neurological Surgeons; Congress of Neurological Surgeons; Joint Section on Neurotrauma and Critical Care, AANS/CNS. Guidelines for the Management of Severe Traumatic Brain Injury." *J Neurotrauma*, 24(Suppl 1): S59–64.

Brines, Michael L, et al. 2000. "Erythropoietin Crosses the Blood-Brain Barrier to Protect against Experimental Brain Injury." *Proceedings of the National Academy of Sciences* 97(19): 10526–31.

Bullock, M Ross, et al. 2006. "Surgical Management of Depressed Cranial Fractures." *Neurosurgery*, 58(suppl_3): S2-56.

Burke, Allan M, Donald O Quest, Shu Chien, and Cesare Cerri. 1981. "The Effects of Mannitol on Blood Viscosity." *Journal of neurosurgery*, 55(4): 550–53.

Byts, Nadiya, et al. 2008. "Essential Role for Stat5 in the Neurotrophic but Not in the Neuroprotective Effect of Erythropoietin." *Cell Death & Differentiation*, 15(4): 783–92.

Canty, Allana L, David H K Shum, Harvey S Levin, and Raymond C K Chan. 2014. "Memory Impairments after Traumatic Brain Injury."

Cekic, Milos, Sarah M Cutler, Jacob W VanLandingham, and Donald G Stein. 2011. "Vitamin D Deficiency Reduces the Benefits of Progesterone Treatment after Brain Injury in Aged Rats." *Neurobiology of aging*, 32(5): 864–74.

Cerami, Anthony, Michael L Brines, Pietro Ghezzi, and Carla J Cerami. 2001. "Effects of Epoetin Alfa on the Central Nervous System." In *Seminars in Oncology*, Elsevier, 66–70.

Cernak, Ibolja, et al. 2004. "The Pathobiology of Moderate Diffuse Traumatic Brain Injury as Identified Using a New Experimental Model of Injury in Rats." *Neurobiology of disease*, 17(1): 29–43.

Chesnut, Randall M et al. 2012. "A Trial of Intracranial-Pressure Monitoring in Traumatic Brain Injury." *New England Journal of Medicine*, 367(26): 2471–81.

Compagnone, Christian et al. 2007. "The Management of Patients with Intradural Post-Traumatic Mass Lesions: A Multicenter Survey of Current Approaches to Surgical Management in 729 Patients Coordinated by the European Brain Injury Consortium." *Neurosurgery*, 61(suppl_1): 1183–92.

Conte, Valeria, et al. 2004. "Vitamin E Reduces Amyloidosis and Improves Cognitive Function in Tg2576 Mice Following Repetitive Concussive Brain Injury." *Journal of neurochemistry*, 90(3): 758–64.

Cook, Naomi L, Corinna Van Den Heuvel, and Robert Vink. 2009. "Are the Transient Receptor Potential Melastatin (TRPM) Channels Important in Magnesium Homeostasis Following Traumatic Brain Injury?" *Magnesium research*, 22(4): 225–34.

Cope, Elise C et al. 2011. "Zinc Supplementation Provides Behavioral Resiliency in a Rat Model of Traumatic Brain Injury." *Physiology & behaviour*, 104(5): 942–47.

Cottenceau, Vincent et al. 2011. "Comparison of Effects of Equiosmolar Doses of Mannitol and Hypertonic Saline on Cerebral Blood Flow and Metabolism in Traumatic Brain Injury." *Journal of neurotrauma*, 28(10): 2003–12.

Darby, Joseph M, Howard Yonas, Donald W Marion, and Richard E Latchaw. 1988. "Local 'Inverse Steal' Induced by Hyperventilation in Head Injury." *Neurosurgery*, 23(1): 84–88.

Digicaylioglu, Murat, and Stuart A Lipton. 2001. "Erythropoietin-Mediated Neuroprotection Involves Cross-Talk between Jak2 and NF-κB Signalling Cascades." *Nature*, 412(6847): 641–47.

Drosos, G I et al. 2012. "Mechanical Characterization of Bone Graft Substitute Ceramic Cements." *Injury*, 43(3): 266–71.

Dujovny, M et al. 1997. "Post-Cranioplasty Cerebrospinal Fluid Hydrodynamic Changes: Magnetic Resonance Imaging Quantitative Analysis." *Neurological research*, 19(3): 311–16.

Fay, T. 1943. "Observation on Generalized Refrigeration in Cases of Severe Cerebral Trauma." *Assoc Res Nerv Dis Proc*, 24: 611–19.

Feldman, Zeev, et al. 1992. "Effect of Head Elevation on Intracranial Pressure, Cerebral Perfusion Pressure, and Cerebral Blood Flow in Head-Injured Patients." *Journal of neurosurgery*, 76(2): 207–11.

Fu, Terence S, Ruwei Jing, Wayne W Fu, and Michael D Cusimano. 2016. "Epidemiological Trends of Traumatic Brain Injury Identified in the Emergency Department in a Publicly-Insured Population, 2002-2010." *PloS one*, 11(1): e0145469.

Gentner, Bernhard et al. 2009. "Stable Knockdown of MicroRNA *in Vivo* by Lentiviral Vectors." *Nature methods*, 6(1): 63–66.

Ghezzi, P, and M Brines. 2004. "Erythropoietin as an Anti-apoptotic, Tissue-Protective Cytokine." *Cell death & differentiation*, 11(1): S37–44.

Girgis, Haymen, et al. 2013. "Effects of Selective and Non-Selective Cyclooxygenase Inhibition against Neurological Deficit and Brain Oedema Following Closed Head Injury in Mice." *Brain Research*, 1491: 78–87.

Gladstone, Hayes B, Michael W McDermott, and Darren D Cooke. 1995. "Implants for Cranioplasty." *Otolaryngologic Clinics of North America*, 28(2): 381–400.

Goldstein, Lee E et al. 2012. "Chronic Traumatic Encephalopathy in Blast-Exposed Military Veterans and a Blast Neurotrauma Mouse Model." *Science translational medicine*, 4(134): 134ra60-134ra60.

Greenberg, M S. 2006. "Handbook of Neurosurgery. 6-Th Ed." *New York*: 289–365.

Guyot, L L, and D B Michael. 2000. "Post-Traumatic Hydrocephalus." *Neurological research*, 22(1): 25–28.

Haar, Cole Vonder, Gail D Anderson, and Michael R Hoane. 2011. "Continuous Nicotinamide Administration Improves Behavioral Recovery and Reduces Lesion

Size Following Bilateral Frontal Controlled Cortical Impact Injury." *Behavioural brain research*, 224(2): 311–17.

Hall, Edward D, et al. 2005. "Spatial and Temporal Characteristics of Neurodegeneration after Controlled Cortical Impact in Mice: More than a Focal Brain Injury." *Journal of neurotrauma*, 22(2): 252–65.

Hasselblatt, Martin, Hannelore Ehrenreich, and Anna-Leena Sirén. 2006. "The Brain Erythropoietin System and Its Potential for Therapeutic Exploitation in Brain Disease." *Journal of neurosurgical anesthesiology*, 18(2): 132–38.

Honeybul, Stephen, et al. 2018. "A Randomised Controlled Trial Comparing Autologous Cranioplasty with Custom-Made Titanium Cranioplasty: Long-Term Follow-Up." *Acta neurochirurgica*, 160(5): 885–91.

Honeybul, Stephen, and Kwok M Ho. 2011. "Long-Term Complications of Decompressive Craniectomy for Head Injury." *Journal of neurotrauma*, 28(6): 929–35.

Huijben, Jilske A et al. 2020. "Changing Care Pathways and Between-Center Practice Variations in Intensive Care for Traumatic Brain Injury across Europe: A CENTER-TBI Analysis." *Intensive care medicine*, 46(5): 995–1004.

Hutchinson, P, and A Kolias. 2010. "Protocol 14PRT/6944: Randomised Evaluation of Surgery with Craniectomy for Patients Undergoing Evacuation of Acute Subdural Haematoma (RESCUE-ASDH)–ISRCTN87370545."

Hyder, Adnan A., et al. 2007. "The Impact of Traumatic Brain Injuries: A Global Perspective." *NeuroRehabilitation*, 22(5): 341–53. http://www.ncbi.nlm.nih.gov/pubmed/18162698.

Jelkmann, Wolfgang. 1992. "Erythropoietin: Structure, Control of Production, and Function." *Physiological reviews*, 72(2): 449–89.

Jia, Yu et al. 2014. "EPO-Dependent Activation of PI3K/Akt/FoxO3a Signalling Mediates Neuroprotection in *in Vitro* and *in Vivo* Models of Parkinson's Disease." *Journal of Molecular Neuroscience*, 53(1): 117–24.

Jolliffe, Laura, Natasha A Lannin, Dominique A Cadilhac, and Tammy Hoffmann. 2018. "Systematic Review of Clinical Practice Guidelines to Identify Recommendations for Rehabilitation after Stroke and Other Acquired Brain Injuries." *BMJ Open*, 8(2): e018791. https://bmjopen.bmj.com/lookup/doi/10.1136/bmjopen-2017-018791.

Keddie, Stephen, and Lebur Rohman. 2012. "Reviewing the Reliability, Effectiveness and Applications of Licox in Traumatic Brain Injury." *Nursing in critical care*, 17(4): 204–12.

Klinger, Daniel R et al. 2014. "Autologous and Acrylic Cranioplasty: A Review of 10 Years and 258 Cases." *World neurosurgery*, 82(3–4): e525–30.

Kostron, Herwig, et al. 1984. "Treatment of the Traumatic Cerebral Vasospasm with the Calciumchannel Blocker Nimodipine: A Preliminary Report." *Neurological research*, 6(1–2): 29–32.

Langham, Julia, et al. 2003. "Calcium Channel Blockers for Acute Traumatic Brain Injury." *Cochrane Database of Systematic Reviews*, (4).

Lazaridis, Christos, and Marek Czosnyka. 2012. "Cerebral Blood Flow, Brain Tissue Oxygen, and Metabolic Effects of Decompressive Craniectomy." *Neurocritical care*, 16(3): 478–84.

Lee, Jin Hwan, et al. 2014. "Therapeutic Effects of Pharmacologically Induced Hypothermia against Traumatic Brain Injury in Mice." *Journal of neurotrauma*, 31(16): 1417–30.

Ley, Eric J, et al. 2011. "Diabetic Patients with Traumatic Brain Injury: Insulin Deficiency Is Associated with Increased Mortality." *Journal of Trauma and Acute Care Surgery*, 70(5): 1141–44.

Long, Joseph B, et al. 2009. "Blast Overpressure in Rats: Recreating a Battlefield Injury in the Laboratory." *Journal of neurotrauma*, 26(6): 827–40.

Low, Chyi Yeu David et al. 2013. "Post-Traumatic Hydrocephalus after Ventricular Shunt Placement in a Singaporean Neurosurgical Unit." *Journal of Clinical Neuroscience*, 20(6): 867–72.

Maas, Andrew I., et al. 2010. "Common Data Elements for Traumatic Brain Injury: Recommendations From the Interagency Working Group on Demographics and Clinical Assessment." *Archives of Physical Medicine and Rehabilitation*, 91(11): 1641–49. https://linkinghub.elsevier.com/retrieve/pii/S0003999310007185.

Maes, Michael, et al. 1994. "Hypozincemia in Depression." *Journal of Affective Disorders*, 31(2): 135–40.

Mangat, Halinder S et al. 2015. "Hypertonic Saline Reduces Cumulative and Daily Intracranial Pressure Burdens after Severe Traumatic Brain Injury." *Journal of neurosurgery*, 122(1): 202–10.

Marbacher, Serge, Robert H Andres, Ali-Reza Fathi, and Javier Fandino. 2008. "Primary Reconstruction of Open Depressed Skull Fractures with Titanium Mesh." *Journal of craniofacial surgery*, 19(2): 490–95.

Marklund, Niklas, and Lars Hillered. 2011. "Animal Modelling of Traumatic Brain Injury in Preclinical Drug Development: Where Do We Go from Here?" *British journal of pharmacology*, 164(4): 1207–29.

Marmarou, A, Abd-Elfattah Foda, and van den Brink MA. 1994. "W., Campbell, J., Kita, H. and Demetradou, K., A New Model of Diffuse Brain Injury in Rats." *J. Neurosurg*, 80: 291–300.

Marmarou, Anthony, et al. 1996. "Posttraumatic Ventriculomegaly: Hydrocephalus or Atrophy? A New Approach for Diagnosis Using CSF Dynamics." *Journal of neurosurgery*, 85(6): 1026–35.

Maroon, Joseph C, Darren B LePere, Russell L Blaylock, and Jeffrey W Bost. 2012. "Postconcussion Syndrome: A Review of Pathophysiology and Potential Nonpharmacological Approaches to Treatment." *The Physician and sportsmedicine*, 40(4): 73–87.

McClain, Craig J, et al. 1986. "Serum and Urine Zinc Response in Head-Injured Patients." *Journal of neurosurgery*, 64(2): 224–30.

McIntosh, T K. "Nobel l, Andrews B., and Faden, AI (1987). Traumatic Brain Injury in the Rat: Characterization of a Midline Fluidpercussion Model." *Cent. Nerv. Syst. Trauma*, 4: 119–34.

McIntosh, T K, R Vink, and L Yamakami Noble. "I., Fernyak, S., Soares, H. and Faden, AI (1989)." *Neuroscience*, 28: 233–44.

Mullan, Sean, Anthony J Raimondi, and Charas Suwanwela. 1961. "Effect of Hypothermia upon Cerebral Injuries in Dogs: Some Observations Made in Cases of Experimental Injury at 28-30 Centigrade." *Archives of neurology*, 5(5): 545–51.

Nichol, Alistair, et al. 2015. "Erythropoietin in Traumatic Brain Injury (EPO-TBI): A Double-Blind Randomised Controlled Trial." *The Lancet*, 386(10012): 2499–2506.

Paoletti, P, S Pezzotta, and G Spanu. 1983. "Diagnosis and Treatment of Post-Traumatic Hydrocephalus." *Journal of neurosurgical sciences*, 27(3): 171–75.

Peterson, Todd C et al. 2015. "A Combination Therapy of Nicotinamide and Progesterone Improves Functional Recovery Following Traumatic Brain Injury." *Journal of neurotrauma*, 32(11): 765–79.

Petroni, Gustavo et al. 2010. "Early Prognosis of Severe Traumatic Brain Injury in an Urban Argentinian Trauma Center." *Journal of Trauma and Acute Care Surgery*, 68(3): 564–70.

Polin, Richard S, et al. 1997. "Decompressive Bifrontal Craniectomy in the Treatment of Severe Refractory Posttraumatic Cerebral Edema." *Neurosurgery*, 41(1): 84–94.

Ponce, Lucido L, Jovany Cruz Navarro, Osama Ahmed, and Claudia S Robertson. 2013. "Erythropoietin Neuroprotection with Traumatic Brain Injury." *Pathophysiology*, 20(1): 31–38.

Prince, Carolyn, and Maya E Bruhns. 2017. "Evaluation and Treatment of Mild Traumatic Brain Injury: The Role of Neuropsychology." *Brain sciences*, 7(8): 105.

Rahme, Ralph, et al. 2010. "Decompressive Craniectomy Is Not an Independent Risk Factor for Communicating Hydrocephalus in Patients with Increased Intracranial Pressure." *Neurosurgery*, 67(3): 675–78.

Schuss, Patrick, et al. 2012. "Cranioplasty after Decompressive Craniectomy: The Effect of Timing on Postoperative Complications." *Journal of neurotrauma*, 29(6): 1090–95.

Sen, Ananda P, and Anil Gulati. 2010. "Use of Magnesium in Traumatic Brain Injury." *Neurotherapeutics*, 7(1): 91–99.

Srinivasan, Visish M et al. 2014. "The History of External Ventricular Drainage: Historical Vignette." *Journal of neurosurgery*, 120(1): 228–36.

Stocchetti, N, C Mattioli, and A Paparella. 1993. "Bedside Assessment of CO2 Reactivity in Head Injury: Changes in CBF Estimated by Changes in ICP and Cerebral Extraction of Oxygen." *J Neurotrauma*, 10(suppl): 187.

Tandelilin, Eduardus. 2010. "Scholar (6)." *Portofolio dan Investasi: Teori dan aplikasi, Kanisius*.

Tang, Huiling, et al. 2015. "Progesterone and Vitamin D Combination Therapy Modulates Inflammatory Response after Traumatic Brain Injury." *Brain injury*, 29(10): 1165–74.

Ten, Vadim S, and Anatoly Starkov. 2012. "Hypoxic-Ischemic Injury in the Developing Brain: The Role of Reactive Oxygen Species Originating in Mitochondria." *Neurology research international*, 2012.

Thompson, Hilaire J, et al. 2005. "Lateral Fluid Percussion Brain Injury: A 15-Year Review and Evaluation." *Journal of neurotrauma*, 22(1): 42–75.

Torbic, Heather, et al. 2013. "Use of Anti-epileptics for Seizure Prophylaxis after Traumatic Brain Injury." *American journal of health-system pharmacy*, 70(9): 759–66.

Turner-Stokes, Lynne, et al. 2015. "Multi-Disciplinary Rehabilitation for Acquired Brain Injury in Adults of Working Age." *Cochrane Database of Systematic Reviews*. http://doi.wiley.com/10.1002/14651858.CD004170.pub3.

Vergouwen, Mervyn D I, Marinus Vermeulen, and Yvo BWEM Roos. 2006. "Effect of Nimodipine on Outcome in Patients with Traumatic Subarachnoid Haemorrhage: A Systematic Review." *The Lancet Neurology*, 5(12): 1029–32.

Vonder Haar, Cole, Michael A Emery, and Michael R Hoane. 2012. "Chronic Folic Acid Administration Confers No Treatment Effects in Either a High or Low Dose Following Unilateral Controlled Cortical Impact Injury in the Rat." *Restorative neurology and neuroscience*, 30(4): 291–302.

Wagner, Simone, et al. 2001. "Suboptimum Hemicraniectomy as a Cause of Additional Cerebral Lesions in Patients with Malignant Infarction of the Middle Cerebral Artery." *Journal of neurosurgery*, 94(5): 693–96.

Wahls, Terry, Linda Rubenstein, Michael Hall, and Linda Snetselaar. 2014. "Assessment of Dietary Adequacy for Important Brain Micronutrients in Patients Presenting to a Traumatic Brain Injury Clinic for Evaluation." *Nutritional neuroscience*, 17(6): 252–59.

Walcott, Brian P, et al. 2011. "Craniectomy for Malignant Cerebral Infarction: Prevalence and Outcomes in US Hospitals." *PloS one*, 6(12): e29193.

Wang, David Z, Deepak S Nair, and Arun V Talkad. 2011. "Acute Decompressive Hemicraniectomy to Control High Intracranial Pressure in Patients with Malignant MCA Ischemic Strokes." *Current treatment options in cardiovascular medicine*, 13(3): 225–32.

Williams, A J, and J A Hartings. 2005. "Lu Xc, Rolli Ml, Dave JR, Tortella Fc." *Characterization of a new rat model of penetrating ballistic brain injury. J Neurotrauma*, 22: 313–31.

Wu, Aiguo, Zhe Ying, and Fernando Gomez-Pinilla. 2010. "Vitamin E Protects against Oxidative Damage and Learning Disability after Mild Traumatic Brain Injury in Rats." *Neurorehabilitation and neural repair*, 24(3): 290–98.

Xia, Xiaoyu, et al. 2017. "Effects of 10 Hz Repetitive Transcranial Magnetic Stimulation of the Left Dorsolateral Prefrontal Cortex in Disorders of Consciousness." *Frontiers in neurology*, 8: 182.

Xiao, Guomin, et al. 2008. "Improved Outcomes from the Administration of Progesterone for Patients with Acute Severe Traumatic Brain Injury: A Randomized Controlled Trial." *Critical care*, 12(2): 1–10.

Xiong, Ye et al. 2012. "Neuroprotective and Neurorestorative Effects of Thymosin B4 Treatment Initiated 6 Hours after Traumatic Brain Injury in Rats." *Journal of neurosurgery*, 116(5): 1081–92.

Xiong, Ye, Asim Mahmood, and Michael Chopp. 2013. "Animal Models of Traumatic Brain Injury." *Nature Reviews Neuroscience*, 14(2): 128–42.

Yu, Xiaobing, et al. 2002. "Erythropoietin Receptor Signalling Is Required for Normal Brain Development." *Development*, 129(2): 505–16.

Chapter 2

Concepts of Neurorehabilitation in Neurotrauma

V. Arvind Kumar, MS, MCh
and Rajesh Alugolu*, MS, MCh
Department of Neurosurgery, Nizam's Institute of Medical Sciences, Punjagutta, Hyderabad, India

Abstract

Neurorehabilitation aims to maximize the physical, psychological and social functioning of an individual. The process of rehabilitation in traumatic brain injury runs in anti-clockwise starting from the severest form to near normalcy taking small strides towards betterment. Historically, the primary goal following neurotrauma was survival which gradually evolved into reducing disability whereby the patient could return to his workplace. This can be achieved by the following approaches: to minimize disability, acquiring new skills and strategies and altering physical and social environment so that a given disability carries minimal handicap. Considering the heterogeneity of physical, cognitive, behavioral and psychosocial sequelae after TBI, rehabilitation program needs to have an individualized and focused approach on the patients' aims, needs, resources, and deficits. The existing literature regarding the use of these interventions is inadequate, however some of the interventions that have been used include neurofeedback, transcranial magnetic stimulation and transcranial direct current stimulation.

Keywords: neurorehabilitation, concepts

---

* Correspondence Author's Email: drarajesh1306@gmail.com.

In: Rehabilitation in Neurotrauma
Editors: VD Sinha, Amit Chakraborty, Jitin Bajaj et al.
ISBN: 978-1-68507-787-7

Introduction

Historically, the primary goal following neurotrauma was survival which gradually evolved into reducing disability whereby the patient could return to his workplace (Ritchie et al., 2014). Studies have shown that return to work is directly related to the severity of injury with rates ranging from 12.5 to 70% for moderate to severe TBI and 100% for mild TBI (Vuadens, Arnold, and Bellmann 2006). Cognitive deficit after TBI is the most important factor which determines the ability of a person to return to his workplace (Zarshenas et al., 2019). Neurorehabilitation takes into account not only the disability but also the handicap that the individual suffers and ranges from early rehabilitation of patients with impaired consciousness to support and reintegration of patients to their social and professional environments (Oberholzer and Müri 2019). Disability is perhaps the most devastating outcome of neurotrauma given its financial and psychosocial implications. Each year, out of 1.4 million people who suffer neurotrauma almost 124,000 people are expected to have long term disability (Zaloshnja et al., 2008). Data on the economic impact of this problem are scarce, but estimates of the Center of Disease Control put it around 56 billion U.S. dollars, annually (Leo and McCrea 2016). Neurorehabilitation aims to maximize the physical, psychological and social functioning of an individual. This can be achieved by the following approaches: to minimize disability, acquiring new skills and strategies and altering physical and social environment so that a given disability carries minimal handicap (Barnes and Radermacher 2003).

Rehabilitation in Neurotrauma

The process of rehabilitation in traumatic brain injury runs in anti-clockwise starting from the severest form to near normalcy taking small strides towards betterment. In severe traumatic brain injury, the usual sequence is coma, disturbed consciousness, post-traumatic agitation and amnesia and finally, recovery of function (Andriessen, Jacobs, and Vos 2010, Zarshenas et al., 2019). In milder forms of TBI though, symptoms such as headache, dizziness, fatigue, sleep disturbances, and balance problems are common complaints and persist for long. Clinical conditions like paroxysmal sympathetic hyperactivity, posttraumatic hydrocephalus, and posttraumatic neuroendocrine dysfunctions are frequently encountered during various phases of rehabilitation. Experimental studies of animals by Oliff et al., 1998

(Oliff et al., 1998) and studies of patients with stroke by Liepert et al., 2000 (Liepert et al., 2000) demonstrated that brain plasticity is activity driven, and according a study by Zhu et al.,2007 the potential to enhance brain plasticity and improve functional recovery is greater in the early stages of recovery after injury (Zhu et al., 2007).

Process of Neurorehabilitation

The entire process of rehabilitation is dynamic and the caregivers have to work closely with the disabled person and their relatives. This involves the following steps:

a. Giving accurate information about the nature of disability, natural history and prognosis
b. Giving due importance to the needs and perceptions of the disabled person and family
c. Interdisciplinary approach
d. Setting realistic goals (Zarshenas et al., 2019).

The goals of rehabilitation need to be patient specific. Once a realistic and achievable goal is established, sub goals can be planned in order to meet the final objective (Dobkin 2003). If for example the long term goal is to walk without assistance then short term goals can be set like sitting without support followed by standing with support followed by standing without support subsequently followed by walking with aid and finally walking without aid.

Components of Rehabilitation Programme

Rehabilitation is the process of enabling an individual to cope with family, friends, work and leisure as independently as possible (Barnes 2003). Impairment, disability and handicap are the keywords of rehabilitation. Impairment is defined as any loss or abnormality of psychological, physiological or anatomical structure or function (Wood 2009). Disability is any restriction or lack of activity resulting from an impairment to perform an activity in the manner or in the range considered normal for people of the same age, sex, and culture (Wood 2009). Handicap is the disadvantage for a given individual resulting from impairment or disability that limits or prevents the fulfilment of a role that would otherwise be normal for that individual (Wood 2009). A holistic rehabilitation program consists of cognitive rehabilitation, individual and group rehabilitation, vocational rehabilitation and family psychotherapy. Out of this neurorehabilitation primarily details with cognitive rehabilitation.

Neurorehabilitation Team

A neurorehabilitation team typically consists of a specialized nursing team, physiotherapists, occupational and speech therapists, neuropsychologists, and physicians; optionally, it could include nutritionists, social workers, and recreational/vocation therapists. The team regularly meets to reassess the patient's state and progress and to discuss treatment goals. Frequent education of the patient and his family is suggested in order to improve the understanding of the treatment plan and possible outcomes (Oberholzer and Müri 2019).

Inclusion Criteria for Rehabilitation

The Canadian INESSS-ONF "Clinical Practice Guideline for the Rehabilitation of Adults with Moderate to Severe TBI" defines that "Rehabilitation programs should have clearly stated admission criteria, which include a traumatic brain injury diagnosis, medical stability, the ability to improve through the rehabilitation process, the ability to learn and engage in rehabilitation and sufficient tolerance for therapy duration." (Lamontagne et al., 2018).

Phases of Neurorehabilitation

Neurological rehabilitation consists of several phases: They are based on the severity of the neurological injuries and their symptoms. The phase in which the patient is determines the treatment (Knecht, Hesse, and Oster 2011).

Phase A – Acute Treatment: Intensive care unit.

Phase B – Early Rehabilitation: The patient's consciousness is usually still severely impaired. Intensive care treatment options are still needed.

Rehabilitative measures are intended to improve the state of consciousness. Inclusion criteria: Permanent ventilation is no longer required, circulation is stable, injuries have been treated, no intracranial pressure.

Phase C – Further Rehabilitation: The patient can already actively participate in the therapy, but still needs to be cared for with high nursing effort. The rehabilitation aims at partial mobilization.

Phase D – Medical Rehabilitation: Starts after completion of the early mobilization and represents medical rehabilitation in the traditional sense. The patient is largely independent in the activities of daily living, s/he possibly needs some technical aid. The patient is able to participate in therapy physically and mentally for several hours a day. She or he is cooperative and is able to be without professional supervision for several hours during the day.

Phase E – Secondary Rehabilitation: This is mostly about professional, social, and domestic reintegration. The treatment results are to be maintained.

Phase F – Activating Rehabilitation: Continuing measures to support, maintain, or improve function.

Timing, Dose and Outcomes of Rehabilitation

According to recent research, rehabilitation after severe TBI should start in the acute phase of hospital care to optimize patient's outcomes and recovery potential (Lamontagne et al., 2018). Khan and associates (2002) reported that implementation of an integrated TBI program reduced the average hospital stay from 30.5 to 12 days (Khan, Khan, and Feyz 2002). Mackay and associates (1992) concluded that "aggressive rehabilitation during acute hospitalization" contributed to a shorter total rehabilitation stay for the group that received acute rehabilitation. They also observed a greater functional capacity in the group that received early treatment, which resulted in a higher employment rate for that group. In a study by Choi and associates (2008), 135 consecutive survivors of severe TBI were studied in a multimodal early rehabilitation unit at a Level I trauma center. Almost two thirds of the patients improved and had a good clinical outcome, and one third reached independence in the activities of daily living. (Choi et al., 2008) Frequency and duration are readily definable for stroke rehabilitation in terms of number of sessions per day or per week, and the time period, in days or weeks, over which the intervention is delivered. Amount however, is harder to quantify. Amount can be quantified as number of repetitions or the number of minutes of active therapy. (Lang, Lohse, and Birkenmeier 2015) While each parameter of dose can influence outcomes, data are accumulating to suggest that amount may be the primary parameter, with frequency and duration as secondary parameters. These data come largely from studies of constraint-induced movement therapy (CIMT), within which task-specific practice is a critical component (Kwakkel et al., 2015).

There has been a general understanding of rehabilitation that more practice is likely better. This vague understanding is largely derived from several decades of testing experimental interventions at arbitrarily-set doses and by comparing higher-dose experimental interventions against lower-dose control interventions (Wolf et al., 2007).The idea that more may be better was further supported by the results of the multi-site, Phase III LEAPS trial. In the LEAPS trial, the groups that received more therapy sessions of locomotor training or home physical therapy had substantially better mobility outcomes compared to the group that received fewer therapy sessions (Duncan et al., 2011). Zhu et al. (Zhu et al., 2007) compared more intensive (4 h/day) to conventional (2 h/d) rehabilitation in 68 patients. A significantly greater number of patients with a more intensive programme reached maximal Functional Independent Measure (FIM) and Glasgow Outcome Scale (GOS) scores within three months with no significant effects at later points in time.The percentage of productive patients (those involved in full- or part-time employment, studying, household management, supported or sheltered work, work trials, voluntary work) was higher in those patients who receive neuropsychologic rehabilitation group (89%) than in the matched control group (55%) receiving conventional clinical care and rehabilitation (Sarajuuri et al., 2005).The likelihood of being productive was greater among patients who were employed or studying at the time of injury, which is in line with previous findings in studies attempting to predict employment outcome after TBI (Ponsford et al., 1995).

Conclusion

Several new technologies that help in neuromodulation have been tried in neurorehabilitation. The existing literature regarding the use of these interventions is inadequate, however some of the interventions that have been used include neurofeedback (Munivenkatappa et al., 2014), transcranial magnetic stimulation (Chantsoulis et al., 2015, George 2010) and transcranial direct current stimulation: (Chantsoulis et al., 2015, Nitsche and Paulus 2000). Considering the heterogeneity of physical, cognitive, behavioural and psychosocial sequelae after TBI, rehabilitation programme needs to have an individualized and focused approach on the patients' aims, needs, resources, and deficits. Furthermore early and adequate neuropsychologically oriented rehabilitation programs can improve psychosocial functioning in terms of productivity in postacute patients with significant TBI. It seems that comprehensive rehabilitation does overcome handicaps and improve outcome.

Conflict of Interest

None.

Source of Funding

Self.

References

Andriessen, T. M., B. Jacobs, and P. E. Vos. 2010. "Clinical characteristics and pathophysiological mechanisms of focal and diffuse traumatic brain injury." *J. Cell Mol. Med.* 14 (10):2381-92. doi: 10.1111/j.1582-4934.2010.01164.x.

Barnes, M. P. 2003. "Principles of neurological rehabilitation." *Journal of Neurology, Neurosurgery & Psychiatry* 74 (suppl 4):iv3. doi: 10.1136/jnnp.74.suppl_4.iv3.

Barnes, Michael P, and Harriet Radermacher. 2003. *Community rehabilitation in neurology*: Cambridge University Press.

Chantsoulis, Marzena, Andrzej Mirski, Anna Rasmus, Yury Kropotov, and Maria Pachalska. 2015. *"Neuropsychological rehabilitation for traumatic brain injury patients."*

Choi, J. H., M. Jakob, C. Stapf, R. S. Marshall, A. Hartmann, and H. Mast. 2008. "Multimodal early rehabilitation and predictors of outcome in survivors of severe traumatic brain injury." *J. Trauma.* 65 (5):1028-35. doi: 10.1097/TA.0b013e31815eba9b.

Dobkin, Bruce H. 2003. *The clinical science of neurologic rehabilitation*. Vol. 67: Oxford University Press.

Duncan, P. W., K. J. Sullivan, A. L. Behrman, S. P. Azen, S. S. Wu, S. E. Nadeau, B. H. Dobkin, D. K. Rose, J. K. Tilson, S. Cen, and S. K. Hayden. 2011. "Body-weight-supported treadmill rehabilitation after stroke." *N. Engl. J. Med.* 364 (21):2026-36. doi: 10.1056/NEJMoa1010790.

George, M. S. 2010. "Transcranial magnetic stimulation for the treatment of depression." *Expert Rev. Neurother.* 10 (11):1761-72. doi: 10.1586/ern.10.95.

Khan, S., A. Khan, and M. Feyz. 2002. "Decreased Length of stay, cost savings and descriptive findings of enhanced patient care resulting from and integrated traumatic brain injury programme." *Brain Inj.* 16 (6):537-54. doi: 10.1080/02699050110119862.

Knecht, S., S. Hesse, and P. Oster. 2011. "Rehabilitation after stroke." *Dtsch Arztebl. Int.* 108 (36):600-6. doi: 10.3238/arztebl.2011.0600.

Kwakkel, Gert, Janne M. Veerbeek, Erwin E. H. van Wegen, and Steven L. Wolf. 2015. "Constraint-induced movement therapy after stroke." *The Lancet. Neurology* 14 (2):224-234. doi: 10.1016/S1474-4422(14)70160-7.

Lamontagne, Marie-Eve, Judith Gargaro, Pascale Marier-Deschênes, Catherine Truchon, Mark Theodore Bayley, Shawn Marshall, Corinne Kagan, Anabèle Brière, and Bonnie Swaine. 2018. "A survey of perceived implementation gaps for a clinical practice guideline for the rehabilitation of adults with moderate to severe traumatic brain injury." *The Journal of head trauma rehabilitation* 33 (5):306-316.

Lang, C. E., K. R. Lohse, and R. L. Birkenmeier. 2015. "Dose and timing in neurorehabilitation: prescribing motor therapy after stroke." *Curr. Opin. Neurol.* 28 (6):549-55. doi: 10.1097/wco.0000000000000256.

Leo, Peter, and Michael McCrea. 2016. "Epidemiology." In *Translational Research in Traumatic Brain Injury*, edited by Daniel Laskowitz and Gerald Grant. Boca Raton (FL): CRC Press/Taylor and Francis Group.

Liepert, J., H. Bauder, H. R. Wolfgang, W. H. Miltner, E. Taub, and C. Weiller. 2000. "Treatment-induced cortical reorganization after stroke in humans." *Stroke* 31 (6):1210-6. doi: 10.1161/01.str.31.6.1210.

Munivenkatappa, A., J. Rajeswaran, B. Indira Devi, N. Bennet, and N. Upadhyay. 2014. "EEG Neurofeedback therapy: Can it attenuate brain changes in TBI?" *NeuroRehabilitation* 35 (3):481-4. doi: 10.3233/nre-141140.

Nitsche, M. A., and W. Paulus. 2000. "Excitability changes induced in the human motor cortex by weak transcranial direct current stimulation." *J. Physiol.* 527 Pt 3 (Pt 3):633-9. doi: 10.1111/j.1469-7793.2000.t01-1-00633.x.

Oberholzer, M., and R. M. Müri. 2019. "Neurorehabilitation of Traumatic Brain Injury (TBI): A Clinical Review." *Med. Sci. (Basel)* 7 (3). doi: 10.3390/medsci7030047.

Oliff, H. S., N. C. Berchtold, P. Isackson, and C. W. Cotman. 1998. "Exercise-induced regulation of brain-derived neurotrophic factor (BDNF) transcripts in the rat hippocampus." *Brain Res. Mol. Brain Res.* 61 (1-2):147-53. doi: 10.1016/s0169-328x(98)00222-8.

Ponsford, J. L., J. H. Olver, C. Curran, and K. Ng. 1995. "Prediction of employment status 2 years after traumatic brain injury." *Brain Inj.* 9 (1):11-20. doi: 10.3109/02699059509004566.

Ritchie, Linda, Valerie A Wright-St Clair, Justin Keogh, and Marion Gray. 2014. "Community integration after traumatic brain injury: a systematic review of the clinical implications of measurement and service provision for older adults." *Archives of Physical Medicine and Rehabilitation* 95 (1):163-174.

Sarajuuri, J. M., M. L. Kaipio, S. K. Koskinen, M. R. Niemelä, A. R. Servo, and J. S. Vilkki. 2005. "Outcome of a comprehensive neurorehabilitation program for patients with traumatic brain injury." *Arch. Phys. Med. Rehabil.* 86 (12):2296-302. doi: 10.1016/j.apmr.2005.06.018.

Vuadens, P, P Arnold, and A Bellmann. 2006. "Return to work after a traumatic brain injury: a difficult challenge." In *Vocational rehabilitation*, 143-163. Springer.

Wolf, S. L., H. Newton, D. Maddy, S. Blanton, Q. Zhang, C. J. Winstein, D. M. Morris, and K. Light. 2007. "The Excite Trial: relationship of intensity of constraint induced movement therapy to improvement in the wolf motor function test." *Restor. Neurol. Neurosci.* 25 (5-6):549-62.

Wood, P. N. H. 2009. World Health Organization International Classification of Impairments, Disabilities and Handicaps. Office of Publications, WHO, Geneva.

Zaloshnja, E., T. Miller, J. A. Langlois, and A. W. Selassie. 2008. "Prevalence of long-term disability from traumatic brain injury in the civilian population of the United States, 2005." *J. Head Trauma. Rehabil.* 23 (6):394-400. doi: 10.1097/01.HTR.0000341435.52004.ac.

Zarshenas, Sareh, Angela Colantonio, Seyed Mohammad Alavinia, Susan Jaglal, Laetitia Tam, and Nora Cullen. 2019. "Predictors of discharge destination from acute care in patients with traumatic brain injury: a systematic review." *The Journal of head trauma rehabilitation* 34 (1):52-64.

Zhu, X. L., W. S. Poon, C. C. Chan, and S. S. Chan. 2007. "Does intensive rehabilitation improve the functional outcome of patients with traumatic brain injury (TBI)? A randomized controlled trial." *Brain Inj.* 21 (7):681-90. doi: 10.1080/02699050701468941.

Chapter 3

Essential Neuroimaging in Rehabilitation

Md Moshiur Rahman*, MS

Neurosurgery Department, Holy Family Red Crescent Medical College, Dhaka, Bangladesh

Abstract

A growing number of neuroimaging investigations focus on rehabilitation-related issues. For interpreting this emerging field of study, a basic familiarity with neuroimaging techniques is required. Scientists have explored brain activities in new and intriguing ways because of the fast-evolving neuroimaging area. These methodologies have improved cognitive rehabilitation research by critically evaluating alterations across both behavior and associated brain anatomy and functioning. Some of the most common approaches for capturing changes in speaking, cognition, concentration, and motor skills are functional magnetic resonance imaging (fMRI), systemic MRI, diffusion-weighted imaging, and electroencephalography. Among other advancements in neuroimaging research, rest-state coherence and evolutionary algorithms are paving the way for new techniques to evaluate rehabilitation-related modifications at a global communications level. Innovative methods combined with traditional clinical assessment and standard quantitative metrics provide the rehabilitation clinician with various tools to learn more about the type and scope of the fundamental neurophysiology.

* Corresponding Author's Email: dr.tutul@yahoo.com.

In: Rehabilitation in Neurotrauma
Editors: VD Sinha, Amit Chakraborty, Jitin Bajaj et al.
ISBN: 978-1-68507-787-7

Introduction

Since the debut of computed tomography (CT) in the 1970s, neuroimaging's ability to capture conformational neurology following the onset of some sort of neurodegenerative illness has vastly increased. Initially, neuroimaging was primarily used for descriptive reasons, that is, to establish the occurrence of a disorder and its approximate location. Early detection of traumatic brain injury (TBI) and stroke was significantly improved by neuroimaging, resulting in a higher proportion of people surviving these neurological events and, as a result, a higher number of people in need of neurorehabilitation. However, neuroimaging for diagnostic and descriptive purposes to discover anomalies did not necessarily modify how neurorehabilitation therapies were delivered. The main focus of neuroimaging in the early days was primarily lesion location (Kertesz, 1994). This was mainly owing to the lack of accurate numerical processes for the "measurement system" of cognitive function apart from crude measurement results such as the size and thickness of a lesion, which had to be done by hand (Bigler, Yeo, & Turkheimer, 1989). While knowing that a hemorrhage had happened and where it was located was undoubtedly helpful, this information was not entirely related to the clinical practice that would be recommended during recovery.

Neuroimaging in Rehabilitation

As neuroimaging technology progressed in parallel with much more digital hardware and improved operating systems, researchers began to look at 3d digital metrics like the diameter of damage and connect this with treatment outcomes (Beloosesky, Streifler, Burstin, & Grinblat, 1995; Levin et al. 1997; Turkheimer, Yeo, & Bigler, 1990). On the other hand, these measurements could only provide a stable, exclusively physical representation of the brain damage at best. Advances in video processing techniques, resolution, responsiveness to disease, and methods to quantify physiological and malignant neuroanatomy became widely available until the time of the revolution, allowing researchers to gain insight into some of the underlying pathophysiology. This special issue will focus on new computer vision and projection approaches that use neuroimaging that gives accurate anatomical information. Complex methods such as diffusion tensor and relaxed state functional MRI can be used to identify these morphometric characteristics and compare them to a big sample group and the actual interconnection of tissues such as the cerebral cortex. Wilde et al. (E. A. Wilde, J. V. Hunter, & E. D. Bigler, 2012) discuss the essential acquisition and analytic methodologies currently accessible for imaging examinations of patients taking interventional treatments, such as visual quantification and structural and functional neuroimaging in rehabilitation results. Voelbel et al. (Voelbel, Genova, Chiaravalotti, & Hoptman, 2012) discuss DTI uses in neurorehabilitation, whereas another study showed how DTI findings could be used to predict memory rehabilitation (Strangman et al. 2012) Benson and colleagues look at how DTI can be used to assess and plan treatment for minor traumatic brain injury. Few studies highlight the efficacy of DTI to provide neurorehabilitation clinicians with information about route integrity. As emphasized by Wilde and colleagues (E. A. Wilde, Hunter, & E. D. Bigler, 2012) from their research on neuroimaging in juvenile neurorehabilitation, advances in connectivity knowledge are crucial to comprehending damaged neuromotor, neurosensory, cognitive, and psychosocial impacts.

Aspects of Neuroimaging

Experts from a range of professions can now explore the electrochemical, morphological, and skills of the brain in sound and pathological conditions in a couple of areas through modern diagnostic tools. The electroencephalograph, which detects brain function, was one of the first technologies for visualizing neurological processes. EEG involves placing electrodes, or sensitive electrical activity recorders, and along the brain's exterior to detect and monitor the cumulative responses of individuals throughout the prefrontal cortex. EEG technique is especially effective at studying resting and comatose stages and detecting and classifying epilepsy in patients. Since it provides rapid timing of neural activity, EEG has a good resolution but a limited image quality because it gets impulses from millions of synapses. Regardless, researchers continue using EEG to help explain the electromagnetic pathways of a number of brain illnesses caused by neurodegenerative or psychiatric factors. EEG is a cost-effective and quick way to detect variations in localized cognitive ability due to a particular therapy or mental stimulation in recovery. Computed scanning, also known as computed axial tomography, is a technique for examining the brain that includes passing X-ray photons through the brain at distinct viewpoints to obtain a three-dimensional representation of the skull. They can quickly calculate the diameter and placement of neurons since different tissue types absorb X-rays differently. CT scans are beneficial for locating acute cerebral masses and are reasonably affordable. Magnetic resonance imaging (MRI) is the most widely used neuroimaging technique for investigating brain structure today (MRI).

In contrast to CT scans, which employ X-rays, MRI depends on the hydrogen ion concentration atoms in the skull that have positively and negatively sides that act as magnets in the transmitter coil by the MR device. In the context of the MR device's magnetic field, atoms coordinate in their orientation, which is subsequently thrown over by radio wave impulses given by the sensor. As the ions reconnect to their polarized relaxed state, they release energy captured by the machine and used to build a three-dimensional image of the skull. MR imaging has a high level of detail in its capacity to discern between different types of tissue and fluid, allowing it to rebuild the brain's structure precisely. Brain tissue density, intense morphometry using surface forms, and regional volumetrics are among the indicators that can be calculated using MRI methodological approaches. DTI is becoming an increasingly common way of thinking about the interconnections and linkages between brain regions and how these are disrupted in the setting of disorder. Functional neuroimaging differs from structural neuroimaging in that it can assess quick biological processes associated with an individual's brain activities utilizing available brain sequences. Using these tools, modern scientists recognize the disorder usually results from scattered neural circuits rather than single brain units. PET became one of the first structural imaging procedures involving the use of implanted radioisotopes effective in tagging various substances to monitor the metabolic activity of the brain. PET's intrusive nature, the high cost of generating radioactive isotopes, and limited spatial resolution have made widespread adoption difficult. In recent years, the development of functional magnetic resonance imaging (fMRI) has expedited the growth of functioning neuroimaging. The hypothesis underpinning functional magnetic resonance imaging (fMRI) is that neural synapses cause fast changes in brain metabolism. FMRI is an excellent system detection of cerebral blood flow enzyme activity fluctuations to identify cognitive function to specific regions. Recent advances in engineering and physics are pushing the current standards of in vivo imaging techniques ahead. Modern high-field strength MRI scanners, on the other hand, have superconducting magnets that produce fields ranging from 7 to 9 Tesla, resulting in pictures with improved spatial resolution and tissue contrast (Nowogrodzki, 2018). The problem is that these machines are relatively costly to acquire and run, which limits their application. One of the most intriguing breakthroughs in neuroimaging is a modern statistical technique that allows the evaluation of theories related to global social cognition and interconnection. Using either neurological information present in MR images, quantitative approaches for analyzing neural correlates, such as practical and integrated networking tools, generate connectivity maps throughout the brain (Farahani, Karwowski, & Lighthall, 2019).

Neuroimaging Techniques from Rehabilitation Literature

Current neuroimaging technologies can define a variety of aspects of cerebral function and its environs in the setting of injuries, and their use in rehabilitation, in particular, has grown in recent years. A range of imaging techniques, like fMRI, structural magnetic resonance imaging (sMRI), resting-state functional connectivity (rs-fcMRI), and electroencephalography (EEG), can be used to assess the impact of cognitive rehabilitation on the structural and functional brain. The volume of studies suggesting the use of fMRI to assess wound healing or replacement has increased in recent years. Hubacher et al. (Hubacher et al. 2015) used functional MRI methods in conjunction with rs-fMRI to investigate the treatment of working memory deficiencies associated with multiple sclerosis. Both fMRI activation and procedural sedation were performed at baseline and follow-up visits, with a 2-month psychotherapy behavioral rehabilitation program supplemented by home exercise. Increased activation in frontal areas was associated with cognitive improvements in name and memory ability in the repaired group over time. Postoperative scanning revealed an overall rise and broad stimulation compared to the control group.

Furthermore, fMRI has been used to determine the efficacy of rehabilitation in patients with aging and neurodegenerative diseases. Mnemonics, semantics, and expanded practice were used to reinforce learning in weekly hour-long sessions. In posttreatment fMRI scans, enhanced stimulation in bilaterally prefrontal areas and bilateral striatum was detected. These studies recommend using functional imaging methods to capture neuronal function during therapy because of its possible higher exposure to underlying alterations due to plasticity.

Diffusion-weighted scanning has become a popular way to assess underlying white matter health and structural network integrity (Voelbel et al. 2012). After ten weeks of memory training, Engvig et al. (Engvig et al. 2012) established the accuracy of DTI in identifying a continuous change in a healthy aging group. They discovered that alterations in white matter structure were connected to enhancements in recognition ability after treatment, implying that intact white matter in such locations was linked to essential cognitive networking devices. As evaluated by DTI, white matter stability is a marker of perfect ideas in robust, ordinarily developing people. Therefore this makes medical rationale (Chung et al. 2018). DTI measurements in determining excellent versus bad responses to intellectual therapeutic intervention and function improvement are becoming more evidence-based.

Neuroimaging Techniques

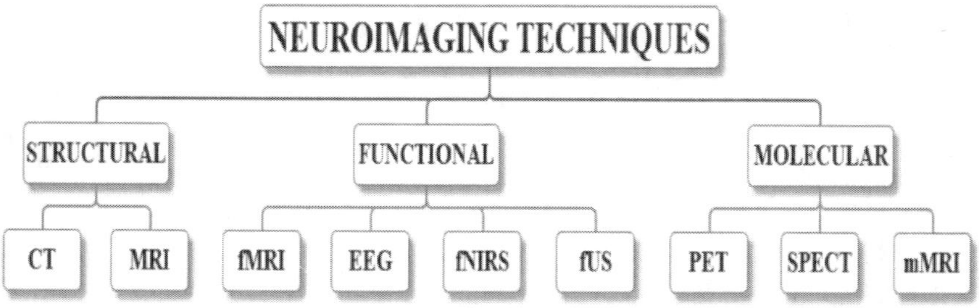

Figure 1. Classification of neuroimaging techniques.

Table 1. Different types of neuroimaging techniques

	Image/Data Quality	Temporal Resolution	Spatial Resolution	Mobility Tolerance	Scale	Safety	Cost
MRI	High	Low (~30s)	Very-High (3-6 mm)	Medium	Bulky	High	High
fMRI	High	Low (~30s)	Very-High (3-6 mm)	Medium	Bulky	High	High
X-Ray	Low	Medium (1s-10s)	Very-High (1 mm)	Low	Bulky	Low*	Low
CT-Scan	Low	Medium (10s)	Very-High (1mm)	Low	Bulky	Low*	Low
Ultrasound	Low	Hi (~1ms)	Depends on the probe element width	Low	Medium	Very-High	Low
PET	High	Low (30s-40s)	High (5mm)	Very-high	Bulky	Low*	Very-high (1-2M$)
SPECT	Medium	Very-Low	Medium (1cm)	Medium	Bulky	Low	High (0.5-1M$)
MEG	Medium	Very-High (~1ms)	Low (1cm - 2cm)	Medium	Bulky	Low	High
EEG/ERP	Medium	Very-High (~1ms)	Medium (1cm)	Low	Small	High	Low
fNIRS	High	High (0.5s-1s)	Low-Medium (0.5cm-2cm)	Medium	Small	Very-High	Very-low

The advantages and disadvantages of the following investigative procedures are based on their strengths and limits. We compare and contrast the various approaches in terms of invasiveness, task capability, geographical resolution, etc. The measured activity's image quality refers to how accurately it is positioned inside the cortex, whereas the spectral resolution relates to how closely the person perceives matches the time of genuine cell activity.

MEG

Magnetoencephalography is a method that makes use of the cosmic rays that exist in all lifeforms. These energies are discovered in conjunction with the brain's inherent magnetic fields. The visible magnetic fields change as cationic streams fluctuate during brain function. Dendritic activation in the cerebral cortex's cell bodies is assumed to be the source of the quantifiable neural signals in MEG (Hämäläinen, Hari, Ilmoniemi, Knuutila, & Lounasmaa, 1993). As a result, this method provides a direct indication of cellular activity. Using the MEG technique, sensors outside the skull monitor the electromagnetic field (Lounasmaa, Hämäläinen, Hari, & Salmelin, 1996). The magnetic field's nature is responsible for this pattern. When the thumb is pointed in the direction of flow, the gravitational flux circles around it in the tip of the fingers, following the "right-hand rule." If the current is vertical of the skull, the gravitational flux will be vertical of the head. The MEG technique can be used to conduct a wide range of behavioral assessments (Henry, 2006; Lounasmaa et al. 1996). Resting brain activity can also be measured using baseline investigations with no task. The "inverse problem" is one consideration in MEG analysis. Although provided the flows inside the skull, the fields outside the head may be calculated without ambiguity; the opposite issue has a no better approach. The thread will run parallel to the head's surface and will not pass through the detection coils. If the stream is symmetrical, the electric force will escape and penetrate the skull. This induced area is a billionth of the size of the earth's magnetic field (Lounasmaa et al. 1996). For a significant signal to be produced out of this flow, the patient and the MEG equipment would be in a field-protected environment.

Positron Emission Tomography (PET)

PET (positron emission tomography) is a technique that uses a fluorescent compound to produce images. Isotopes of carbon, nitrogen, oxygen, and fluorine are frequently utilized in PET research. These isotopes have a short half-life, usually 1 - 2 minutes to two hours. PET entails combining this element with a clinically relevant chemical and injecting or breathing the mixture into the individual. The chemical build of the molecule and the biochemical and blood circulation demands of the brain cause it to concentrate in specific brain locations. When the molecule emits a positron, these locations are detected. When this positron collides with a nearby (1–2 mm) electron, it is annihilated, creating two gamma rays that are almost 180 degrees apart. When two oppositely directed gamma rays collide and hit two photodetectors coincidently and collinearly, the PET scanner identifies them. The PET picture is built on these sorts of detection.

Because a wide range of chemicals can be used, PET can be used to assess the flow of blood, tissue perfusion, neural activity, and neuroreceptor or synapse physiology. PET has a spatial resolution of around 4-5 mm (Cherry & Phelps, 2002). PET investigations benefit from providing a wide range of data thanks to the different labeled compounds accessible. A downside of this technology is that it exposes the victim to radiation, making repeated scanning impossible. Because of this flaw, work recurrence and completing several activities in a single session are limited. Such data can be displayed in various ways, such as maps showing the marked substance's distribution or patterns of challenge fluctuations in cognitive function, similar to MEG.

TMS

Transcranial magnetic stimulation is a one-of-a-kind technology for studying brain activity. TMS activates neurons by producing alternating energy underneath tissue, contrasting techniques of imaging that observe complex organic brain function. Such an approach could trace cognitive function, clarify neural circuits implicated in executive function, and perhaps provide medication as a clinical treatment by modulating cognitive function. Electricity flows through this line, generating a gravity force that flows painlessly and unimpeded through the scalp and skull into the head beneath. Because the activity is produced rather than monitored, the technique's temporal resolution must be viewed differently. Regardless of the type of coil, the spread of spinal fluid, and other factors, the solution ranges from centimeters to millimeters (Walsh & Cowey, 2000).

MRI

As the name implies, magnetic resonance imaging (MRI) uses high electromagnetic waves to produce images of live cells, making use of properties unique to brain tissues and avoiding the use of radiation. MRI can provide details on a variety of atoms. However, the fraction of interest is hydrogen, namely hydrogen linked to water. The magnetic field of the earth is roughly 0.00005 T (Buxton, 2009). Magnetic fields of 1.5 to 3 T are standard in architectural MRI machines. The scanner creates images by adjusting magnetic field gradients and oscillating electromagnetic fields using the stress-related set for the properties of hydrogen atoms (Huettel, Song, & McCarthy, 2004). The quantity and vicinity of hydrogen atoms in cellular organelles, like tendons, malignancies, and greyish or white matter in the skull, can discriminate between tissue types using pulse sequences.

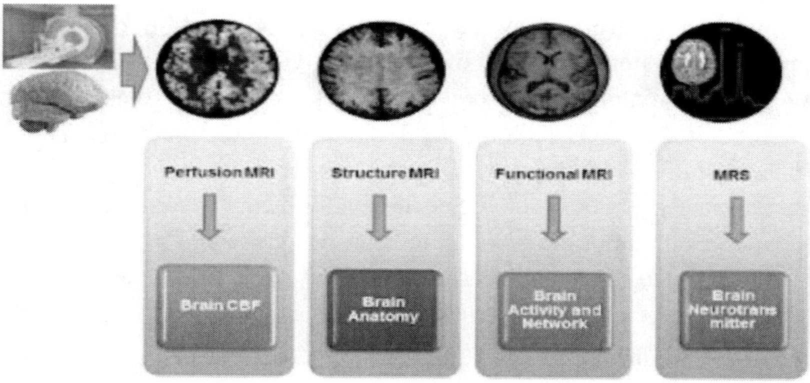

Figure 2. Multimodal neuroimaging approaches.

BOLD Contrast Method

The BOLD contrast approach is an indirect measure of brain activity because it is dependent on the cortical thickness to brain activity. Blood flow increases with brain activity, which has been known since the late 1800s. In 1936, it was found that the magnetic characteristics of hemoglobin largely depend upon what is coupled to oxygen. Hemoglobin that has been deoxygenated is electric, whereas oxygenated hemoglobin is not (DeYoe, Bandettini, Neitz, Miller, & Winans, 1994). The ratio between the two kinds of hemoglobin changes as brain activity rises. In the 1990s, it was discovered that utilizing the BOLD wave; this phenomenon might be used to assess cognitive abilities (Ogawa, Lee, & Barrere, 1993). Both the regional electric potential (Logothetis, Pauls, Augath, Trinath, & Oeltermann, 2001) and the synaptic discharge velocity were shown to have substantial correlations with the BOLD signal (Mukamel et al. 2005). The balance of oxygen consumption and oxygen supply in the brain's microvasculature determines the BOLD contrast in a given brain area. BOLD contrast images employ the signal to indicate how and where intense cognitive function originates throughout a sensory activity, such as fingertip taps or watching a lighting pattern. Such technology is similar to traditional MRI. However, the BOLD fMRI imaging sequence is more reactive to plasma characteristics.

Indications from Neuroimaging and Electrophysiology in Recovery

Neuroplasticity determines the cortex's and non-affected brain's ability to recover development strategy following brain loss or disease. During a cortex lesion in the neuromotor areas, neighboring preserved brain tissues and related fields endure alterations required to reestablish proper motor function. At present, rehabilitation techniques aim to promote recovery by using the brain's intrinsic capacity for constructive remodeling following neurological injury or disease. The authors offer information from many nervous system disorders and repair types to show how neuroimaging and electrophysiological data are beginning to shape and inform rehabilitation approaches.

Clinical Utility of TBI Functional Neuroimaging

Five important clinical goals whose achievement would considerably benefit from functional neuroimaging research based on the Evidence are following:

1. Differentiating between patients who are vegetative, minimally cognizant, and locked-in.
2. Developing creative approaches to help people with TBI recover their motor skills.

3. Identifying ways to improve clinical care to help people with memory problems.
4. Finding ways to reduce the loss of cognitive control following a brain injury through therapy.
5. Developing clinical ways to help people with personality disorders and mental health issues.

In the case of the first clinical goal, knowing whether a patient is vegetative, minimally cognizant, or locked-in is critical for establishing essential communication and designing appropriate clinical care for patients who appear to be unresponsive. Reducing motor impairments in TBI patients is crucial for the second goal because it can allow TBI survivors to resume normal daily activities and minimize caregiver assistance. Memory deficiencies and the reversal of cognitive control deterioration are particularly essential rehabilitation goals, partially because improvements in life quality, resumption of meaningful employment, and other purposes sometimes necessitate substantial intellectual ability recovery. Finally, reintegrating TBI survivors into society, achieving and maintaining emotional stability, and avoiding social disputes can be made more accessible by addressing personality changes and mental health consequences.

TBI Recovery: What Can Be Learned From Neuroimaging?

The cerebral implications of plasticity linked with TBI are being revealed and monitored using functional neuroimaging approaches like PET and fMRI. Furthermore, data collected from neuroimaging techniques can be used to examine the effectiveness of different treatment methods. For instance, functional neuroimaging is used to tailor the decision, planning, and customization of cognitive rehabilitation services for individuals. Ultimately, after TBI, the functional MRI has revealed persistent abnormalities in the head in multiple frontal cortical areas that are routinely engaged in controlling behavioral performance. This research has looked chiefly at single time points and hasn't evaluated specific TBI rehabilitation therapies (Kim, Park, Ko, Jang, & Lee, 2004).

Other Central Nervous System Diseases and Neuroimaging

Recent research has looked at the links between rehabilitation, recovery, and brain function in various central nervous system illnesses. In these studies, cortical rearrangement has been intensively examined, essentially using fMRI, to assess the ability for restoration in people with multiple sclerosis and Alzheimer's disease (Lustig & Buckner, 2004; Morgen et al. 2006; Ukkonen, Dastidar, Heinonen, Laasonen, & Elovaara, 2003; Wang et al. 2006). According to data from the latest report, patients with MS are unable to enhance the activation of the cerebral sensory cortex through active learning, according to data from the latest news that used functional magnetic resonance imaging to scan cognitive abilities throughout measuring the reactivity of patients with MS to mental knowledge (Ukkonen et al. 2003). This observation of diminished neuroplastic change connected with competent task performance could point to a type of plasticity unique to MS patients (Lustig & Buckner, 2004). MS may cause transsynaptic degeneration in brain areas that don't appear to be impacted. Because MS is a white matter illness, this could be the case. It's possible that neuroimaging-based plasticity is pointing to functional brain tissue remodelling over MS-related skeletal muscle damage; white matter plasticity has yet to be discovered. As a result, the cortical areas may be unable to recruit regularly. Even though there is a tiny body of research on the use of neuroimaging to investigate MS rehabilitation, these results suggest that a limited capacity to elicit training-dependent neurocognitive alteration may obstruct healing. To determine whether this is the case, more trials are required. Implicit memory was found to be intact using fMRI, demonstrating that in people with Alzheimer's disease, both actions and attitude for this type of knowledge may be affected. For example, Lustig and Buckner (Lustig & Buckner, 2004) used fMRI to demonstrate that people with mild dementia can regularly use the cerebral cortex. Advances in neuroimaging have changed how we think about and explore human cognitive abilities, malfunction, and recovery. Neuroimaging data is becoming useful in the search for pathways that underpin dysfunction and regulate therapeutic responses. Early signs suggest that certain molecular breakthroughs would spur the creation of even more specific, cognitively influenced medicines, allowing for better therapeutic individualization. Brain Imaging is a topical and crucial thing that provides a venue for integrating cutting-edge neuroimaging technology with rehabilitation.

Three independent clinical studies of the system are administered among the studies using MRI-based neuroimaging to explore comprehension in the multiple sclerosis population. Parisi et al. examine rested phase brain activity fMRI pre and post-computer-assisted cognitive rehabilitation in a randomized controlled experiment (Parisi et al. 2014). Leavitt and colleagues investigated resting-state functional connectivity in a controlled trial. However, they utilized a psychological instead of a computer-based intervention (Leavitt et al. 2014). The study by Dobryakova and colleagues examines the impact of memory restoration following medication in people with MS using fMRI (Dobryakova et al. 2018). Traumatic brain damage is the subject of many investigations and review papers. New biomarkers are being developed all the time, and they will add to the information base. The tailored rehabilitation diagnostics and therapies of the future are made possible by neuroimaging and other complementary techniques.

Conclusion

Preliminary budget proposals, conflicting legal requirements throughout nations and organizations, which aggravate required collaboration, and conventional stereotypes that classify this amount of people with consciousness disorders are just a few of the challenges researchers currently face (Owen, Doyon, Dagher, Sadikot, & Evans, 1998). When weighed against the expected positive effects of neuroimaging, electrophysiologic, and cognitive screening tools, as well as the establishment of successful neurorehabilitative therapies, these tremendous difficulties seem insignificant. Overall, increased research efforts focusing on consciousness disorders and removing numerous barriers to conducting this study could result in a "massive leap" in benefits for informed primary care supporting critically head-injured patients. There is an urgent need for a new conceptualization for study with people who have cognitive issues.

References

Beloosesky, Y., Streifler, J. Y., Burstin, A., & Grinblat, J. (1995). The importance of brain infarct size and location in predicting outcome after stroke. *Age Ageing, 24*(6), 515-518. doi:10.1093/ageing/24.6.515.

Bigler, E. D., Yeo, R. A., & Turkheimer, E. (1989). Neuropsychological function and brain imaging *Neuropsychological function and brain imaging* (pp. 1-12): Springer.

Buxton, R. B. (2009). *Introduction to functional magnetic resonance imaging: principles and techniques*: Cambridge university press.

Cherry, S. R., & Phelps, M. E. (2002). Imaging brain function with positron emission tomography *Brain mapping: The methods* (pp. 485-511): Elsevier.

Chung, S., Fieremans, E., Kucukboyaci, N. E., Wang, X., Morton, C. J., Novikov, D. S., Lui, Y. W. (2018). Working Memory And Brain Tissue Microstructure: White Matter Tract Integrity Based On Multi-Shell Diffusion MRI. *Scientific Reports, 8*(1), 3175. doi:10.1038/s41598-018-21428-4.

DeYoe, E. A., Bandettini, P., Neitz, J., Miller, D., & Winans, P. (1994). Functional magnetic resonance imaging (FMRI) of the human brain. *J Neurosci Methods, 54*(2), 171-187. doi:10.1016/0165-0270(94)90191-0.

Dobryakova, E., Hulst, H. E., Spirou, A., Chiaravalloti, N. D., Genova, H. M., Wylie, G. R., & DeLuca, J. (2018). Fronto-striatal network activation leads to less fatigue in multiple sclerosis. *Mult Scler, 24*(9), 1174-1182. doi:10.1177/1352458517717087.

Engvig, A., Fjell, A. M., Westlye, L. T., Moberget, T., Sundseth, Ø., Larsen, V. A., & Walhovd, K. B. (2012). Memory training impacts short-term changes in aging white matter: a longitudinal diffusion tensor imaging study. *Hum Brain Mapp, 33*(10), 2390-2406. doi:10.1002/hbm.21370.

Farahani, F. V., Karwowski, W., & Lighthall, N. R. (2019). Application of Graph Theory for Identifying Connectivity Patterns in Human Brain Networks: A Systematic Review. *Frontiers in Neuroscience, 13*(585). doi:10.3389/fnins.2019.00585.

Hämäläinen, M., Hari, R., Ilmoniemi, R. J., Knuutila, J., & Lounasmaa, O. V. (1993). Magnetoencephalography---theory, instrumentation, and applications to noninvasive studies of the working human brain. *Reviews of Modern Physics, 65*(2), 413-497. doi:10.1103/RevModPhys.65.413.

Henry, J. C. (2006). Electroencephalography: Basic Principles, Clinical Applications, and Related Fields, Fifth Edition. *Neurology, 67*(11), 2092. doi:10.1212/01.wnl.0000243257.85592.9a.

Hubacher, M., DeLuca, J., Weber, P., Steinlin, M., Kappos, L., Opwis, K., & Penner, I. K. (2015). Cognitive rehabilitation of working memory in juvenile multiple sclerosis-effects on cognitive functioning, functional MRI and network related connectivity. *Restor Neurol Neurosci, 33*(5), 713-725. doi:10.3233/rnn-150497.

Huettel, S. A., Song, A. W., & McCarthy, G. (2004). *Functional magnetic resonance imaging* (Vol. 1): Sinauer Associates Sunderland, MA.

Kertesz, A. E. (1994). *Localization and neuroimaging in neuropsychology*: Academic Press.

Kim, Y. H., Park, J. W., Ko, M. H., Jang, S. H., & Lee, P. K. (2004). Plastic changes of motor network after constraint-induced movement therapy. *Yonsei Med J, 45*(2), 241-246. doi:10.3349/ymj.2004.45.2.241.

Leavitt, V. M., Wylie, G., Krch, D., Chiaravalloti, N., DeLuca, J., & Sumowski, J. F. (2014). Does slowed processing speed account for executive deficits in multiple sclerosis? Evidence from neuropsychological performance and structural neuroimaging. *Rehabil Psychol, 59*(4), 422-428. doi:10.1037/a0037517.

Levin, H. S., Mendelsohn, D., Lilly, M. A., Yeakley, J., Song, J., Scheibel, R. S., Bruce, D. (1997). Magnetic resonance imaging in relation to functional outcome of pediatric closed head injury: a test of the Ommaya-Gennarelli model. *Neurosurgery, 40*(3), 432-440; discussion 440-431. doi:10.1097/00006123-199703000-00002.

Logothetis, N. K., Pauls, J., Augath, M., Trinath, T., & Oeltermann, A. (2001). Neurophysiological investigation of the basis of the fMRI signal. *Nature, 412*(6843), 150-157. doi:10.1038/35084005.

Lounasmaa, O. V., Hämäläinen, M., Hari, R., & Salmelin, R. (1996). Information processing in the human brain: magnetoencephalographic approach. *Proc Natl Acad Sci USA, 93*(17), 8809-8815. doi:10.1073/pnas.93.17.8809.

Lustig, C., & Buckner, R. L. (2004). Preserved neural correlates of priming in old age and dementia. *Neuron, 42*(5), 865-875. doi:10.1016/j.neuron.2004.04.002.

Morgen, K., Sammer, G., Courtney, S. M., Wolters, T., Melchior, H., Blecker, C. R., Vaitl, D. (2006). Evidence for a direct association between cortical atrophy and cognitive impairment in relapsing-remitting MS. *Neuroimage, 30*(3), 891-898. doi:10.1016/j.neuroimage.2005.10.032.

Mukamel, R., Gelbard, H., Arieli, A., Hasson, U., Fried, I., & Malach, R. (2005). Coupling between neuronal firing, field potentials, and FMRI in human auditory cortex. *Science, 309*(5736), 951-954. doi:10.1126/science.1110913.

Nowogrodzki, A. (2018). The world's strongest MRI machines are pushing human imaging to new limits. *Nature, 563*(7729), 24-26. doi:10.1038/d41586-018-07182-7.

Ogawa, S., Lee, T. M., & Barrere, B. (1993). The sensitivity of magnetic resonance image signals of a rat brain to changes in the cerebral venous blood oxygenation. *Magn Reson Med, 29*(2), 205-210. doi:10.1002/mrm.1910290208.

Owen, A. M., Doyon, J., Dagher, A., Sadikot, A., & Evans, A. C. (1998). Abnormal basal ganglia outflow in Parkinson's disease identified with PET. Implications for higher cortical functions. *Brain, 121 (Pt 5)*, 949-965. doi:10.1093/brain/121.5.949.

Parisi, L., Rocca, M. A., Mattioli, F., Copetti, M., Capra, R., Valsasina, P., Filippi, M. (2014). Changes of brain resting state functional connectivity predict the persistence of cognitive rehabilitation effects in patients with multiple sclerosis. *Mult Scler, 20*(6), 686-694. doi:10.1177/1352458513505692.

Strangman, G. E., O'Neil-Pirozzi, T. M., Supelana, C., Goldstein, R., Katz, D. I., & Glenn, M. B. (2012). Fractional anisotropy helps predicts memory rehabilitation outcome after traumatic brain injury. *NeuroRehabilitation, 31*(3), 295-310. doi:10.3233/nre-2012-0797.

Turkheimer, E., Yeo, R. A., & Bigler, E. D. (1990). Basic relations among lesion laterality, lesion volume and neuropsychological performance. *Neuropsychologia, 28*(10), 1011-1019. doi:10.1016/0028-3932(90)90136-c.

Ukkonen, M., Dastidar, P., Heinonen, T., Laasonen, E., & Elovaara, I. (2003). Volumetric quantitation by MRI in primary progressive multiple sclerosis: volumes of plaques and atrophy correlated with neurological disability. *Eur J Neurol, 10*(6), 663-669. doi:10.1046/j.1468-1331.2003.00617.x.

Voelbel, G. T., Genova, H. M., Chiaravalotti, N. D., & Hoptman, M. J. (2012). Diffusion tensor imaging of traumatic brain injury review: implications for neurorehabilitation. *NeuroRehabilitation, 31*(3), 281-293. doi:10.3233/nre-2012-0796.

Walsh, V., & Cowey, A. (2000). Transcranial magnetic stimulation and cognitive neuroscience. *Nature Reviews Neuroscience, 1*(1), 73-80. doi:10.1038/35036239.

Wang, L., Zang, Y., He, Y., Liang, M., Zhang, X., Tian, L., Li, K. (2006). Changes in hippocampal connectivity in the early stages of Alzheimer's disease: evidence from resting state fMRI. *Neuroimage, 31*(2), 496-504. doi:10.1016/ j.neuroimage.2005.12.033.

Wilde, E. A., Hunter, & Bigler, E. D. (2012). Pediatric traumatic brain injury: neuroimaging and neurorehabilitation outcome. *NeuroRehabilitation, 31*(3), 245-260. doi:10.3233/nre-2012-0794.

Wilde, E. A., Hunter, J. V., & Bigler, E. D. (2012). A primer of neuroimaging analysis in neurorehabilitation outcome research. *NeuroRehabilitation, 31*(3), 227-242. doi:10.3233/nre-2012-0793.

Chapter 4

Neural Plasticity and Functional Recovery

Nazmin Ahmed*

Department of Neurosurgery, Ibrahim Cardiac Hospital and Research Institute, Shahbag, Dhaka, Bangladesh

Abstract

The brain has a remarkable ability to remodel itself in response to various sensory inputs. This has been demonstrated in many research publications and the number of these research works is increasing. During early development, this plastic characteristic of the brain is mostly limited to a short period of time which was the traditional view of the plastic nature. However, examples show that neuroplasticity's existence, outside of these finite periods between starting and ending, have existed for some time. In recent times, a better knowledge of several regulators that modify and underpin plasticity has begun to emerge. Through this chapter, we show shreds of evidence to prove that neuroplasticity's mechanisms are highly variable across persons and throughout the life span. This irregularity is caused by several factors, like neuromodulator systems, sex, age, brain disease, inhibitory network function, and psychological attributes. We also discuss the evidence of how neuroplasticity is controlled in both healthy and diseased brains. We propose that our ability to connect brain plasticity in order to develop personalized translational approaches for learning and recovery succeeding brain disease or injury will be improved by our understanding of the individual variances' existence within the diverse mechanisms which control experience-dependent neuroplasticity.

Keywords: neuroplasticity, functional recovery

---

* Corresponding Author's Email: nazmin.bsmmu@gmail.com.

In: Rehabilitation in Neurotrauma
Editors: VD Sinha, Amit Chakraborty, Jitin Bajaj et al.
ISBN: 978-1-68507-787-7

Introduction

Brown and Sherrington stimulated chimps' motor cortex in 1912, proposing the concept of a dynamically structured cerebral cortex (T. G. Brown and Sherrington 1912). Neural plasticity is the central nervous system's (CNS) adaptability with the changing environment or lesions. CNS may modify overall cognitive strategies in order to efficaciously adapt to new challenges like attention and behavioral compensation (Bury and Jones 2002), unmasking the hidden networks (Fridman et al. 2004), employ new/different neural networks (Heuninckx, Wenderoth, and Swinnen 2008), or change in the potency of neural network connections in the particular brain regions, performing a specific task like language, movement, hearing, vision, etc. (Grefkes et al. 2008) may be involved in this property. While conducting both in vivo and in vitro tests, changes in membrane excitability, synaptic plasticity at the cellular level, and structural changes in dendritic and axonal anatomy may be observed in animal as well as human studies (Clarkson et al. 2010; Li et al. 2010).

A growing amount of research enriches our understanding at the cellular and molecular level of neuroplasticity which advances our knowledge in several neurodevelopmental and neurodegenerative disorders. The interindividual variability in different outcomes in neuroplastic process shed light on the complex interaction of neurotransmitters and neuromodulators at the synaptic level along with genetic influence, demographic factors and environmental triggers (Robin et al. 2018; Voss et al. 2017). This complex mechanism plays a pivotal role in functional recovery following CNS injuries such as stroke (Floel and Cohen 2006) and traumatic brain injury (Xiong et al. 2018).

Types of Neuroplasticity

Developmental Plasticity

Developmental plasticity refers to the changes as a result of experience and maturation. During early development, initial synaptogenesis results in the formation of immature neural circuits which undergo synaptic refinement by the complex interaction between neuron and glial cells that leads to elimination of inappropriate connections. This process in known as synaptic pruning where, in addition, strong synapses are reinforced (Robin et al. 2018). Hence, children bear more synaptic connections than adults.

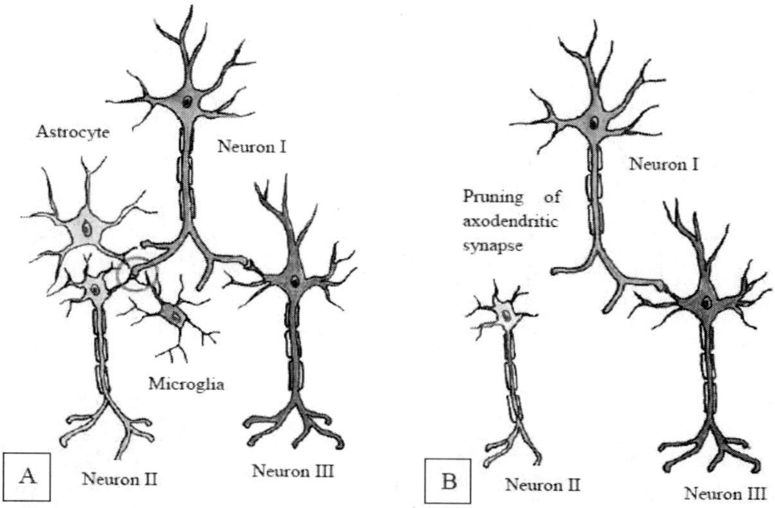

Figure 1. Schematic representation of the complex interaction of neuron with glial cells to maintain synaptic homeostasis. Synaptic remodeling done by the pruning away of an unwanted axodendritic synapse between neuron I and II (A), followed by reinforcement of another axodendritic synapse between neuron I and III(B).

Adaptive Plasticity

The brain reorganizes neurons' way of operation in different regions in response to a deficit. The deficit can occur as a result of brain damage or from birth.

- *Congenital:* Neural plasticity occurs from cradle to grave (Elias and Wagster 2007). The CNS continues to maximize performance during normal human development. Moreover, it learns and adapts to changes in anatomical constraints. For instance, those born blind may have occipital lobes which are used for senses except for vision. This may delineate born blind persons' extraordinary hearing or tactile sensitivity (Voss et al. 2017).
- *Damage from injury:* Whenever a particular area of the brain gets damaged from any pathology, like stroke, other neurons control the

damaged cell's functions. These functions are performed by either sprouting (growth of new dendrites - growth may occur in other parts of the brain adjacent to the damaged area), or rerouting (neurons adjacent to damaged area search for new active connections with healthy neurons) (Li et al. 2010). Rerouting allows the shifting of functions from the damaged area to a healthy area (Vargha-Khadem et al. 1997; Qiu et al. 2017). Moreover, releasing tasks, like running, drinking, etc. helps to form new connections (Heuninckx, Wenderoth, and Swinnen 2008; Hummel et al. 2010). For instance, the substantial recoveries of motor function or language in children, post hemispherectomy, implemented to ameliorate intractable seizures (Vargha-Khadem et al. 1997).

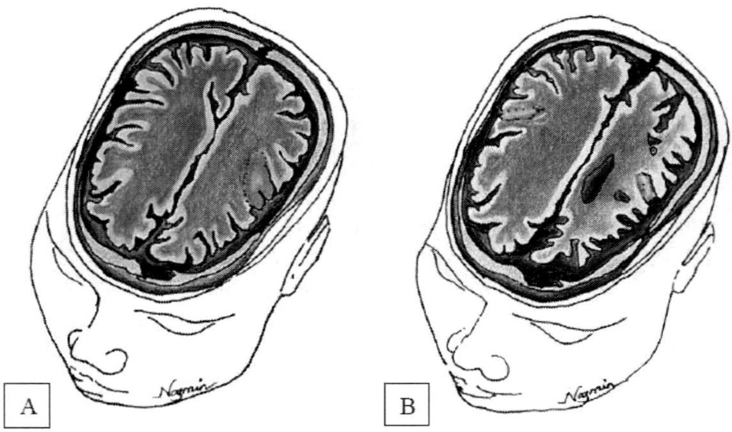

Figure 2. Schematic demonstration of the location of Broca's area in the left cerebral hemisphere of a healthy subject (A); shifting of the area towards right side following traumatic brain injury involving left hemisphere (B).

Cytogenetics

The ability of the human brain to experience neuroplastic changes can be influenced by genetic factors (Pearson-Fuhrhop, Kleim, and Cramer 2009). For instance, a genetic polymorphism (Val66Met) in a brain-derived neurotrophic factor (BDNF) reduces electrophysiological assessments of training-dependent plasticity in the primary motor cortex (Kleim et al. 2006; Cheeran et al. 2008). The conclusion can be drawn from motor learning and recovery of function although it can not be explicitly stated. It needs to be firmly recognized. Interindividual heterogeneity in functional recovery or response to pharmacological or training-based therapies can be partially explained by these considerations. Other pathways being studied include serotonin transporter polymorphisms, catechol-O-methyltransferase gene polymorphisms, and other proteins involved in modifying or regulating neurotransmission. These studies could lead to more individually customized rehabilitative methods for those who have had brain injuries (Pearson-Fuhrhop, Kleim, and Cramer 2009).

Mechanism of Neuroplasticity and the Role of Neuromodulators

Structural changes of neurons and their functional properties can explain the mechanism of plasticity. Synaptic plasticity is the most important among numerous structural changes. It refers to variations in the strength of connections between synapses. There are changes in the protein synthesis inside the cell, alterations in the number of receptors for specific neurotransmitters, and changes in the synaptic efficacy. Neuroplastic changes may be long term (minute to lifetime) or short term (second to a minute). Many existing neural connections are masked by the dominant connections. Following injury, this inhibition is lost which unmasks these connections. These short-term neuroplastic changes are more advantageous than long-term changes. Long-term changes are established only after the formation of new connections. Besides, in this process, neurogenesis plays a vital role. In the hippocampus, neurons can undergo only a limited number of proliferations. Recent studies show some other sites of neuronal proliferation following injury. In contrast, in order to facilitate new synaptic connections, existing neurons can increase their dendritic branches.

The brain, by using adaptive coding, alters the number of resources assigned to a function based on its importance. Depending on a person's particular skills and needs, sensory and motor representations will reorganize. Functional plasticity can be defined as the matching of dynamic reorganization with its inputs. Sometimes the adjacent sensory areas take over those areas that respond to the damaged part of the body, which explains the mechanism of phantom limb ache (Flor, Nikolajsen, and Jensen 2006). Besides, new forms of input are enabled by the plasticity of the brain. For instance, the brain can learn to interpret input from a retinal implant.

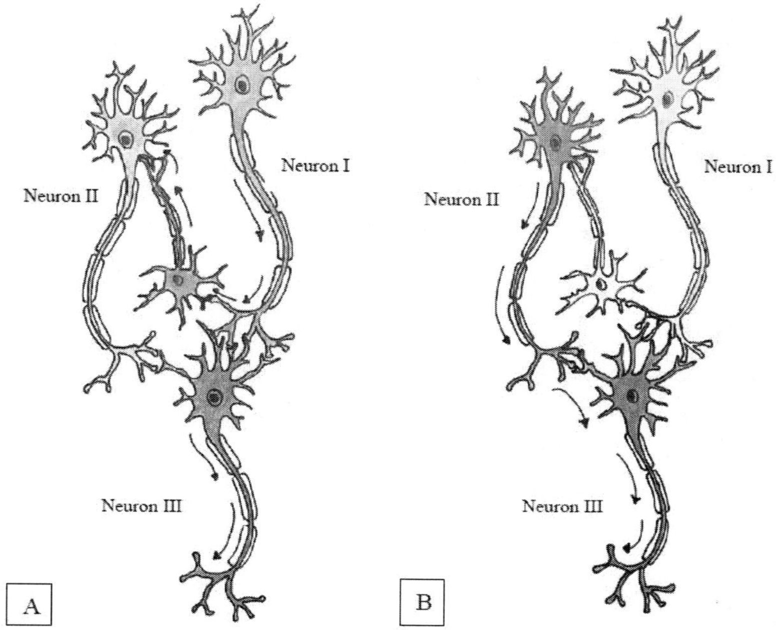

Figure 3. Schematic demonstration of short-term plasticity following disinhibition of the inhibitory neurons (orange) and unmasking the existing connections between neuron II and III (A & B).

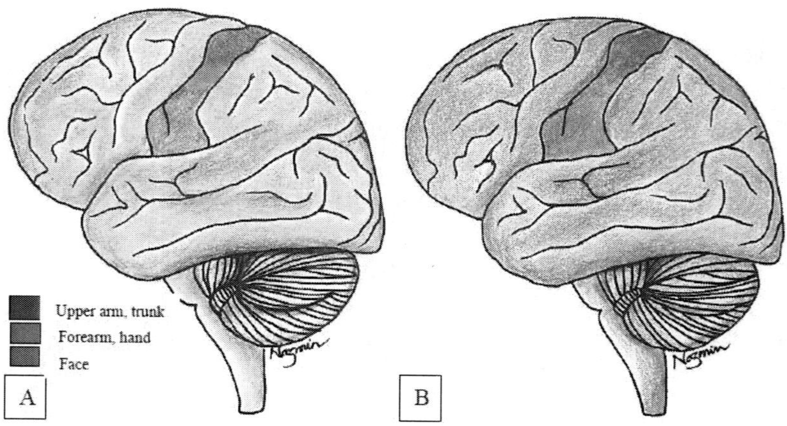

Figure 4. Sensory representation of face, upper limb and trunk in primary sensory cortex of a healthy subject (A); Sensory reorganization after below elbow amputation (B).

Critical Periods, Plasticity Inhibitors and Cellular Brakes

Experience-dependent cortical plasticity is influenced by age. Critical periods can be defined as the vital structural and functional alterations that are likely to happen mostly in the early stage of life in time-limited periods of stimulus-driven plasticity (Knudsen 2004). Sensory representations are calmed with CP closure (Zhang, Bao, and Merzenich 2002; De Villers-Sidani et al. 2007). Inhibitory (GABAergic) cellular networks' maturation and sufficient GABAergic tone maintenance in the cortex are required in this process (Fritschy and Panzanelli 2014). A sequence of plasticity inhibitors and molecular brakes regulate additional modification of these networks and connected cortical plasticity. Functional and structural elements like extracellular matrix components encompass perineuronal nets (PNNs) (Wang and Fawcett 2012), the inhibitory activity of GABAergic interneurons for instance parvalbumin-positive cells (PVC) (Kuhlman et al. 2013), and myelin related proteins (McGee et al. 2005) promote and constrain plasticity. Throughout one's life, the ratio of GABAergic interneurons in the cortex remains largely constant. Yet, with the increase of age, the number of PVC and somatostatin positive (SOMC) interneurons declines. This demonstrates that aging affects different interneuron subtypes distinctively (Ouellet and de Villers-Sidani 2014). Disrupting PNNs (Wang and Fawcett 2012) or down-regulating cortical inhibition (Fagiolini and Hensch 2000) or myelin (McGee et al. 2005) can induce adult brain CP-like plastic remodeling depicting new hope in functional recovery following different CNS insults.

Correlation between Neuroplasticity and Neuro Modulator System

Apart from sensory input, several neuromodulator systems can affect both CPs and adult cortical plasticity by raising neuronal excitability and modulating activity circulation through the cortex (Kirkwood 2007). Early research found that norepinephrine, a major neurotransmitter of the noradrenergic system, is required for ocular dominance column plasticity during the critical time (Kasamatsu, Pettigrew, and Ary 1979). However, research suggested that cortical plasticity requires the balanced action of both noradrenergic and cholinergic networks. This also shows that the two systems are locked in a functional redundancy loop (Bear and Singer 1986). Recent studies have shown that in both humans (Chamoun et al. 2017; Beer, Vartak, and Greenlee 2013) and animal models, the cholinergic system is a strong neuromodulator of attention, learning, and memory (Herrero et al. 2008; Hasselmo and Sarter 2011).

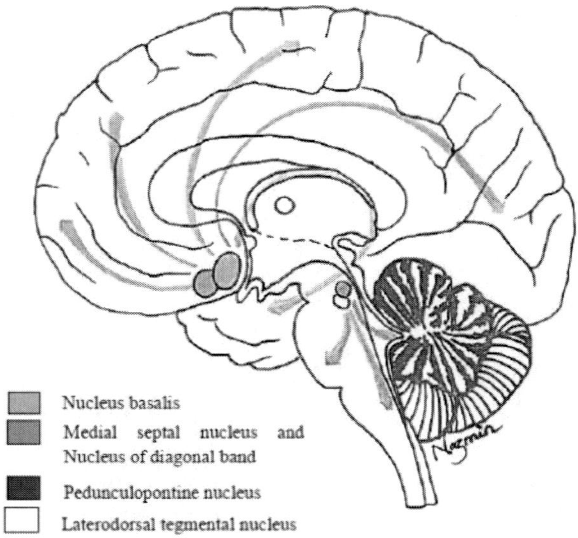

Figure 5. Schematic illustration demonstrates a brief idea about the gating mechanism of neuroplasticity where cholinergic (from nucleus basalis and medial septal nucleus and nucleus of diagonal band in the basal forebrain) and dopaminergic (pedunculopontine nucleus and laterodorsal tegmental nucleus) systems combined play a pivotal role in neuroplastic process to promote functional recovery.

These findings highlight plasticity's main gating mechanisms in the adult sensory cortex whereas neuromodulator systems play a critical role. Moreover, these highlight their vital role in shaping cognitive abilities and cortical function. Certainly, a noteworthy effect of learning and the cortical processing of stimuli observed on rates by stimulating the basal forebrain from where the cholinergic neurons project to the cortex (Kang et al. 2014; Kang and Vaucher 2009) and neurochemically boosting cholinergic transmission (Voss et al. 2016) have been seen. Beside this, it is seen that modulation of plasticity within the sensory cortex (Hui et al. 2009) and enhancement of visual perceptual performance (Noudoost and Moore 2011) are attributed to the stimulation of the dopaminergic system. These findings open up exciting research possibilities that could aid in the development of strategies to increase neuroplasticity in the aftermath of brain damage or in the case of learning challenges. To put it another way, the efficacy of the dopaminergic and cholinergic systems fluctuates throughout time. The maturity of these systems has been linked to cognitive ability.

Moreover, animal studies have found that sex steroids can modulate dopaminergic neurotransmission (Booze et al. 1999). Estrogen increases a baseline dopamine release, striatal dopamine synthesis, and the behavioral and neurochemical response to d-amphetamines significantly (Becker 1999). Previous research has discovered a rather strong link between dopamine receptors and individual differences in self-reported novelty-seeking personality (Norbury and Husain 2015). Furthermore, there are individual variances in sensation-seeking behaviors that are linked to dopamine activity in the brain (Derringer et al. 2010).

Evaluation of Neuroplasticity

Some of the technologies are playing a vital role in the noninvasive evaluation of neuroplastic processes which are related to the recovery of function following CNS lesions. They are positron emission tomography (PET), magnetic resonance imaging (MRI), functional MRI (fMRI), magnetoencephalography (MEG), structural (specifically diffusion tensor imaging, DTI), direct current stimulation, electroencephalography (EEG), and transcranial magnetic stimulation (TMS). These approaches provide information on the potential relationship between anatomical connectivity (DTI), functional activity in specific brain areas, interactions between neural networks (fMRI) and specific behavior, the recovery process, and therapeutic responses (Sharma, Classen, and Cohen 2013).

The existence of resting-state networks is proven by Model "free" analysis using multivariate statistical approaches like independent component analysis and principal component analysis (De Luca et al. 2006). Changes in resting networks may be lost in traditional fMRI study methods. In traditional fMRI studies, one condition (task) is compared to a control condition (most commonly rest). The analysis of dynamic changes in neural networks has been the focus of a lot of research. Even so, there is substantial evidence that motor training can result in structural alterations. Gray matter density changes were measured using voxel-based morphometry (Smith et al. 2007; Wrigley et al. 2009) and DTI was used to assess white matter (Johansen-Berg and Rushworth 2009). A recent study shows the constraints in keeping fMRI data. This includes induced therapy, which is a potential treatment for regaining motor function after a stroke and has caused increased matter density in the damaged hemisphere (Gauthier et al. 2008). Moreover, in our current framework of understanding, it is difficult to predict the increases in gray matter density in the nonaffected hemisphere.

Unlike MRI approaches, MEG and EEG offer millisecond-by-millisecond study of activity in functional networks related to behavior (Pantev et al. 2009). As a result, they can provide information on serial processing or the timing of neuroplastic changes in ways that imaging approaches can't. Furthermore, MEG and EEG can provide crucial information on brain network activity. Moreover, this data is delivered with a high level of temporal precision (Fujioka et al. 2006).

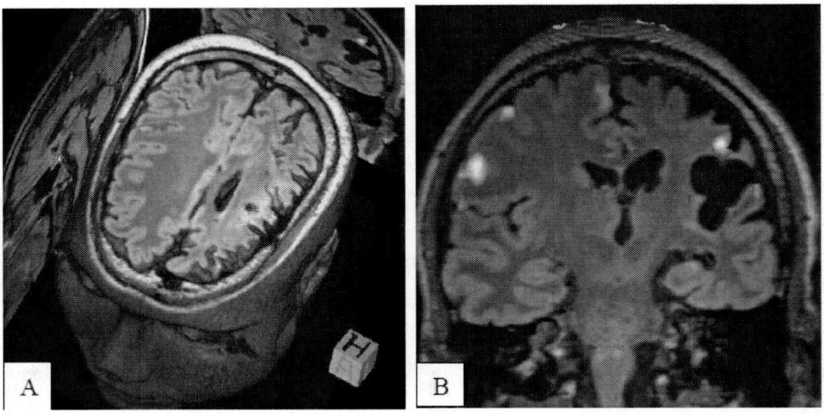

Figure 6. A 32-year-old-male with preceding history of childhood head injury, sustained right sided weakness for 15 years and recurrent episodes of complex partial seizure for 21 years. fMRI was realized using standard multitasking paradigm which demonstrated robust cortical activation in the right motor cortices while relatively poor cortical activation in the left side due to left hemiatrophy. Right frontal lobe activation is noted for native language hence confirming the presence of Broca's area in the right side.

Outcome of Neuroplasticity

Neuroplasticity is a ubiquitous phenomenon. In the outcome of the neuroplastic process, there is interindividual variability. Genetic influence, environmental modifications, age, and pattern of stimulus- all of them are responsible for the outcome. Positive outcomes include the acquisition of new abilities, enhanced aging brain function, greater cognition, more efficient connection between the sensory and motor pathways, a slowdown of the pathogenic process, increasing sensory loss recovery, increased motor control, and improved memory. Adaptive plasticity is the most prevalent type of plasticity examined, and it is generally referred to as a positive consequence (Cohen et al. 1997; Lee 2009). Beside this, it even results in harmful consequences like maladaptive performance of particular tasks or sensory experiences, like impaired performance of the activities of daily living, decline in brain function, altered motor control, and amplified perception of pain etc (Flor, Nikolajsen, and Jensen 2006; Sharma, Classen, and Cohen 2013). This concept is cited as the functional relevance of neuroplasticity.

Future Hope to Treat the Imbalance of Neuromodulator System and Therapeutic Targets to Modulate Plasticity

With significant neuromodulator disparities, several neuropathological conditions exist. One of the hallmark pathophysiological aspects of schizophrenia and Parkinson's disease, for example, is the disruption of dopaminergic networks. Disturbances in the cholinergic and noradrenergic systems, on the other hand, have been linked to Alzheimer's disease and other types of dementia. Perceptual impairments, which are possibly initiated or worsened by neuromodulatory imbalances, often have a connection with these neuropathological conditions. For example, besides lacking higher-order processes in schizophrenia, lacking can be identified throughout the cortex at the early sensory processing level (Javitt 2015). Schizophrenia, in particular, has been linked, in recent years, to a range of low-level auditory dysfunctions as evidenced by electrophysiological, behavioral, and structural metrics (Javitt and Sweet 2015). However, there is an indication that visual cortex plasticity may perhaps also be negotiated with the disease (Çavuş et al. 2012).

In order to target the neuromodulator systems related to neuropathological disorders, explicitly, quite a lot of medications have been developed. As a result, it has an impact on sensory processes as well as brain plasticity. These medications might theoretically be used to target the sensory plasticity mechanism in healthy adults. Furthermore, these medications could be combined with training to protect against natural aging-related perceptual losses. For example, it is seen that occipital cortical responsiveness in rats (Kang, Huppé-Gourgues, and Vaucher 2015) and visual perceptual learning in humans (Rokem and Silver 2010) is significantly improved by cholinergic antagonists. These learning effects can endure for several months after cholinergic stimulation has stopped, according to new research (Rokem and Silver 2013). Through the intake of cholinesterase inhibitors like rivastigmine or donepezil (Colovic et al. 2013), cholinergic functions can also be intensified. These medications are now being utilized to treat various forms of dementia and Alzheimer's disease (Birks 2006).

Beside the application of various pharmacological agents, Sharma and his colleagues proposed another strategy to modulate neuroplasticity. It plays an adaptive function to facilitate and performs a maladaptive function to downregulate it (Sharma, Classen, and Cohen 2013). In both animal and human environments, a variety of treatments have been tested. In humans, pharmacological treatments such as amphetamine, L-dopa, or selective serotonin reuptake inhibitors (SSRIs) (Floel and Cohen 2010) as well as motor training procedures may result in behavioral benefits as well as cortical reconfiguration (Tardy et al. 2006). To improve function by combining traditional training protocols with action observation (Stefan et al. 2005), motor imaging (Sharma et al. 2009), and focused attention (Stefan, Wycislo, and Classen 2004) are proposed in new rehabilitative paradigms (Nelissen, Luppino, and Vanduffel 2009).

In addition to noninvasive approaches for plasticity modification, invasive cortical stimulation with epidural electrodes over the main motor cortex has been reported to have therapeutic benefits in both people and animal models following stroke (J. A. Brown et al. 2006; Plow et al. 2009). It causes clear effects on somatosensory motor functions due to manipulation of somatosensory input while hand anesthesia in healthy humans brings about rises in excitability and improved tactile discrimination in the non-anesthetized hand. Following this principle, somatosensory stimulation of the median, ulnar, and/or radial nerves at the wrist causes significant increases in fMRI activation and cortical excitability in the stimulated hand motor cortical representations (Ridding et al. 2001), as well as comparable short-term electrophysiological beneficial effects on paretic hand functions and the documented correction of abnormalities in interhemispheric interactions between the primary motor cortices (Floel et al. 2008; Celnik et al. 2007; Sheffler et al. 2006). Results of those studies are consistent, which open a new hope in neurorehabilitation to promote functional recovery.

Future Research Aspects

More research is needed to better understand how to modify aging and disease-related plastic changes in the sensory cortex. It will then offer us improved behavioral training paradigms or tailor stimulus exposure to create the aimed behavioral and functional outcome measures. Without precisely establishing a connection with behavior, it will be difficult to determine if the reorganization is adaptive or maladaptive. When procedures allow for functional perturbation of special relevance to show causation, studies focusing on this goal will be critical.

Individual characteristics such as gender, age, drug usage, and pathological conditions must all be taken into account when developing tailored treatments for memory, learning, and recovery from brain injury and disease. Neuromodulator systems, in particular, differ greatly from person to person. This is most apparent when a wide range of interindividual changeability in the effects of dopaminergic, cholinergic, and noradrenergic drugs, irrespective of the anticipated outcome measure is considered (Keers and Aitchison 2010; Turner, Park, and Pirmohamed 2015).

Conclusion

In the last decade, we've made significant progress in our knowledge of the CNS's ability to rearrange in response to changes in the environment and lesions. This knowledge led to improvements in our understanding of both action and cognition systems in health and sickness. An understanding of these neuroplastic principles is gradually leading to the creation of more reasonable, hypothesis-driven techniques to improve function recovery.

References

Bear, Mark F., and Wolf Singer. 1986. "Modulation of Visual Cortical Plasticity by Acetylcholine and Noradrenaline." *Nature* 320 (6058): 172–76. https://doi.org/10.1038/320172a0.

Becker, Jill B. 1999. "Gender Differences in Dopaminergic Function in Striatum and Nucleus Accumbens." *Pharmacology Biochemistry and Behavior* 64 (4): 803–12. https://doi.org/10.1016/S0091-3057(99)00168-9.

Beer, Anton L., Devavrat Vartak, and Mark W. Greenlee. 2013. "Nicotine Facilitates Memory Consolidation in Perceptual Learning." *Neuropharmacology* 64: 443–51. https://doi.org/10.1016/j.neuropharm.2012.06.019.

Birks, J. 2006. "Cholinesterase Inhibitors for Alzheimer's Disease. [Review] [47 Refs] BT - Cochrane Database of Systematic Reviews."

Booze, Rosemarie M., Marian A. Welch, Marcie L. Wood, Katharyn A. Billings, Stephanie R. Apple, and Charles F. Mactutus. 1999. "Behavioral Sensitization Following Repeated Intravenous Nicotine Administration: Gender Differences and Gonadal Hormones." *Pharmacology Biochemistry and Behavior* 64 (4): 827–39. https://doi.org/10.1016/S0091-3057(99)00169-0.

Brown, Jeffrey A., Helmi L. Lutsep, Martin Weinand, and Steven C. Cramer. 2006. "Motor Cortex Stimulation for the Enhancement of Recovery from Stroke: A Prospective, Multicenter Safety Study." *Neurosurgery* 58 (3): 464–71. https://doi.org/10.1227/01.NEU.0000197100.63931.04.

Brown, Thomas Graham, and Charles Scott Sherrington. 1912. "On the Instability of a Cortical Point." *Proceedings of the Royal Society of London. Series B, Containing Papers of a Biological Character* 85 (579): 250–77. https://doi.org/10.1098/rspb.1912.0050.

Bury, Scott D., and Theresa A. Jones. 2002. "Unilateral Sensorimotor Cortex Lesions in Adult Rats Facilitate Motor Skill Learning with the 'Unaffected' Forelimb and Training-Induced Dendritic Structural Plasticity in the Motor Cortex." *Journal of Neuroscience* 22 (19): 8597–8606. https://doi.org/10.1523/jneurosci.22-19-08597.2002.

Çavuş, Idil, Robert M.G. Reinhart, Brian J. Roach, Ralitza Gueorguieva, Timothy J. Teyler, Wesley C. Clapp, Judith M. Ford, John H. Krystal, and Daniel H. Mathalon. 2012. "Impaired Visual Cortical Plasticity in Schizophrenia." *Biological Psychiatry* 71 (6): 512–20. https://doi.org/10.1016/j.biopsych.2012.01.013.

Celnik, Pablo, Friedhelm Hummel, Michelle Harris-Love, Rebecca Wolk, and Leonardo G. Cohen. 2007. "Somatosensory Stimulation Enhances the Effects of Training Functional Hand Tasks in Patients With Chronic Stroke." *Archives of Physical Medicine and Rehabilitation* 88 (11): 1369–76. https://doi.org/10.1016/j.apmr.2007.08.001.

Chamoun, Mira, Frédéric Huppé-Gourgues, Isabelle Legault, Pedro Rosa-Neto, Daniela Dumbrava, Jocelyn Faubert, and Elvire Vaucher. 2017. "Cholinergic Potentiation Improves Perceptual-Cognitive Training of Healthy Young Adults in Three Dimensional Multiple Object Tracking." *Frontiers in Human Neuroscience* 11. https://doi.org/10.3389/fnhum.2017.00128.

Cheeran, Binith, Penelope Talelli, Francesco Mori, Giacomo Koch, Antonio Suppa, Mark Edwards, Henry Houlden, Kailash Bhatia, Richard Greenwood, and John C. Rothwell. 2008. "A Common Polymorphism in the Brain-Derived Neurotrophic Factor Gene (BDNF) Modulates Human Cortical Plasticity and the Response to RTMS." *Journal of Physiology* 586 (23): 5717–25. https://doi.org/10.1113/jphysiol.2008.159905.

Clarkson, Andrew N., Ben S. Huang, Sarah E. MacIsaac, Istvan Mody, and S. Thomas Carmichael. 2010. "Reducing Excessive GABA-Mediated Tonic Inhibition Promotes

Functional Recovery after Stroke." *Nature* 468 (7321): 305–9. https://doi.org/10.1038/nature09511.

Cohen, Leonardo G., Pablo Celnik, Alvaro Pascual-Leone, Brian Corwell, Lala Faiz, James Dambrosia, Manabu Honda, et al. 1997. "Functional Relevance of Cross-Modal Plasticity in Blind Humans." *Nature* 389 (6647): 180–83. https://doi.org/10.1038/38278.

Colovic, Mirjana B., Danijela Z. Krstic, Tamara D. Lazarevic-Pasti, Aleksandra M. Bondzic, and Vesna M. Vasic. 2013. "Acetylcholinesterase Inhibitors: Pharmacology and Toxicology." *Current Neuropharmacology* 11 (3): 315–35. https://doi.org/10.2174/1570159x11311030006.

Derringer, Jaime, Robert F. Krueger, Danielle M. Dick, Scott Saccone, Richard A. Grucza, Arpana Agrawal, Peng Lin, et al. 2010. "Predicting Sensation Seeking From Dopamine Genes." *Psychological Science* 21 (9): 1282–90. https://doi.org/10.1177/0956797610380699.

Elias, Jeffrey W., and Molly V. Wagster. 2007. "Developing Context and Background Underlying Cognitive Intervention/ Training Studies in Older Populations." *Journals of Gerontology - Series B Psychological Sciences and Social Sciences* 62 (SPEC. ISSUE 1): 5–10. https://doi.org/10.1093/geronb/62.special_issue_1.5.

Fagiolini, Michela, and Takao K. Hensch. 2000. "Inhibitory Threshold for Critical-Period Activation in Primary Visual Cortex." *Nature* 404 (6774): 183–86. https://doi.org/10.1038/35004582.

Floel, Agnes, and Leonardo G. Cohen. 2006. "Translational Studies in Neurorehabilitation: From Bench to Bedside." *Cognitive and Behavioral Neurology* 19 (1): 1–10. https://doi.org/10.1097/00146965-200603000-00001.

———. 2010. "Recovery of Function in Humans: Cortical Stimulation and Pharmacological Treatments after Stroke." *Neurobiology of Disease* 37 (2): 243–51. https://doi.org/10.1016/j.nbd.2009.05.027.

Floel, Agnes, Friedhelm Hummel, Julie Duque, Stefan Knecht, and Leonardo G. Cohen. 2008. "Influence of Somatosensory Input on Interhemispheric Interactions in Patients with Chronic Stroke." *Neurorehabilitation and Neural Repair* 22 (5): 477–85. https://doi.org/10.1177/1545968308316388.

Flor, Herta, Lone Nikolajsen, and Troels Staehelin Jensen. 2006. "Phantom Limb Pain: A Case of Maladaptive CNS Plasticity?" *Nature Reviews Neuroscience* 7 (11): 873–81. https://doi.org/10.1038/nrn1991.

Fridman, Esteban A., Takashi Hanakawa, Melissa Chung, Friedhelm Hummel, Ramon C. Leiguarda, and Leonardo G. Cohen. 2004. "Reorganization of the Human Ipsilesional Premotor Cortex after Stroke." *Brain* 127 (4): 747–58. https://doi.org/10.1093/brain/awh082.

Fritschy, Jean Marc, and Patrizia Panzanelli. 2014. "GABAA Receptors and Plasticity of Inhibitory Neurotransmission in the Central Nervous System." *European Journal of Neuroscience* 39 (11): 1845–65. https://doi.org/10.1111/ejn.12534.

Fujioka, Takako, Bernhard Ross, Ryusuke Kakigi, Christo Pantev, and Laurel J. Trainor. 2006. "One Year of Musical Training Affects Development of Auditory Cortical-Evoked Fields in Young Children." *Brain* 129 (10): 2593–2608. https://doi.org/10.1093/brain/awl247.

Gauthier, Lynne V., Edward Taub, Christi Perkins, Magdalene Ortmann, Victor W. Mark, and Gitendra Uswatte. 2008. "Remodeling the Brain: Plastic Structural Brain Changes Produced by Different Motor Therapies after Stroke." *Stroke; a Journal of Cerebral Circulation* 39 (5): 1520–25. https://doi.org/10.1161/STROKEAHA.107.502229.

Grefkes, Christian, Dennis A. Nowak, Simon B. Eickhoff, Manuel Dafotakis, Jutta Küst, Hans Karbe, and Gereon R. Fink. 2008. "Cortical Connectivity after Subcortical Stroke Assessed with Functional Magnetic Resonance Imaging." *Annals of Neurology* 63 (2): 236–46. https://doi.org/10.1002/ana.21228.

Hasselmo, Michael E., and Martin Sarter. 2011. "Modes and Models of Forebrain Cholinergic Neuromodulation of Cognition." *Neuropsychopharmacology* 36 (1): 52–73. https://doi.org/10.1038/npp.2010.104.

Herrero, J. L., M. J. Roberts, L. S. Delicato, M. A. Gieselmann, P. Dayan, and A. Thiele. 2008. "Acetylcholine Contributes through Muscarinic Receptors to Attentional Modulation in V1." *Nature* 454 (7208): 1110–14. https://doi.org/10.1038/nature07141.

Heuninckx, Sofie, Nicole Wenderoth, and Stephan P. Swinnen. 2008. "Systems Neuroplasticity in the Aging Brain: Recruiting Additional Neural Resources for Successful Motor Performance in Elderly Persons." *Journal of Neuroscience* 28 (1): 91–99. https://doi.org/10.1523/JNEUROSCI.3300-07.2008.

Hui, Gabriel K., Kwan L. Wong, Candice M. Chavez, Matthew I. Leon, Kinna M. Robin, and Norman M. Weinberger. 2009. "Conditioned Tone Control of Brain Reward Behavior Produces Highly Specific Representational Gain in the Primary Auditory Cortex." *Neurobiology of Learning and Memory* 92 (1): 27–34. https://doi.org/10.1016/j.nlm.2009.02.008.

Hummel, Friedhelm C., Kirstin Heise, Pablo Celnik, Agnes Floel, Christian Gerloff, and Leonardo G. Cohen. 2010. "Facilitating Skilled Right Hand Motor Function in Older Subjects by Anodal Polarization over the Left Primary Motor Cortex." *Neurobiology of Aging* 31 (12): 2160–68. https://doi.org/10.1016/j.neurobiolaging.2008.12.008.

Javitt, Daniel C. 2015. "Neurophysiological Models for New Treatment Development in Schizophrenia: Early Sensory Approaches." *Annals of the New York Academy of Sciences* 1344 (1): 92–104. https://doi.org/10.1111/nyas.12689.

Javitt, Daniel C., and Robert A. Sweet. 2015. "Auditory Dysfunction in Schizophrenia: Integrating Clinical and Basic Features." *Nature Reviews Neuroscience* 16 (9): 535–50. https://doi.org/10.1038/nrn4002.

Johansen-Berg, Heidi, and Matthew F.S. Rushworth. 2009. "Using Diffusion Imaging to Study Human Connectional Anatomy." *Annual Review of Neuroscience* 32: 75–94. https://doi.org/10.1146/annurev.neuro.051508.135735.

Kang, Jun Il, Marianne Groleau, Florence Dotigny, Hugo Giguère, and Elvire Vaucher. 2014. "Visual Training Paired with Electrical Stimulation of the Basal Forebrain Improves Orientation-Selective Visual Acuity in the Rat." *Brain Structure and Function* 219 (4): 1493–1507. https://doi.org/10.1007/s00429-013-0582-y.

Kang, Jun Il, Frédéric Huppé-Gourgues, and Elvire Vaucher. 2015. "Pharmacological Mechanisms of Cortical Enhancement Induced by the Repetitive Pairing of Visual/Cholinergic Stimulation." *PLoS ONE* 10 (10). https://doi.org/10.1371/journal.pone.0141663.

Kang, Jun Il, and Elvire Vaucher. 2009. "Cholinergic Pairing with Visual Activation Results in Long-Term Enhancement of Visual Evoked Potentials." *PLoS ONE* 4 (6). https://doi.org/10.1371/journal.pone.0005995.

Kasamatsu, Takuji, John D. Pettigrew, and Marylouise Ary. 1979. "Restoration of Visual Cortical Plasticity by Local Microperfusion of Norepinephrine." *Journal of Comparative Neurology* 185 (1): 163–81. https://doi.org/10.1002/cne.901850110.

Keers, Robert, and Katherine J. Aitchison. 2010. "Gender Differences in Antidepressant Drug Response." *International Review of Psychiatry* 22 (5): 485–500. https://doi.org/10.3109/09540261.2010.496448.

Kirkwood, Alfredo. 2007. "Neuromodulation of Cortical Synaptic Plasticity." *Monoaminergic Modulation of Cortical Excitability*, 209–16. https://doi.org/10.1007/978-0-387-72256-6_14.

Kleim, Jeffrey A., Sheila Chan, Erin Pringle, Kellan Schallert, Vincent Procaccio, Richard Jimenez, and Steven C. Cramer. 2006. "BDNF Val66met Polymorphism Is Associated with Modified Experience-Dependent Plasticity in Human Motor Cortex." *Nature Neuroscience* 9 (6): 735–37. https://doi.org/10.1038/nn1699.

Knudsen, Eric I. 2004. "Sensitive Periods in the Development of the Brain and Behavior." *Journal of Cognitive Neuroscience* 16 (8): 1412–25. https://doi.org/10.1162/0898929042304796.

Kuhlman, Sandra J., Nicholas D. Olivas, Elaine Tring, Taruna Ikrar, Xiangmin Xu, and Joshua T. Trachtenberg. 2013. "A Disinhibitory Microcircuit Initiates Critical-Period Plasticity in the Visual Cortex." *Nature* 501 (7468): 543–46. https://doi.org/10.1038/nature12485.

Lee, Jonathan L.C. 2009. "Reconsolidation: Maintaining Memory Relevance." *Trends in Neurosciences* 32 (8): 413–20. https://doi.org/10.1016/j.tins.2009.05.002.

Li, Songlin, Justine J. Overman, Diana Katsman, Serguei V. Kozlov, Christopher J. Donnelly, Jeffery L. Twiss, Roman J. Giger, Giovanni Coppola, Daniel H. Geschwind, and S. Thomas Carmichael. 2010. "An Age-Related Sprouting Transcriptome Provides Molecular Control of Axonal Sprouting after Stroke." *Nature Neuroscience* 13 (12): 1496–1506. https://doi.org/10.1038/nn.2674.

Luca, M. De, C. F. Beckmann, N. De Stefano, P. M. Matthews, and S. M. Smith. 2006. "FMRI Resting State Networks Define Distinct Modes of Long-Distance Interactions in the Human Brain." *NeuroImage* 29 (4): 1359–67. https://doi.org/10.1016/j.neuroimage.2005.08.035.

McGee, Aaron W., Yupeng Yang, Quentin S. Fischer, Nigel W. Daw, and Stephen H. Strittmatter. 2005. "Neuroscience: Experience-Driven Plasticity of Visual Cortex Limited by Myelin and Nogo Receptor." *Science* 309 (5744): 2222–26. https://doi.org/10.1126/science.1114362.

Nelissen, Koen, Giuseppe Luppino, and Wim Vanduffel. 2009. "Observing Others : Multiple Action Representation in the Frontal Lobe Observing Others : Multiple Action Representation in the Frontal Lobe." *October* 332 (2005). https://doi.org/10.1126/science.1115593.

Norbury, Agnes, and Masud Husain. 2015. "Sensation-Seeking: Dopaminergic Modulation and Risk for Psychopathology." *Behavioural Brain Research* 288: 79–93. https://doi.org/10.1016/j.bbr.2015.04.015.

Noudoost, Behrad, and Tirin Moore. 2011. "Control of Visual Cortical Signals by Prefrontal Dopamine." *Nature* 474 (7351): 372–75. https://doi.org/10.1038/nature09995.

Ouellet, Lydia, and Etienne de Villers-Sidani. 2014. "Trajectory of the Main GABAergic Interneuron Populations from Early Development to Old Age in the Rat Primary Auditory Cortex." *Frontiers in Neuroanatomy* 8 (JUN). https://doi.org/10.3389/fnana.2014.00040.

Pantev, Christo, Claudia Lappe, Sibylle C. Herholz, and Laurel Trainor. 2009. "Auditory-Somatosensory Integration and Cortical Plasticity in Musical Training." *Annals of the New York Academy of Sciences* 1169: 143–50. https://doi.org/10.1111/j.1749-6632.2009.04588.x.

Pearson-Fuhrhop, Kristin M., Jeffrey A. Kleim, and Steven C. Cramer. 2009. "Brain Plasticity and Genetic Factors." *Topics in Stroke Rehabilitation* 16 (4): 282–99. https://doi.org/10.1310/tsr1604-282.

Plow, Ela B., James R. Carey, Randolph J. Nudo, and Alvaro Pascual-Leone. 2009. "Invasive Cortical Stimulation to Promote Recovery of Function after Stroke: A Critical Appraisal." *Stroke* 40 (5): 1926–31. https://doi.org/10.1161/STROKEAHA.108.540823.

Qiu, Wei Hong, Hui Xiang Wu, Qing Lu Yang, Zhuang Kang, Zhao Cong Chen, Kui Li, Guo Rong Qiu, Chun Qing Xie, Gui Fang Wan, and Shao Qiong Chen. 2017. "Evidence of Cortical Reorganization of Language Networks after Stroke with Subacute Broca's Aphasia: A Blood Oxygenation Level Dependent-Functional Magnetic Resonance Imaging Study." *Neural Regeneration Research* 12 (1): 109–17. https://doi.org/10.4103/1673-5374.198996.

Ridding, Michael C., Darrin R. McKay, Philip D. Thompson, and Timothy S. Miles. 2001. "Changes in Corticomotor Representations Induced by Prolonged Peripheral Nerve Stimulation in Humans." *Clinical Neurophysiology* 112 (8): 1461–69. https://doi.org/10.1016/S1388-2457(01)00592-2.

Robin, Laurie M., José F. Oliveira da Cruz, Valentin C. Langlais, Mario Martin-Fernandez, Mathilde Metna-Laurent, Arnau Busquets-Garcia, Luigi Bellocchio, et al. 2018. "Astroglial CB1 Receptors Determine Synaptic D-Serine Availability to Enable Recognition Memory." *Neuron* 98 (5): 935-944.e5. https://doi.org/10.1016/j.neuron.2018.04.034.

Rokem, Ariel, and Michael A. Silver. 2010. "Cholinergic Enhancement Augments Magnitude and Specificity of Visual Perceptual Learning in Healthy Humans." *Current Biology* 20 (19): 1723–28. https://doi.org/10.1016/j.cub.2010.08.027.

———. 2013. "The Benefits of Cholinergic Enhancement during Perceptual Learning Are Long-Lasting." *Frontiers in Computational Neuroscience*, no. MAY. https://doi.org/10.3389/fncom.2013.00066.

Sharma, Nikhil, Joseph Classen, and Leonardo G. Cohen. 2013. "Neural Plasticity and Its Contribution to Functional Recovery." *Handbook of Clinical Neurology* 110: 3–12. https://doi.org/10.1016/B978-0-444-52901-5.00001-0.

Sharma, Nikhil, Lucy H. Simmons, P. Simon Jones, Diana J. Day, T. Adrian Carpenter, Valerie M. Pomeroy, Elizabeth A. Warburton, and Jean Claude Baron. 2009. "Motor

Imagery after Subcortical Stroke: A Functional Magnetic Resonance Imaging Study." *Stroke* 40 (4): 1315–24. https://doi.org/10.1161/STROKEAHA.108.525766.

Sheffler, Lynne R., Maureen T. Hennessey, Gregory G. Naples, and John Chae. 2006. "Peroneal Nerve Stimulation versus an Ankle Foot Orthosis for Correction of Footdrop in Stroke: Impact on Functional Ambulation." *Neurorehabilitation and Neural Repair* 20 (3): 355–60. https://doi.org/10.1177/1545968306287925.

Smith, Charles D., Himachandra Chebrolu, David R. Wekstein, Frederick A. Schmitt, and William R. Markesbery. 2007. "Age and Gender Effects on Human Brain Anatomy: A Voxel-Based Morphometric Study in Healthy Elderly." *Neurobiology of Aging* 28 (7): 1075–87. https://doi.org/10.1016/j.neurobiolaging.2006.05.018.

Stefan, Katja, Leonardo G. Cohen, Julie Duque, Riccardo Mazzocchio, Pablo Celnik, Lumy Sawaki, Leslie Ungerleider, and Joseph Classen. 2005. "Formation of a Motor Memory by Action Observation." *Journal of Neuroscience* 25 (41): 9339–46. https://doi.org/10.1523/JNEUROSCI.2282-05.2005.

Stefan, Katja, Matthias Wycislo, and Joseph Classen. 2004. "Modulation of Associative Human Motor Cortical Plasticity by Attention." *Journal of Neurophysiology* 92 (1): 66–72. https://doi.org/10.1152/jn.00383.2003.

Tardy, Jean, Jérémie Pariente, Anne Leger, Sophie Dechaumont-Palacin, Angélique Gerdelat, Vincent Guiraud, Fabrice Conchou, et al. 2006. "Methylphenidate Modulates Cerebral Post-Stroke Reorganization." *NeuroImage* 33 (3): 913–22. https://doi.org/10.1016/j.neuroimage.2006.07.014.

Turner, Richard M., B. Kevin Park, and Munir Pirmohamed. 2015. "Parsing Interindividual Drug Variability: An Emerging Role for Systems Pharmacology." *Wiley Interdisciplinary Reviews: Systems Biology and Medicine* 7 (4): 221–41. https://doi.org/10.1002/wsbm.1302.

Vargha-Khadem, Faraneh, Lucinda J. Carr, Elizabeth Isaacs, Edward Brett, Christopher Adams, and Mortimer Mishkin. 1997. "Onset of Speech after Left Hemispherectomy in a Nine-Year-Old Boy." *Brain* 120 (1): 159–82. https://doi.org/10.1093/brain/120.1.159.

Villers-Sidani, Etienne De, Edward F. Chang, Shaowen Bao, and Michael M. Merzenich. 2007. "Critical Period Window for Spectral Tuning Defined in the Primary Auditory Cortex (A1) in the Rat." *Journal of Neuroscience* 27 (1): 180–89. https://doi.org/10.1523/JNEUROSCI.3227-06.2007.

Voss, Patrice, Maryse Thomas, You Chien Chou, José Miguel Cisneros-Franco, Lydia Ouellet, and Etienne De Villers-Sidani. 2016. "Pairing Cholinergic Enhancement with Perceptual Training Promotes Recovery of Age-Related Changes in Rat Primary Auditory Cortex." *Neural Plasticity* 2016. https://doi.org/10.1155/2016/1801979.

Voss, Patrice, Maryse E. Thomas, J. Miguel Cisneros-Franco, and Étienne de Villers-Sidani. 2017. "Dynamic Brains and the Changing Rules of Neuroplasticity: Implications for Learning and Recovery." *Frontiers in Psychology* 8 (OCT). https://doi.org/10.3389/fpsyg.2017.01657.

Wang, Difei, and James Fawcett. 2012. "The Perineuronal Net and the Control of Cns Plasticity." *Cell and Tissue Research* 349 (1): 147–60. https://doi.org/10.1007/s00441-012-1375-y.

Wrigley, P. J., S. M. Gustin, P. M. Macey, P. G. Nash, S. C. Gandevia, V. G. Macefield, P. J. Siddall, and L. A. Henderson. 2009. "Anatomical Changes in Human Motor Cortex and Motor Pathways Following Complete Thoracic Spinal Cord Injury." *Cerebral Cortex* 19 (1): 224–32. https://doi.org/10.1093/cercor/bhn072.

Xiong, Liu Lin, Yue Hu, Piao Zhang, Zhuo Zhang, Li Hong Li, Guo Dong Gao, Xin Fu Zhou, and Ting Hua Wang. 2018. "Neural Stem Cell Transplantation Promotes Functional Recovery from Traumatic Brain Injury via Brain Derived Neurotrophic Factor-Mediated Neuroplasticity." *Molecular Neurobiology* 55 (3): 2696–2711. https://doi.org/10.1007/s12035-017-0551-1.

Zhang, Li I., Shaowen Bao, and Michael M. Merzenich. 2002. "Disruption of Primary Auditory Cortex by Synchronous Auditory Inputs during a Critical Period." *Proceedings of the National Academy of Sciences of the United States of America* 99 (4): 2309–14. https://doi.org/10.1073/pnas.261707398.

Chapter 5

Economic Dynamics in Neurorehabilitation

Gaurav Jain* and V. D. Sinha
Neurosurgery, SMS Medical College and Hospital, Jaipur, India

Abstract

The neurological diseases lead to suffering and have an impact on the humans in many ways, personal, social, economic and demographic. Global burden of Neurological illnesses has become more prominent as a result of increase in the lifespan of those affected and the lifestyle changes which have resulted in an increase in neurological non-communicable illnesses (NCDs). India is bearing the weight of the neurological illnesses and coping with their after effects like mortality, morbidity, disability making a portion of society dependent over others. Neurorehabilitation forms an important of rehabilitative service for the neurological disorder's disabilities affecting mobility, cognition and behaviour, leading to pain, functional as well as consciousness level changes. The amount of human resource hours gone in their management, as well as the cost of treatment, has a negative effect on the annual GDP of our country and thereby individual economic productivity. Effective Neuro-rehabilitation helps reducing the overall cost of care and leads to improvement in both human suffering and financial terms.

Keywords: neurorehabilitation, economic loss, disability, traumatic brain injury (TBI)

---

*Corresponding Author's Email: drgauravjain9@gmail.com.

In: Rehabilitation in Neurotrauma
Editors: VD Sinha, Amit Chakraborty, Jitin Bajaj et al.
ISBN: 978-1-68507-787-7

Introduction

Neuronal health is one of most precious resources of mankind for human activity and progression, demanding all care and resources. Even a slight change in the neuronal performance can lead to a significant effect on the functioning and execution by humans in their physical, cognitive, socioeconomic domains of life. So neuronal care, support and repair if needed are important for our race on earth.

Global Scenario

The neurological diseases lead to suffering and have an impact on the humans in many ways, personal, social, economic and demographic. In the recent years, the change in the epidemiology of neurological diseases from infectious to non communicable disorders and their increasing incidence have caused a concern world over. In the 2015 study of global burden of diseases, injuries, and risk factors (GBD), the term socioeconomic demographics was coined in place of the Socio-demographic Index (SDI), which is a better scale to measure the impact of neurological illnesses and which was further analysed in 2016 study(Feigin et al. 2019, The 2016). The frequency, fatalities, years of life lost (YLLs), years lived with disability (YLDs), and disability-adjusted life-years (DALYs) as per age and sex for 15 neurological conditions, which included brain and spinal cord trauma, were calculated from 195 countries from 1990 to 2016(Shakir and Norrving 2017). Neurological disorders are the major cause of disability, with 276 million DALYs and 116% of global DALYs. They lead to around 9 million deaths and 16•5 percent of global deaths, making them the second important cause of mortality after heart disease. Global burden by neurological illnesses has become more prominent as a result of increase in the lifespan of those affected and an increase in neurological non-communicable illnesses (NCDs) due to the modern lifestyle changes. (Vos et al. 2017). Every country has the responsibility to work in the direction for the betterment and cure of its citizens suffering from various diseases. The burden which these neurological disorders put on the nations and their health-care systems take a toll on their population and economic growth. The national and regional demands can be difficult to meet, and as each country has its own resources and health-care system to cope with this growing demand, the GBD study gave the most detailed picture of neurological illnesses experienced by every country. The size of global, regional, and national disease-specific burdens will help us manage the situation efficiently, not only in terms of social development but also in terms of economic growth of the country.

Indian Scenario

India, with 1.3 billion people, is still a developing country, but it has made significant economic development in recent years. Although healthcare is a huge sector, but India's Gross Domestic Product (GDP) contribution is still modest, and it must be expanded in order to develop a healthy and prosperous society. India is plagued by communicable diseases, dietary problems and, like the rest of the world, an increasing incidence of non-communicable diseases (NCD) (Srinath Reddy et al. 2005). India is bearing the weight of the neurological illnesses and coping with their after effects like mortality, morbidity, disability making a portion of society dependent over others. The progressive degeneration and prolong nature of these neurological conditions along with limited as well as expensive treatment options for many of them, further increases the suffering of the nation. The amount of human resource hours gone in their management, as well as the cost of treatment, has a negative effect on the individual economic productivity and on the annual GDP of our country as well. Some recent developments in diagnostic and therapeutic modalities have changed the clinical scenario, assuring early diagnosis and specific treatment leading to better outcome in few diseases, but we are still in the developmental phase for most of the diseases to control or treat.

The first detail estimates of the burden of neurological disorders in every state of India was stated in The India State-Level Disease Burden Initiative, published in The Lancet Global Health on 14 July 2021 (Singh et al. 2021). The neurological disorders included were categorised as non-communicable (stroke, headache disorders, epilepsy, cerebral palsy, Alzheimer's disease and other dementias, brain and central nervous system cancer, Parkinson's disease, multiple sclerosis, motor neuron diseases, and other neurological disorders), communicable disorders (encephalitis, meningitis, and tetanus), and injury-related disorders (traumatic brain injuries and spinal cord injuries).In India, neurological illnesses account for 10% of the total disease burden. Non-communicable neurological disorders contributed 82.8% of total DALYs attributable to all neurological illnesses in India in 2019, communicable neurological disorders contributed 12.8%, and trauma-related neurological disorders contributed 6.0 percent. When considering severe disability (individuals requiring help daily) neurological causes account for approximately 40% of the cases and the complex disability with physical, cognitive and behavioural impairments majority of them have the neurological origin (Greenwood 2001). India, with a mix of urban and rural population, have always portrayed urban India being the real victim of neurological diseases. In the recent times better data collection and its analysis has revealed that rural India is the major sufferer, having a ratio of 1.85:1 with the urban India. This is an eye-opener, and an important figure in regards to planning and governance needed to deal with the morbidity as well the economic slowing it can have on the country's GDP (Gourie-Devi et al. 2004). The economic burden due to the neurological disorders not only comprise the treatment cost but comprises of long list due to its collateral effect on family, caregiver, loss of employment of patient and family, travelling and many other expenses met in the long course of the disease (Gourie-Devi et al. 2004). They can be summarised as in Table 1.

Table 1. Economic burden of neurological disorder needing neurehabilitation

Direct cost	Indirect costs	Intangible costs
• outpatient care	• Unemployment of patient	• Attributable to pain
• drugs	• under-employment	• Disability
• emergency admissions	• income lost by family members / Care-giver	• Suffering of patient
• in-patient care	• disability-associated issues	• Suffering of Care-giver
• expenses for transport particularly from remote areas to centres of healthcare and hospitals	• excess mortality	• Stress to Care-giver
• Neuro-rehabilitation • Physical therapy • Speech therapy • Cognitive therapy • Psychosocial therapy • Magnetic stimulation • Electric stimulation		• Loss of happiness
• Gadgets for rehabilitation		• Suffering of next Generation deprived from education due to economic issues
		• Debt in family
		• Social Stigma for family

Road Traffic Accidents (RTA) Scenario

Our country, which is now moving at a great pace to become a developed nation has witnessed economic growth and development. The automobiles industry has developed many times and it has increased the incidence of RTA many times than before. The government of India, Ministry of Road Transport and Highways (MoRTH) estimates around 4.5 lakhs road accidents occurring yearly, leading to 1.5 lakhs deaths. The economic cost of these road accidents is weighed as 0.77% of the GDP. Majority of these victims (76.2%) are in their economically productive lifespan i.e., working- age group of 18-45 years and the sole supporters to their families(MORTH 2019). The economic impact due to the loss of economically productive lives is estimated to be around 3.14% of Gross Domestic Product (GDP), which is quite under reported. India accounts for 11% of the global deaths only due to RTA, highest in the world. In an earlier study done in 1995 by government of India, it was estimated that cost of road traffic crash injuries in India was 3.2% of GDP, which acted as a hindrance in progress. The 2019 World Bank report, titled 'Guide for Road Safety Opportunities and Challenges: Low- and Middle-Incom e Countries Country Profiles', concludes that the road accident and serious injury has an negative impact on India's GDP of around 7.5%, which comes out as Rs. 12.9 lakh crore, for the year 2016. This value included the cost inculcated by medical expenses, legal fees, property damage, insurance costs, and loss of output due to death. The risk of a road accident is three times greater in low-income countries than high-income countries. Though the developed and developing worlds get affected differently but the cost has to be borne by citizens (Bank 2021). Unsafe roads and vehicles, violation of traffic rules, fear of being a good Samaritan, improper pre-hospital care by the first responders and delay in reaching to a competent health facility are few of the contributing reasons to the suffering and loss. We are improving on these pitfalls but still have to tread a long way. The lack of specialists in emergency management, transportation facilities, neurologists, neurosurgeons, physiotherapists along with unavailability of facilities at peripheral areas, the morbidity and mortality rise to a great extent.

The poor daily wage workers who travel to their workplace are the victims of road crash in almost half of the cases and so termed as Vulnerable Road Users (VRUs). They are the contributors to national GDP as well with their work in industries and daily earnings for their households. The mortality and morbidity occurring has an immense effect on the household of each of the affected individual, and as per the world bank`s report at least seven months of income is lost. This financial crunch pushes all the non-poor householdsinto poverty and the poor ones into a cycle of poverty and debt. Women suffer a lot in these affected families of victims bearing the household as well as the economic responsibilities. They often take up extra work, along with the care giving activities for the affected person. This burden is equal in both poor and richhouseholds. About 50% of women were severely affected by the loss of household incomeafter a crash and about40% of women had to change their working patternspost-accident, while around11% reported taking up extra workto deal with the financial crisis(Bank 2021). Theincome declinefor low-incomerural households was the maximum (56%) compared to low-income urban (29.5%) and high-income rural households (39.5%) as per the World Bank report for the Indian states. The death rate in India due to RTA has increased by 40% from 2003 to 2008. India is expected to have the maximum numbers of automobiles by 2050, even more than USA, which will be a leading cause to neurological morbidity and mortality leading to human suffering and hampering the financial status of India.

RTA is among the major causes of head injuries and related TBI in India as well as across world. WHO estimates that by 2030 RTA fatalities will emerge as fifth biggest killer, to claim around 24 lakhs lives yearly worldover! Among these 90% will be occurring in developing countries of Asia-pacific region, mostly in low or middle income group families and among the economically productive age group(Bank 2021). Thus on the bigger picture it is evident that the neurological conditions be it non-communicable, infectious or Traumatic, cause a lot of human suffering and economic loss to the country and act as a hindrance to growth, prosperity and happiness. Thus, we all must work against these challenges and reduce the suffering and proceed towards a prosperous and caring society. While keeping prevention and good treatment in mind we must focus on rehabilitation for improving the future prospect of these victims, and for this part neurorehabilitation will be a major role player.

Neurorehabilitation

Neurorehabilitation is a comprehensive rehabilitation including physio-therapy, speech therapy, occupational therapy, neurophysiological support which help the patient to improve in his functional aspect and return to normalcy or near normalcy earlier, by tapping the 'neuroplastic' quality of the brain. Neurorehabilitation is an interdisciplinary approach needing the dedicated efforts of different sectors, professions, patients and community to manage complex condition-related disability (Khan et al. 2017). Neurorehabilitation is an important form of rehabilitative service for the neurological disorders related disabilities affecting mobility, cognition and behavior thereby leading to pain, disturbance of consciousness and other functions (Hewer and Tennant 2002). Neurological disability may result from a combination of neuronal impairments and on the worse part a single impairment may lead to multiple disabilities. Disability assessment includes severity as well as involvement of different aspects. There have been only a few reports published stating the magnitude and severity of disability consequent to neurological disorders. Studies by Taly and Chaudhuri et al. [24] and Prabhakar et al. suggested that after discharge, patients with varying severity of disability, some of the patients showed improvement at an interval of few months (Prabhakar, Chopra, and Pershad 1991). An isolated study with community survey as a component of Bangalore Urban Rural Neuroepidemiological survey (BURN), stated that neurological disorders with significant disability were two times more common in the rural region as compared to the urban (Gururaj, Gourie-Devi, and Taly 1998). Thus rural India needs more neurorehabilitation than urban, but at the same time the availability of family members ready to give time and care to the victim in rural area is high and holds as an advantage for them despite poor resources and facilities. Rehabilitation is usually done for motor, sensory, cognitive deficits, but the psychosocial rehabilitation along with proper use of community utilization may be the key to better outcome (Prakashi and Gourie-Devi 1988).

Challenges

Neurological rehabilitation services in developing countries like India pose a great challenge considering the limited resources and manpower. Currently, neurological rehabilitation with a multidisciplinary team is confined to only a few major cities in the country. To limit the disability and improve upon our country`s future prospect and unhindered growth, providing neurorehabilitation services to all should be the goal. There are some limitations in regards to this, like unavailability of resources both human and infrastructure as well as the exorbitant cost. We should make policies to overcome these. India has only 5,000 qualified physiotherapists to cater to lakhs of patients requiring their dedicated services in comparison with the recommended one for every 10,000 citizens. As per WHO norms currently we are short of 95,000 physiotherapists in India (Bank 2021). Also the neurologists to population ratio is too low than the developed countries with only 2500 neurologists serving the india population, unlike the developed countries with ratio of one to two neurologists per 20000 to 100000 people.

The disparity remains with certain areas of the world having no neurologist even now and USA having one neurologist per 26200 and Africa with one per 5,009,908 (Bergen 2002, Bower and Zenebe 2005, Singh et al. 2021).Similarly India has approximately more than 3500 neurosurgeons and increasing as colleges and hospitals are being recognised for MCh/DNB Neurosurgery training program, with an approved seats of more than 190/year (Raj and Agrawal 2018). So as we need around 5000 neurologists to take care of our citizens, we also need neurosurgeons and neurorehabilitators and physiotherapists to match this huge demand of the world`s greatest democracy. The infrastructure for the patients is available in big cities and towns unlike the small towns or nearby villages. Specific machinery or gadgets for neurorehabilitation is required in some cases, but therapies particularly involving speech, occupational and cognition require specialised trained professionals which are not available in lower tier cities and peripheral areas. Employing these professionals also adds to the cost. Neurorehablitation is a long process and may need 6-18 months, which makes the stay at a hospital or specialisedcentre practically not feasible due to the exorbitant cost involved as well the time constraints in regards to the care taker or family members. Moreover the scarcity of beds make it necessary to discharge the patient early when stabilized, to vacate and making it available to new patients(Zorowitz and Ward 2014). Our country has heavy burden of stroke, TBI occupying hospital beds for long durations in government as well as in private setups. As a routine protocol, hospital stay is permitted for a reasonable period till the required medical or surgical intervention is needed and discharge is planned once the patient stabilizes and no hospital intervention is needed. A flowchart representation of the process can easily be explained to all for motivating (Table 2). Initial neurorehabilitation can be done in the form of physiotherapy and stimulation techniques like music or familiar voices. Patient is then sent home or to a step-down centre for care as per the need. Few of the patients require prolonged and continuous medical care due to acquired infections, family or psychological issues. In general, to accommodate the huge load, sometimes the discharge is prioritized or speeded up in some cases which stabilize early.

The cost for the hospital stay in days, infections acquired due to lack of physiotherapy or care and other changing needs, which is met by the government or the patient himself at a private setup. The financial pressure continues later too if the patient is dependent or needs assistance for daily

Table 2. A flowchart representation of the process for a person with disability post neurological problem

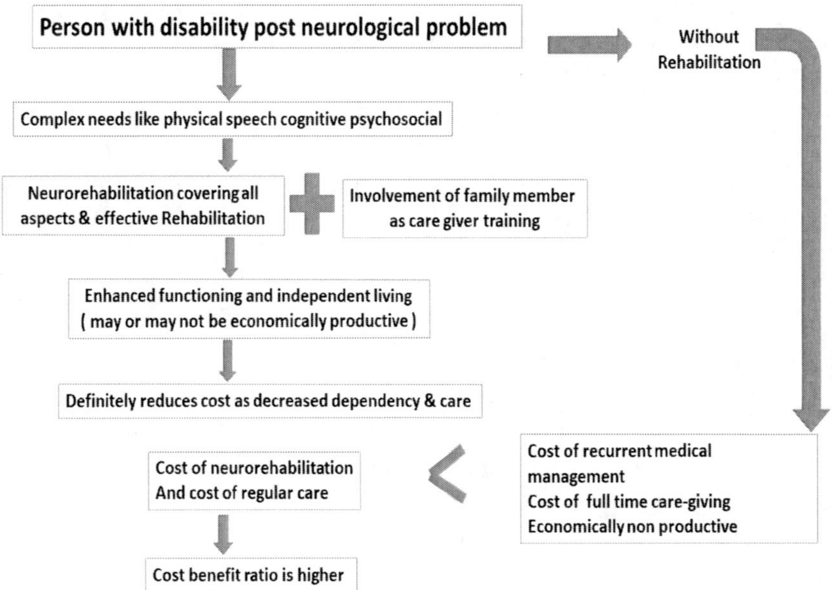

routine and cannot be economically productive. The time period post deficit witnesses continuous and changing medical needs of the patient, with or without neurorehabilitation, which also have financial implications. But the medical needs, infections and daily care requirement increases when neurorehabilitation is not undertaken and leads to higher as well as prolonged financial burden.To have an overview of the cost what a single neurological disease can have Thomas et al. conducted a study on Economic burden of epilepsy in six medical centres in 6 different states of India(Thomas et al. 2001). The study concluded that the annual cost of epilepsy treatment per patient was around Rs.13755, and estimating it for the country it escalated to a huge figure of Rs. 68.75 billion. Also, an important eyeopener in this study was that the indirect costs, in the form of travel to the distantly located hospitals and the consequent loss of productivity amounted to 14% of the total annual cost. We don't have much studies of this kind for other neurological conditions but similar travel expense can be taken in consideration for other neurological conditions needing treatment at a distant centre or hospital. Though better treatment has improved the outcome, but providing neurological care at the community level that is “doorstep” care will help considerably to cut on the cost and give relief to the patient and family. Thus prevention, cure, doorstep availability of medical care by nursing and medical professional may help to unburden our country and have an exponential economic growth. Thus we need proper assessment, planning and as well as good execution with a regular feedback check. In a study done in USA the cost for hospitalisation on an average came out to be 2200$ weekly and total of 2.2 million $ for each covered life whereas if the patient received early neurorehabilitation and remained in the centre for even 6-18 months the cost came out to be 0.45 million $ which is much less and comforting(Ward et al. 2012).

OUR Experience

Our institute SMS Medical College and Hospital, at Jaipur, India is a very high-volume centre for traumatic brain and spine injury in India and Asian region. Looking to the huge load of suffering we need quick treatment as well early discharge to accommodate all the patients. So with the good adequate neurosurgical services going on round the clock, we initiated a planned neurorehabilitation programme for early stabilisation of patient and their discharge. The neurorehabilitation centre was made near to the neurosurgical ward, so that the patients could get easy neurorehabilitation services and the family members were trained under supervision since the beginning our neurosurgical team and by the therapists for the required therapy. They were explained the importance and the economic benefits as well. The care-giver was also constantly instructed by our neurosurgical team, inclusive of round the clock residents and consultants for even basic therapies like chest and limb physiotherapy. We started a study in this regard in 2016 and is still continuing at present with 6897 cases registered, who receive neurorehabilitation in the ward through the same pattern. As the study is yet not concluded though we can wisely comment that we achieved early stabilisation of patients and improvement in cognitive as well as motor functions. Early discharge was possible and no readmissions in view of rehabilitation occurred. Though the improvement varies as per the prior disability but a few were seen walking to the OPD by themselves in a month’s time as well. The stabilised patients could be discharged with the family member or care-giver as a personal and all-time available therapist even in the remotest of villages.We have seen better results on follow-up and good improvement in functional life in follow-up periods of few months. This led to better management of the beds and creation of vacancy for the new sufferers. Similarly in India we can tackle the huge burden with good and early neurorehabilitation starting at the hospital during the primary stay. Involvement and training of the family members who are going to be the care taker, which usually happens in Indian scenario, can fulfil the deficit of the professional to some extent at periphery. So hereby, we conclude that minimising the hospital stay, by early physiotherapy and care of the patient, thereby preventing infections like pneumonia and bedsores, and improving the disability as well as suffering by neurorehabilitation can lead to betterment on humanitarian as well as financial grounds. This is the reason why we stress upon the importance of apt and early execution of neurorehabilitation.

Delivery of Services

Another aspect of concern is the delivery of the NR services and making it widely available. Few of the proposals are already in channel to make efforts at rural, community centre, satellite clinics, district centre and tertiary care centre for wide coverage. It might take few years but the benefit will be enormous in terms of decreasing suffering and minimizing financial loss as well. As proposed by Gourie Devi et al. for the neurology services being available at doorstep (Gourie-Devi et al. 2004), a similar model can be used for the neurorehabilitation services also.

Rural Model

70% of India's population lives in the villages and rural burden of neurological diseases is twice. Therefore, making these facilities available at the village level would avoid the costs for travel, loss of wages and most importantly delay in treatment. I must stress upon, here comes the role of training to family members, who will be acting as trained neurorehabilitators till the time professional services reach to the villages.

CommunityHealth Centre Model

Our country has a great setup of CHC (Community Health Centres) which are attached to various medical colleges and medical institutions. These centres act with their own staff for general healthcare and immunization programs. They also interact with peripheral health centres and reach out to interior villages and can be a great workforce if trained to deliver neurorehabilitation services and also to teach the family members.

Satellite Clinics

Satellite clinics attached to the apex centres with clinical experts along with the facilities of the peripheral hospitals and the help offered by various NGOs can be very helpful in forming a link between periphery and tertiary centre.

District Model

In nearly 718 districts of our country, each has atleast 45000 to 60000 people suffering from various neurological disorders. A district model can function as an independent administrative unit, developing the rehabilitation activities with help of specialised personnel and also act as a monitoring and data managing centre.

TertiaryCentre

Neurology care is available in medical colleges and private hospitals in big cities, which may be considered as regional centres. Government centres with advanced state-of-the-art facilities are now available in Apex centres. Urgent need is to increase these centres in government sector since affordability is a major concern. We see an increasing number of hospitals in the private sector offering excellent care but at a prohibitive cost.

Tele-Neurorehabilitation (TNR)

Tele-medicine is a way of connecting with the patient and family virtually over the video conference through various applications available in market either using mobile or computer. The 74.9 crore mobile and internet users at present in India, including rural India, make the technical and operational use easier even in a developing country like India. Soon the users in rural India will be surpassing the urban internet usage as per the study by Internet & Mobile Association of India (IAMAI), and total users by 2025 would be around 90 crores. It was recently used well in the Covid-19 era throughout India for tele-medical consultation and had good results. It appears to be an alternative and innovative way for connecting the needy patients with the health-care providers through real-time video. The rehabilitation specialist of a particular centre can provide consultation and advise for referral whenever required, to a higher centre. Also it can be helpful for the monitoring and observing the care giver, whether he/she is giving correct therapy and as well can be trained further (Khanna et al. 2018).

Care Giver Burden

We have focused on the rehabilitation and improving functionality of the patient, and we advocated the need of family member to be a trained as a care giver for economic reasons and for wide reach in villages. Simultaneously we must not forget that the responsibility which the Caregiver takes on, may lead to him into physical, psychological, financial and social problems (Singh et al. 2021). Caregiver may become the second victim of the disease, due to their involvement in the care of patients and, in particular, the level of stress they undertake. They often have to take on this responsibility suddenly with minimal preparation or guidance, though with some support from healthcare systems (Gourie-Devi et al. 2004). This concept of caregiver burden and his needs in the setting of community neurorehabilitation should be considered while planning, and structuring interventions. While deciding for a global approach towards the management of care, one must take into consideration the requirements of the family and caregivers along with that of patients.These caregivers should be supported so as to decrease their stress and increase their ability to cope up during the whole process (Greenwood 2001).

Role of Leadership

The leaders of the world have shown their commitment towards prevention of road traffic accidents and some wise steps have been taken. At global level Brasilia Declaration on Road Safety (2015) as well as the United Nations (UN) declared 2011-2020 as the decade of action for Road Safety. India was also a signatory to the Declaration plan, in the effort to reduce the global deaths and injuries from road traffic accidents, to decrease them to half by 2030. UN also declared Global Road Safety Week, celebrated every two years (held from 6-12 May 2019) to spread awareness. The Indian Government has made the Motor Vehicles Amendment Act, 2019, which hikes the penalties for traffic violations, defective vehicles, juvenile driving, etc. It also includes a Motor Vehicle Accident Fund with compulsory insurance cover to all the road users in India as well as protection of good Samaritans. Similarly, the plan to increase the medical professionals and availability of facilities in terms of more colleges, centres at districts and towns as well as strengthening of community and primary health care centres are all on board. This will help in providing better services and improving the outcome and functional state of patient. The cost involved will be high but the suffering will be reduced, also if the rehabilitative services could be provided through this plan it will be cost effective leading to more and early return to normalcy and economically productive life in many patients. Areas that require action are post-accident care on the spot, emergency care and protocols, insurance and compensation systems. The development agencies, policymakers and respective state governments should prioritize to formulate a complete policy considering the existing system and measures for improvement. For a country to calculate the economic benefit can be cumbersome, so proper and analytical methods should be chosen to identify the change produced by the rehabilitative intervention. More data from new studies are needed to have a proper assessment of all the direct and indirect financial implications. The economics involved is quite intricate and deeper than thought, will include probable earnings and reduced costs to social care as well as the earnings in term of happiness and satisfaction in members of family and society. The economic analyses should also include housing, education, and vocational outcomes and their impact on the family members. The future of the next generation, the children, who are totally dependent, must also be considered. It needs a high level of intellect to assess and execute neurorehabilitation as a cost-effective modality because it involves human suffering, emotions, future generation and money. It has to be balanced in a delicate way to pave the path for a prosperous nation.

Conclusion

A neurological disorder easily makes its morbidity and mortality acceptable to all, though with difficulty. The limited treatment and disability of varying severity leads to human suffering and economic loss which burdens the society. In this scenario the Neuro-rehabilitation programme, which might appear expensive with cost involving the specialists, centres and machinery should be tried. Though it is long way but it has hope for improvement of functionality of patient and his return to normalcy in some if not in all. This small betterment can reduce the suffering a lot and urges us to walk along this less treaded path of neurorehabilitation. Our fellow men with these neurological disorders will be living in the society for many years and early efforts to improve their physical as well as psychological functioning will result in substantial gains of human functions and savings in GDP once they return to productive life. We as medical professionals must ensure this and demonstrate the long-term cost-effectiveness of rehabilitation programme in various studies. The treatment and supportive care if supplemented with neurorehabilitation can give good results. This can encourage our planners to enthusiastically fund and commission neurorehabilitation programme. We also advocate for an approach oriented to saving lives, improvising the functional ability of victims and helping their families to get back to their life, by providing immediate as well as regular financial, medical, legal and neurrehabilitative aid. We all must act together to lessen the human pain as well as help them gaining normalcy while maintaining socio-economic benefit balance.

References

Bank, World. 2021. Traffic Crash Injuries and Disabilities: The Burden on Indian Society. World Bank.

Bergen, D. C. 2002. "Training and distribution of neurologistsworldwide."*J NeurolSci* 198 (1-2):3-7. doi: 10.1016/s0022-510x(02)00071-0.

Bower, J. H., and G. Zenebe. 2005. "Neurologic services in the nations of Africa."*Neurology* 64 (3):412-5. doi: 10.1212/01.wnl.0000150894.53961.e2.

Feigin, Valery L., Emma Nichols, Tahiya Alam, Marlena S. Bannick, Ettore Beghi, Natacha Blake, William J. Culpepper, E. Ray Dorsey, Alexis Elbaz, Richard G. Ellenbogen, James L. Fisher, Christina Fitzmaurice, Giorgia Giussani, Linda Glennie, Spencer L. James, Catherine Owens Johnson, Nicholas J. Kassebaum, Giancarlo Logroscino, Benoît Marin, W. Cliff Mountjoy-Venning, Minh Nguyen, Richard Ofori-Asenso, Anoop P. Patel, Marco Piccininni, Gregory A. Roth, Timothy J. Steiner, Lars Jacob Stovner, Cassandra E. I. Szoeke, Alice Theadom, Stein Emil Vollset, Mitchell Taylor Wallin, Claire Wright, Joseph Raymond Zunt, Nooshin Abbasi, Foad Abd-Allah, Ahmed Abdelalim, Ibrahim Abdollahpour, Victor Aboyans, Haftom Niguse Abraha, Dilaram Acharya, Abdu A. Adamu, Oladimeji M. Adebayo, Abiodun Moshood Adeoye, Jose C. Adsuar, Mohsen Afarideh, Sutapa Agrawal, Alireza Ahmadi, Muktar Beshir Ahmed, Amani Nidhal Aichour, Ibtihel Aichour, Miloud Taki Eddine Aichour, Rufus Olusola Akinyemi, Nadia Akseer, Ayman Al-Eyadhy, Rustam Al-Shahi Salman, Fares Alahdab, Kefyalew Addis Alene, Syed Mohamed Aljunid, Khalid Altirkawi, Nelson Alvis-Guzman, Nahla Hamed Anber, Carl Abelardo T. Antonio, Jalal Arabloo, Olatunde Aremu, Johan Ärnlöv, Hamid Asayesh, Rana Jawad Asghar, Hagos Tasew Atalay, Ashish Awasthi, Beatriz Paulina Ayala Quintanilla, Tambe B. Ayuk, Alaa Badawi, Maciej Banach, Joseph Adel Mattar Banoub, Miguel A. Barboza, Suzanne Lyn Barker-Collo, Till Winfried Bärnighausen, Bernhard T. Baune, Neeraj Bedi, Masoud Behzadifar, Meysam Behzadifar, Yannick Béjot, Bayu Begashaw Bekele, Abate Bekele Belachew, Derrick A. Bennett, Isabela M. Bensenor, Adugnaw Berhane, Mircea Beuran, Krittika Bhattacharyya, Zulfiqar A. Bhutta, Belete Biadgo, Ali Bijani, Nigus Bililign, Muhammad Shahdaat Bin Sayeed, Christopher Kynrint Blazes, Carol Brayne, Zahid A. Butt, Ismael R. Campos-Nonato, Carlos

Cantu-Brito, Mate Car, Rosario Cárdenas, Juan J. Carrero, Félix Carvalho, Carlos A. Castañeda-Orjuela, Franz Castro, Ferrán Catalá-López, Ester Cerin, Yazan Chaiah, Jung-Chen Chang, Irini Chatziralli, Peggy Pei-Chia Chiang, Hanne Christensen, Devasahayam J. Christopher, Cyrus Cooper, Paolo Angelo Cortesi, Vera M. Costa, Michael H. Criqui, Christopher Stephen Crowe, Albertino Antonio Moura Damasceno, Ahmad Daryani, Vanessa De la Cruz-Góngora, Fernando Pio De la Hoz, Diego De Leo, Gebre Teklemariam Demoz, Kebede Deribe, Samath Dhamminda Dharmaratne, Daniel Diaz, Mesfin Tadese Dinberu, Shirin Djalalinia, David Teye Doku, Manisha Dubey, Eleonora Dubljanin, Eyasu Ejeta Duken, David Edvardsson, Ziad El-Khatib, Matthias Endres, Aman Yesuf Endries, Sharareh Eskandarieh, Alireza Esteghamati, Sadaf Esteghamati, Farzaneh Farhadi, Andre Faro, Farshad Farzadfar, Mohammad Hosein Farzaei, Batool Fatima, Seyed-Mohammad Fereshtehnejad, Eduarda Fernandes, Garumma Tolu Feyissa, Irina Filip, Florian Fischer, Takeshi Fukumoto, Morsaleh Ganji, Fortune Gbetoho Gankpe, Miguel A. Garcia-Gordillo, Abadi Kahsu Gebre, Teklu Gebrehiwo Gebremichael, Belayneh K. Gelaw, Johanna M. Geleijnse, Demeke Geremew, Kebede Embaye Gezae, Maryam Ghasemi-Kasman, Mahari Y. Gidey, Paramjit Singh Gill, Tiffany K. Gill, Efrata Tufa Girma, Elena V. Gnedovskaya, Alessandra C. Goulart, Ayman Grada, Giuseppe Grosso, Yuming Guo, Rahul Gupta, Rajeev Gupta, Juanita A. Haagsma, Tekleberhan B. Hagos, Arvin Haj-Mirzaian, Arya Haj-Mirzaian, Randah R. Hamadeh, Samer Hamidi, Graeme J. Hankey, Yuantao Hao, Josep Maria Haro, Hadi Hassankhani, Hamid Yimam Hassen, Rasmus Havmoeller, Simon I. Hay, Mohamed I. Hegazy, Behnam Heidari, Andualem Henok, Fatemeh Heydarpour, Chi Linh Hoang, Michael K. Hole, Enayatollah Homaie Rad, Seyed Mostafa Hosseini, Guoqing Hu, Ehimario U. Igumbor, Olayinka Stephen Ilesanmi, Seyed Sina Naghibi Irvani, Sheikh Mohammed Shariful Islam, Mihajlo Jakovljevic, Mehdi Javanbakht, Ravi Prakash Jha, Yash B. Jobanputra, Jost B. Jonas, Jacek Jerzy Jozwiak, Mikk Jürisson, Amaha Kahsay, Rizwan Kalani, Yogeshwar Kalkonde, Teshome Abegaz Kamil, Tanuj Kanchan, Manoochehr Karami, André Karch, Narges Karimi, Amir Kasaeian, Tesfaye Dessale Kassa, Zemenu Yohannes Kassa, Anil Kaul, Adane Teshome Kefale, Peter Njenga Keiyoro, Yousef Saleh Khader, Morteza Abdullatif Khafaie, Ibrahim A. Khalil, Ejaz Ahmad Khan, Young-Ho Khang, Habibolah Khazaie, Aliasghar A. Kiadaliri, Daniel N. Kiirithio, Anthony S. Kim, Daniel Kim, Young-Eun Kim, Yun Jin Kim, Adnan Kisa, Yoshihiro Kokubo, Ai Koyanagi, Rita V. Krishnamurthi, Barthelemy Kuate Defo, Burcu Kucuk Bicer, Manasi Kumar, Ben Lacey, Alessandra Lafranconi, Van C. Lansingh, Arman Latifi, Cheru Tesema Leshargie, Shanshan Li, Yu Liao, Shai Linn, Warren David Lo, Jaifred Christian F. Lopez, Stefan Lorkowski, Paulo A. Lotufo, Robyn M. Lucas, Raimundas Lunevicius, Mark T. Mackay, Narayan Bahadur Mahotra, Marek Majdan, Reza Majdzadeh, Azeem Majeed, Reza Malekzadeh, Deborah Carvalho Malta, Navid Manafi, Mohammad Ali Mansournia, Lorenzo Giovanni Mantovani, Winfried März, Tivani Phosa Mashamba-Thompson, Benjamin Ballard Massenburg, Kedar K. V. Mate, Colm McAlinden, John J. McGrath, Varshil Mehta, Toni Meier, Hagazi Gebre Meles, Addisu Melese, Peter T. N. Memiah, Ziad A. Memish, Walter Mendoza, Desalegn Tadese Mengistu, Getnet Mengistu, Atte Meretoja, Tuomo J. Meretoja, Tomislav Mestrovic, Bartosz Miazgowski, Tomasz Miazgowski, Ted R. Miller, G. K.

Mini, Erkin M. Mirrakhimov, Babak Moazen, Bahram Mohajer, Naser Mohammad Gholi Mezerji, Moslem Mohammadi, Maryam Mohammadi-Khanaposhtani, Roghayeh Mohammadibakhsh, Mousa Mohammadnia-Afrouzi, Shafiu Mohammed, Farnam Mohebi, Ali H. Mokdad, Lorenzo Monasta, Stefania Mondello, Yoshan Moodley, Mahmood Moosazadeh, Ghobad Moradi, Maziar Moradi-Lakeh, Mehdi Moradinazar, Paula Moraga, Ilais Moreno Velásquez, Shane Douglas Morrison, Seyyed Meysam Mousavi, Oumer Sada Muhammed, Walter Muruet, Kamarul Imran Musa, Ghulam Mustafa, Mehdi Naderi, Gabriele Nagel, Aliya Naheed, Gurudatta Naik, Farid Najafi, Vinay Nangia, Ionut Negoi, Ruxandra Irina Negoi, Charles Richard James Newton, Josephine W. Ngunjiri, Cuong Tat Nguyen, Long Hoang Nguyen, Dina Nur Anggraini Ningrum, Yirga Legesse Nirayo, Molly R. Nixon, Bo Norrving, Jean Jacques Noubiap, Malihe Nourollahpour Shiadeh, Peter S. Nyasulu, Okechukwu Samuel Ogah, In-Hwan Oh, Andrew T. Olagunju, Tinuke O. Olagunju, Pedro R. Olivares, Obinna E. Onwujekwe, Eyal Oren, Mayowa Ojo Owolabi, Mahesh Pa, Amir H. Pakpour, Wen-Harn Pan, Songhomitra Panda-Jonas, Jeyaraj Durai Pandian, Sangram Kishor Patel, David M. Pereira, Max Petzold, Julian David Pillay, Michael A. Piradov, Guilherme V. Polanczyk, Suzanne Polinder, Maarten J. Postma, Richie Poulton, Hossein Poustchi, Swayam Prakash, V. Prakash, Mostafa Qorbani, Amir Radfar, Anwar Rafay, Alireza Rafiei, Fakher Rahim, Vafa Rahimi-Movaghar, Mahfuzar Rahman, Mohammad Hifz Ur Rahman, Muhammad Aziz Rahman, Fatemeh Rajati, Usha Ram, Anna Ranta, David Laith Rawaf, Salman Rawaf, Nickolas Reinig, Cesar Reis, Andre M. N. Renzaho, Serge Resnikoff, Shahab Rezaeian, Mohammad Sadegh Rezai, Carlos Miguel Rios González, Nicholas L. S. Roberts, Leonardo Roever, Luca Ronfani, Elias Merdassa Roro, Gholamreza Roshandel, Ali Rostami, Parisa Sabbagh, Ralph L. Sacco, Perminder S. Sachdev, Basema Saddik, Hosein Safari, Roya Safari-Faramani, Sare Safi, Saeid Safiri, Rajesh Sagar, Ramesh Sahathevan, Amirhossein Sahebkar, Mohammad Ali Sahraian, Payman Salamati, Saleh Salehi Zahabi, Yahya Salimi, Abdallah M. Samy, Juan Sanabria, Itamar S. Santos, Milena M. Santric Milicevic, Nizal Sarrafzadegan, Benn Sartorius, Shahabeddin Sarvi, Brijesh Sathian, Maheswar Satpathy, Arundhati R. Sawant, Monika Sawhney, Ione J. C. Schneider, Ben Schöttker, David C. Schwebel, Soraya Seedat, Sadaf G. Sepanlou, Hosein Shabaninejad, Azadeh Shafieesabet, Masood Ali Shaikh, Raad A. Shakir, Mehran Shams-Beyranvand, Morteza Shamsizadeh, Mehdi Sharif, Mahdi Sharif-Alhoseini, Jun She, Aziz Sheikh, Kevin N. Sheth, Mika Shigematsu, Rahman Shiri, Reza Shirkoohi, Ivy Shiue, Soraya Siabani, Tariq J. Siddiqi, Inga Dora Sigfusdottir, Rannveig Sigurvinsdottir, Donald H. Silberberg, João Pedro Silva, Dayane Gabriele Alves Silveira, Jasvinder A. Singh, Dhirendra Narain Sinha, Eirini Skiadaresi, Mari Smith, Badr Hasan Sobaih, Soheila Sobhani, Moslem Soofi, Ireneous N. Soyiri, Luciano A. Sposato, Dan J. Stein, Murray B. Stein, Mark A. Stokes, Mu'awiyyah Babale Sufiyan, Bryan L. Sykes, P. N. Sylaja, Rafael Tabarés-Seisdedos, Braden James Te Ao, Arash Tehrani-Banihashemi, Mohamad-Hani Temsah, Omar Temsah, Jarnail Singh Thakur, Amanda G. Thrift, Roman Topor-Madry, Miguel Tortajada-Girbés, Marcos Roberto Tovani-Palone, Bach Xuan Tran, Khanh Bao Tran, Thomas Clement Truelsen, Afewerki Gebremeskel Tsadik, Lorainne Tudor Car, Kingsley Nnanna Ukwaja, Irfan Ullah, Muhammad Shariq Usman,

Olalekan A. Uthman, Pascual R. Valdez, Tommi Juhani Vasankari, Rajagopalan Vasanthan, Yousef Veisani, Narayanaswamy Venketasubramanian, Francesco S. Violante, Vasily Vlassov, Kia Vosoughi, Giang Thu Vu, Isidora S. Vujcic, Fasil Shiferaw Wagnew, Yasir Waheed, Yuan-Pang Wang, Elisabete Weiderpass, Jordan Weiss, Harvey A. Whiteford, Tissa Wijeratne, Andrea Sylvia Winkler, Charles Shey Wiysonge, Charles D. A. Wolfe, Gelin Xu, Ali Yadollahpour, Tomohide Yamada, Yuichiro Yano, Mehdi Yaseri, Hiroshi Yatsuya, Ebrahim M. Yimer, Paul Yip, Engida Yisma, Naohiro Yonemoto, Mahmoud Yousefifard, Chuanhua Yu, Zoubida Zaidi, Sojib Bin Zaman, Mohammad Zamani, Hamed Zandian, Zohreh Zare, Yunquan Zhang, Sanjay Zodpey, Mohsen Naghavi, Christopher J. L. Murray, and Theo Vos. 2019. "Global, regional, and national burden of neurological disorders, 1990–2016: a systematic analysis for the Global Burden of DiseaseStudy 2016." *The Lancet Neurology* 18 (5):459-480. doi: 10.1016/S1474-4422(18)30499-X.

Gourie-Devi, M., G. Gururaj, P. Satishchandra, and D. K. Subbakrishna. 2004. "Prevalence of neurological disorders in Bangalore, India: a community-based study with a comparison between urban and rural areas."*Neuroepidemiology* 23 (6):261-8. doi: 10.1159/000080090.

Greenwood, R. 2001. "The future of rehabilitation."*BMJ (Clinicalresearched.)* 323 (7321):1082-1083. doi: 10.1136/bmj.323.7321.1082.

Gururaj, G, M Gourie-Devi, and AB Taly. 1998. "Satishchandra. Epidemiology of neurological disorders and consequent disabilities-Indian Scenerio: Implications for rehabilitationpolicies and programmes."*Neurorehabilitationprinciples and practice. National Institute of Mental Health and Neuro Sciences: Bangalore*:1-35.

Hewer, R. Langton, and A. Tennant. 2002. "The epidemiology of disabling neurological disorders." In *Handbook of Neurological Rehabilitation*. Psychology Press.

Khan, F., B. Amatya, M. P. Galea, R. Gonzenbach, and J. Kesselring. 2017. "Neurorehabilitation: appliedneuroplasticity." *J Neurol* 264 (3):603-615. doi: 10. 1007/s00415-016-8307-9.

Khanna, M., G. S. Gowda, V. I. Bagevadi, A. Gupta, K. Kulkarni, S. Shyam RP, V. Basavaraju, M. B. Ramesh, H. N. Sashidhara, N. Manjunatha, N. K. Channaveerachari, and S. B. Math. 2018. "Feasibility and Utility of Tele-Neurorehabilitation Service in India: Experience from a Quaternary Center." *J Neurosci Rural Pract* 9 (4):541-544. doi: 10.4103/jnrp.jnrp_104_18.

MORTH. 2019. "Road accidents in India 2019." https://morth.nic.in/sites/default/files/RA_Uploading.pdf.

Prabhakar, S, JS Chopra, and D Pershad. 1991. "Physical disability and psychosocial functioning in neurological disorders: A follow up study."*Neurol India* 39:63-6.

Prakashi, R, and M Gourie-Devi. 1988. "Rehabilitation of neurologically disabled persons, Implications for community participation."*Rehabilitation Asia* 29:8-12.

Raj, Ankit, and Amit Agrawal. 2018. "Neurosurgery in India: Success and challenges."*International Journal of Academic Medicine* 4 (1):89.

Shakir, Raad, and Bo Norrving. 2017. "Stroke in ICD-11: the end of a long exile."*The Lancet* 389 (10087):2373. doi: 10.1016/S0140-6736(17)31567-2.

Singh, Gagandeep, Meenakshi Sharma, G. Anil Kumar, N. Girish Rao, Kameshwar Prasad, Prashant Mathur, Jeyaraj D. Pandian, Jaimie D. Steinmetz, Atanu Biswas, Pramod K.

Pal, Sanjay Prakash, P. N. Sylaja, Emma Nichols, Tarun Dua, Harkiran Kaur, Suvarna Alladi, Vivek Agarwal, Sumit Aggarwal, Atul Ambekar, Bhavani S. Bagepally, Tapas K. Banerjee, Rose G. Bender, Sadhana Bhagwat, Stuti Bhargava, Rohit Bhatia, Joy K. Chakma, Neerja Chowdhary, Subhojit Dey, M. Ashworth Dirac, Valery L. Feigin, Atreyi Ganguli, Mahaveer J. Golechha, M. Gourie-Devi, Vinay Goyal, Gaurav Gupta, Prakash C. Gupta, Rajeev Gupta, Gopalkrishna Gururaj, Rajkumar Hemalatha, Panniyammakal Jeemon, Catherine O. Johnson, Pradeep Joshi, Rajni Kant, Amal C. Kataki, Dheeraj Khurana, Rinu P. Krishnankutty, Hmwe H. Kyu, Stephen S. Lim, Rakesh Lodha, Rui Ma, Rajesh Malhotra, Ridhima Malhotra, Matthews Mathai, Ravi Mehrotra, Usha K. Misra, Parul Mutreja, Mohsen Naghavi, Nitish Naik, Minh Nguyen, Anamika Pandey, Priya Parmar, Arokiasamy Perianayagam, Dorairaj Prabhakaran, Goura K. Rath, Nickolas Reinig, Gregory A. Roth, Rajesh Sagar, Mari J. Sankar, K. S. Shaji, R. S. Sharma, Shweta Sharma, Ravinder Singh, M. V. Padma Srivastava, Benjamin A. Stark, Nikhil Tandon, J. S. Thakur, Akhil S. ThekkePurakkal, Sanjeev V. Thomas, Manjari Tripathi, Avina Vongpradith, Han Y. Wunrow, Denis Xavier, D. K. Shukla, K. Srinath Reddy, Samiran Panda, Rakhi Dandona, Christopher J. L. Murray, Theo Vos, R. S. Dhaliwal, and Lalit Dandona. 2021. "The burden of neurological disorders across the states of India: the Global Burden of DiseaseStudy 1990–2019." *The Lancet Global Health* 9 (8):e1129-e1144. doi: 10.1016/S2214-109X(21)00164-9.

Srinath Reddy, K., B. Shah, C. Varghese, and A. Ramadoss. 2005. "Responding to the threat of chronicdiseases in India." *Lancet* 366 (9498):1744-9. doi: 10.1016/s0140-6736(05)67343-6.

The, Lancet. 2016. "GBD 2015: from big data to meaningful change."*Lancet* 388 (10053):1447. doi: 10.1016/S0140-6736(16)31790-1.

Thomas, S. V., P. S. Sarma, M. Alexander, L. Pandit, L. Shekhar, C. Trivedi, and B. Vengamma. 2001. "Economic burden of epilepsy in India." *Epilepsia* 42 (8):1052-60. doi: 10.1046/j.1528-1157.2001.0420081052.x.

Vos, Theo, Amanuel Alemu Abajobir, Kalkidan Hassen Abate, Cristiana Abbafati, Kaja M. Abbas, Foad Abd-Allah, Rizwan Suliankatchi Abdulkader, Abdishakur M. Abdulle, Teshome Abuka Abebo, Semaw Ferede Abera, Victor Aboyans, Laith J. Abu-Raddad, Ilana N. Ackerman, Abdu Abdullahi Adamu, Olatunji Adetokunboh, Mohsen Afarideh, Ashkan Afshin, Sanjay Kumar Agarwal, Rakesh Aggarwal, Anurag Agrawal, Sutapa Agrawal, Hamid Ahmadieh, Muktar Beshir Ahmed, Miloud Taki Eddine Aichour, Amani Nidhal Aichour, Ibtihel Aichour, Sneha Aiyar, Rufus Olusola Akinyemi, Nadia Akseer, Faris Hasan Al Lami, Fares Alahdab, Ziyad Al-Aly, Khurshid Alam, Noore Alam, Tahiya Alam, Deena Alasfoor, Kefyalew Addis Alene, Raghib Ali, Reza Alizadeh-Navaei, Ala'a Alkerwi, François Alla, Peter Allebeck, Christine Allen, Fatma Al-Maskari, Rajaa Al-Raddadi, Ubai Alsharif, Shirina Alsowaidi, Khalid A. Altirkawi, Azmeraw T. Amare, Erfan Amini, Walid Ammar, Yaw Ampem Amoako, Hjalte H. Andersen, Carl Abelardo T. Antonio, Palwasha Anwari, Johan Ärnlöv, Al Artaman, Krishna Kumar Aryal, Hamid Asayesh, Solomon W. Asgedom, Reza Assadi, Tesfay Mehari Atey, Niguse Tadele Atnafu, Sachin R. Atre, Leticia Avila-Burgos, Euripide Frinel G. Arthur Avokphako, Ashish Awasthi, Umar Bacha, Alaa Badawi, Kalpana Balakrishnan, Amitava Banerjee, Marlena S.

Bannick, Aleksandra Barac, Ryan M. Barber, Suzanne L. Barker-Collo, Till Bärnighausen, Simon Barquera, Lars Barregard, Lope H. Barrero, Sanjay Basu, Bob Battista, Katherine E. Battle, Bernhard T. Baune, Shahrzad Bazargan-Hejazi, Justin Beardsley, Neeraj Bedi, Ettore Beghi, Yannick Béjot, Bayu Begashaw Bekele, Michelle L. Bell, Derrick A. Bennett, Isabela M. Bensenor, Jennifer Benson, Adugnaw Berhane, Derbew Fikadu Berhe, Eduardo Bernabé, Balem Demtsu Betsu, Mircea Beuran, Addisu Shunu Beyene, Neeraj Bhala, Anil Bhansali, Samir Bhatt, Zulfiqar A. Bhutta, Sibhatu Biadgilign, Burcu Kucuk Bicer, Kelly Bienhoff, Boris Bikbov, Charles Birungi, Stan Biryukov, Donal Bisanzio, Habtamu Mellie Bizuayehu, Dube Jara Boneya, Soufiane Boufous, Rupert R. A. Bourne, Alexandra Brazinova, Traolach S. Brugha, Rachelle Buchbinder, Lemma Negesa Bulto Bulto, Blair R. Bumgarner, Zahid A. Butt, Lucero Cahuana-Hurtado, Ewan Cameron, Mate Car, Hélène Carabin, Jonathan R. Carapetis, Rosario Cárdenas, David O. Carpenter, Juan Jesus Carrero, Austin Carter, Felix Carvalho, Daniel C. Casey, Valeria Caso, Carlos A. Castañeda-Orjuela, Chris D. Castle, Ferrán Catalá-López, Hsing-Yi Chang, Jung-Chen Chang, Fiona J. Charlson, Honglei Chen, Mirriam Chibalabala, Chioma Ezinne Chibueze, Vesper Hichilombwe Chisumpa, Abdulaal A. Chitheer, Devasahayam Jesudas Christopher, Liliana G. Ciobanu, Massimo Cirillo, Danny Colombara, Cyrus Cooper, Paolo Angelo Cortesi, Michael H. Criqui, John A. Crump, Abel Fekadu Dadi, Koustuv Dalal, Lalit Dandona, Rakhi Dandona, José das Neves, Dragos V. Davitoiu, Barbora de Courten, Diego De De Leo, Barthelemy Kuate Defo, Louisa Degenhardt, Selina Deiparine, Robert P. Dellavalle, Kebede Deribe, Don C. Des Jarlais, Subhojit Dey, Samath D. Dharmaratne, Preet Kaur Dhillon, Daniel Dicker, Eric L. Ding, Shirin Djalalinia, Huyen Phuc Do, E. Ray Dorsey, Kadine Priscila Bender dos Santos, Dirk Douwes-Schultz, Kerrie E. Doyle, Tim R. Driscoll, Manisha Dubey, Bruce Bartholow Duncan, Ziad Ziad El-Khatib, Jerisha Ellerstrand, Ahmadali Enayati, Aman Yesuf Endries, Sergey Petrovich Ermakov, Holly E. Erskine, Babak Eshrati, Sharareh Eskandarieh, Alireza Esteghamati, Kara Estep, Fanuel Belayneh Bekele Fanuel, Carla Sofia E. Sa Farinha, André Faro, Farshad Farzadfar, Mir Sohail Fazeli, Valery L. Feigin, Seyed-Mohammad Fereshtehnejad, João C. Fernandes, Alize J. Ferrari, Tesfaye Regassa Feyissa, Irina Filip, Florian Fischer, Christina Fitzmaurice, Abraham D. Flaxman, Luisa Sorio Flor, Nataliya Foigt, Kyle J. Foreman, Richard C. Franklin, Nancy Fullman, Thomas Fürst, Joao M. Furtado, Neal D. Futran, Emmanuela Gakidou, Morsaleh Ganji, Alberto L. Garcia-Basteiro, Teshome Gebre, Tsegaye Tewelde Gebrehiwot, Ayele Geleto, Bikila Lencha Gemechu, Hailay Abrha Gesesew, Peter W. Gething, Alireza Ghajar, Katherine B. Gibney, Paramjit Singh Gill, Richard F. Gillum, Ibrahim Abdelmageem Mohamed Ginawi, Ababi Zergaw Giref, Melkamu Dedefo Gishu, Giorgia Giussani, William W. Godwin, Audra L. Gold, Ellen M. Goldberg, Philimon N. Gona, Amador Goodridge, Sameer Vali Gopalani, Atsushi Goto, Alessandra Carvalho Goulart, Max Griswold, Harish Chander Gugnani, Rahul Gupta, Rajeev Gupta, Tanush Gupta, Vipin Gupta, Nima Hafezi-Nejad, Gessessew Bugssa Hailu, Alemayehu Desalegne Hailu, Randah Ribhi Hamadeh, Samer Hamidi, Alexis J. Handal, Graeme J. Hankey, Sarah Wulf Hanson, Yuantao Hao, Hilda L. Harb, Habtamu Abera Hareri, Josep Maria Haro, James Harvey, Mohammad Sadegh Hassanvand, Rasmus Havmoeller, Caitlin Hawley, Simon I. Hay, Roderick J. Hay,

Nathaniel J. Henry, Ileana Beatriz Heredia-Pi, Julio Montañez Hernandez, Pouria Heydarpour, Hans W. Hoek, Howard J. Hoffman, Nobuyuki Horita, H. Dean Hosgood, Sorin Hostiuc, Peter J. Hotez, Damian G. Hoy, Aung Soe Htet, Guoqing Hu, Hsiang Huang, Chantal Huynh, Kim Moesgaard Iburg, Ehimario Uche Igumbor, Chad Ikeda, Caleb Mackay Salpeter Irvine, Kathryn H. Jacobsen, Nader Jahanmehr, Mihajlo B. Jakovljevic, Simerjot K. Jassal, Mehdi Javanbakht, Sudha P. Jayaraman, Panniyammakal Jeemon, Paul N. Jensen, Vivekanand Jha, Guohong Jiang, Denny John, Sarah Charlotte Johnson, Catherine O. Johnson, Jost B. Jonas, Mikk Jürisson, Zubair Kabir, Rajendra Kadel, Amaha Kahsay, Ritul Kamal, Haidong Kan, Nadim E. Karam, André Karch, Corine Kakizi Karema, Amir Kasaeian, Getachew Mullu Kassa, Nigussie Assefa Kassaw, Nicholas J. Kassebaum, Anshul Kastor, Srinivasa Vittal Katikireddi, Anil Kaul, Norito Kawakami, Peter Njenga Keiyoro, Andre Pascal Kengne, Andre Keren, Yousef Saleh Khader, Ibrahim A. Khalil, Ejaz Ahmad Khan, Young-Ho Khang, Ardeshir Khosravi, Jagdish Khubchandani, Aliasghar Ahmad Kiadaliri, Christian Kieling, Yun Jin Kim, Daniel Kim, Pauline Kim, Ruth W. Kimokoti, Yohannes Kinfu, Adnan Kisa, Katarzyna A. Kissimova-Skarbek, Mika Kivimaki, Ann Kristin Knudsen, Yoshihiro Kokubo, Dhaval Kolte, Jacek A. Kopec, Soewarta Kosen, Parvaiz A. Koul, Ai Koyanagi, Michael Kravchenko, Sanjay Krishnaswami, Kristopher J. Krohn, G. Anil Kumar, Pushpendra Kumar, Sanjiv Kumar, Hmwe H. Kyu, Dharmesh Kumar Lal, Ratilal Lalloo, Nkurunziza Lambert, Qing Lan, Anders Larsson, Pablo M. Lavados, Janet L. Leasher, Paul H. Lee, Jong-Tae Lee, James Leigh, Cheru Tesema Leshargie, Janni Leung, Ricky Leung, Miriam Levi, Yichong Li, Yongmei Li, Darya Li Kappe, Xiaofeng Liang, Misgan Legesse Liben, Stephen S. Lim, Shai Linn, Patrick Y. Liu, Angela Liu, Shiwei Liu, Yang Liu, Rakesh Lodha, Giancarlo Logroscino, Stephanie J. London, Katharine J. Looker, Alan D. Lopez, Stefan Lorkowski, Paulo A. Lotufo, Nicola Low, Rafael Lozano, Timothy C. D. Lucas, Erlyn Rachelle King Macarayan, Hassan Magdy Abd El Razek, Mohammed Magdy Abd El Razek, Mahdi Mahdavi, Marek Majdan, Reza Majdzadeh, Azeem Majeed, Reza Malekzadeh, Rajesh Malhotra, Deborah Carvalho Malta, Abdullah A. Mamun, Helena Manguerra, Treh Manhertz, Ana Mantilla, Lorenzo G. Mantovani, Chabila C. Mapoma, Laurie B. Marczak, Jose Martinez-Raga, Francisco Rogerlândio Martins-Melo, Ira Martopullo, Winfried März, Manu Raj Mathur, Mohsen Mazidi, Colm McAlinden, Madeline McGaughey, John J. McGrath, Martin McKee, Claire McNellan, Suresh Mehata, Man Mohan Mehndiratta, Tefera Chane Mekonnen, Peter Memiah, Ziad A. Memish, Walter Mendoza, Mubarek Abera Mengistie, Desalegn Tadese Mengistu, George A. Mensah, Tuomo J. Meretoja, Atte Meretoja, Haftay Berhane Mezgebe, Renata Micha, Anoushka Millear, Ted R. Miller, Edward J. Mills, Mojde Mirarefin, Erkin M. Mirrakhimov, Awoke Misganaw, Shiva Raj Mishra, Philip B. Mitchell, Karzan Abdulmuhsin Mohammad, Alireza Mohammadi, Kedir Endris Mohammed, Shafiu Mohammed, Sanjay K. Mohanty, Ali H. Mokdad, Sarah K. Mollenkopf, Lorenzo Monasta, Marcella Montico, Maziar Moradi-Lakeh, Paula Moraga, Rintaro Mori, Chloe Morozoff, Shane D. Morrison, Mark Moses, Cliff Mountjoy-Venning, Kalayu Birhane Mruts, Ulrich O. Mueller, Kate Muller, Michele E. Murdoch, Gudlavalleti Venkata Satyanarayana Murthy, Kamarul Imran Musa, Jean B. Nachega, Gabriele Nagel, Mohsen Naghavi, Aliya

Naheed, Kovin S. Naidoo, Luigi Naldi, Vinay Nangia, Gopalakrishnan Natarajan, Dumessa Edessa Negasa, Ruxandra Irina Negoi, Ionut Negoi, Charles R. Newton, Josephine Wanjiku Ngunjiri, Trang Huyen Nguyen, Quyen Le Nguyen, Cuong Tat Nguyen, Grant Nguyen, Minh Nguyen, Emma Nichols, Dina Nur Anggraini Ningrum, Sandra Nolte, Vuong Minh Nong, Bo Norrving, Jean Jacques N. Noubiap, Martin J. O'Donnell, Felix Akpojene Ogbo, In-Hwan Oh, Anselm Okoro, Olanrewaju Oladimeji, Tinuke Oluwasefunmi Olagunju, Andrew Toyin Olagunju, Helen E. Olsen, Bolajoko Olubukunola Olusanya, Jacob Olusegun Olusanya, Kanyin Ong, John Nelson Opio, Eyal Oren, Alberto Ortiz, Aaron Osgood-Zimmerman, Majdi Osman, Mayowa O. Owolabi, Mahesh Pa, Rosana E. Pacella, Adrian Pana, Basant Kumar Panda, Christina Papachristou, Eun-Kee Park, Charles D. Parry, Mahboubeh Parsaeian, Scott B. Patten, George C. Patton, Katherine Paulson, Neil Pearce, David M. Pereira, Norberto Perico, Konrad Pesudovs, Carrie Beth Peterson, Max Petzold, Michael Robert Phillips, David M. Pigott, Julian David Pillay, Christine Pinho, Dietrich Plass, Martin A. Pletcher, Svetlana Popova, Richie G. Poulton, Farshad Pourmalek, Dorairaj Prabhakaran, Noela M. Prasad, Narayan Prasad, Carrie Purcell, Mostafa Qorbani, Reginald Quansah, Beatriz Paulina Ayala Quintanilla, Rynaz H. S. Rabiee, Amir Radfar, Anwar Rafay, Kazem Rahimi, Afarin Rahimi-Movaghar, Vafa Rahimi-Movaghar, Mohammad Hifz Ur Rahman, Mahfuzar Rahman, Rajesh Kumar Rai, Sasa Rajsic, Usha Ram, Chhabi Lal Ranabhat, Zane Rankin, Puja C. Rao, Paturi Vishnupriya Rao, Salman Rawaf, Sarah E. Ray, Robert C. Reiner, Nikolas Reinig, Marissa B. Reitsma, Giuseppe Remuzzi, Andre M. N. Renzaho, Serge Resnikoff, Satar Rezaei, Antonio L. Ribeiro, Luca Ronfani, Gholamreza Roshandel, Gregory A. Roth, Ambuj Roy, Enrico Rubagotti, George Mugambage Ruhago, Soheil Saadat, Nafis Sadat, Mahdi Safdarian, Sare Safi, Saeid Safiri, Rajesh Sagar, Ramesh Sahathevan, Joseph Salama, Huda Omer Ba Saleem, Joshua A. Salomon, Sundeep Santosh Salvi, Abdallah M. Samy, Juan R. Sanabria, Damian Santomauro, Itamar S. Santos, João Vasco Santos, Milena M. Santric Milicevic, Benn Sartorius, Maheswar Satpathy, Monika Sawhney, Sonia Saxena, Maria Inês Schmidt, Ione J. C. Schneider, Ben Schöttker, David C. Schwebel, Falk Schwendicke, Soraya Seedat, Sadaf G. Sepanlou, Edson E. Servan-Mori, Tesfaye Setegn, Katya Anne Shackelford, Amira Shaheen, Masood Ali Shaikh, Mansour Shamsipour, Sheikh Mohammed Shariful Islam, Jayendra Sharma, Rajesh Sharma, Jun She, Peilin Shi, Chloe Shields, Girma Temam Shifa, Mika Shigematsu, Yukito Shinohara, Rahman Shiri, Reza Shirkoohi, Shreya Shirude, Kawkab Shishani, Mark G. Shrime, Abla Mehio Sibai, Inga Dora Sigfusdottir, Diego Augusto Santos Silva, João Pedro Silva, Dayane Gabriele Alves Silveira, Jasvinder A. Singh, Narinder Pal Singh, Dhirendra Narain Sinha, Eirini Skiadaresi, Vegard Skirbekk, Erica Leigh Slepak, Amber Sligar, David L. Smith, Mari Smith, Badr H. A. Sobaih, Eugene Sobngwi, Reed J. D. Sorensen, Tatiane Cristina Moraes Sousa, Luciano A. Sposato, Chandrashekhar T. Sreeramareddy, Vinay Srinivasan, Jeffrey D. Stanaway, Vasiliki Stathopoulou, Nicholas Steel, Murray B. Stein, Dan J. Stein, Timothy J. Steiner, Caitlyn Steiner, Sabine Steinke, Mark Andrew Stokes, Lars Jacob Stovner, Bryan Strub, Michelle Subart, Muawiyyah Babale Sufiyan, Bruno F. Sunguya, Patrick J. Sur, Soumya Swaminathan, Bryan L. Sykes, Dillon O. Sylte, Rafael Tabarés-Seisdedos, Getachew Redae Taffere, Jukka S. Takala,

Nikhil Tandon, Mohammad Tavakkoli, Nuno Taveira, Hugh R. Taylor, Arash Tehrani-Banihashemi, Tesfalidet Tekelab, Abdullah Sulieman Terkawi, Dawit Jember Tesfaye, Belay Tesssema, Ornwipa Thamsuwan, Katie E. Thomas, Amanda G. Thrift, Tenaw Yimer Tiruye, Ruoyan Tobe-Gai, Mette C. Tollanes, Marcello Tonelli, Roman Topor-Madry, Miguel Tortajada, Mathilde Touvier, Bach Xuan Tran, Suryakant Tripathi, Christopher Troeger, Thomas Truelsen, Derrick Tsoi, Kald Beshir Tuem, Emin Murat Tuzcu, Stefanos Tyrovolas, Kingsley N. Ukwaja, Eduardo A. Undurraga, Chigozie Jesse Uneke, Rachel Updike, Olalekan A. Uthman, Benjamin S. Chudi Uzochukwu, Job F. M. van Boven, Santosh Varughese, Tommi Vasankari, S. Venkatesh, Narayanaswamy Venketasubramanian, Ramesh Vidavalur, Francesco S. Violante, Sergey K. Vladimirov, Vasiliy Victorovich Vlassov, Stein Emil Vollset, Fiseha Wadilo, Tolassa Wakayo, Yuan-Pang Wang, Marcia Weaver, Scott Weichenthal, Elisabete Weiderpass, Robert G. Weintraub, Andrea Werdecker, Ronny Westerman, Harvey A. Whiteford, Tissa Wijeratne, Charles Shey Wiysonge, Charles D. A. Wolfe, Rachel Woodbrook, Anthony D. Woolf, Abdulhalik Workicho, Denis Xavier, Gelin Xu, Simon Yadgir, Mohsen Yaghoubi, Bereket Yakob, Lijing L. Yan, Yuichiro Yano, Pengpeng Ye, Hassen Hamid Yimam, Paul Yip, Naohiro Yonemoto, Seok-Jun Yoon, Marcel Yotebieng, Mustafa Z. Younis, Zoubida Zaidi, Maysaa El Sayed Zaki, Elias Asfaw Zegeye, Zerihun Menlkalew Zenebe, Xueying Zhang, Maigeng Zhou, Ben Zipkin, Sanjay Zodpey, Liesl Joanna Zuhlke, and Christopher J. L. Murray. 2017. "Global, regional, and national incidence, prevalence, and years lived with disability for 328 diseases and injuries for 195 countries, 1990–2016: a systematic analysis for the Global Burden of Disease Study 2016." *The Lancet* 390 (10100):1211-1259. doi: 10.1016/S0140-6736(17)32154-2.

Ward, Anthony B, Christoph Gutenbrunner, Alessandro Giustini, Alain Delarque, Veronika Fialka-Moser, Carlotte Kiekens, Mihai Berteanu, and Nicolas Christodoulou. 2012. "A position paper on physical & rehabilitation medicine programmes in post-acute settings union of European Medical Specialists Section of Physical & Rehabilitation Medicine (in conjunction with the European Society of Physical & Rehabilitation Medicine)."*Journal of rehabilitation medicine* 44 (4):289-298.

Zorowitz, Richard D., and Anthony B. Ward. 2014. "The rehabilitation team and the economics of neurological rehabilitation." In *Textbook of Neural Repair and Rehabilitation: Volume 2: Medical Neurorehabilitation*, edited by Gert Kwakkel, Leonardo G. Cohen, Michael E. Selzer, Robert H. Miller and Stephanie Clarke, 278-288. Cambridge: Cambridge University Press.

Chapter 6

Prognostication in Traumatic Brain Injury

V. G. Ramesh*, **MCh, DNB**
Department of Neurosurgery, Chettinad Hospital and Research Institute, Chettinad Academy of Research and Education, Chennai, India

Abstract

Prediction of outcome in traumatic brain injury (TBI), is challenging, due to the complexity and continuously changing nature of the pathology and the facilities available in a particular set up. Various prognostic models have evolved over a period time, incorporating different sets of prognostic factors and are still evolving. This chapter highlights the various prognostic models that have evolved so far. Madras Head Injury Prognostic Scale (MHIPS), TBI-IMPACT model, CRASH model, GCS-PA charts are some of the recent models which find easy application. Prognostication in TBI helps not only for family counseling, but also for planning appropriate treatment strategies to improve the outcome.

Keywords: prognosis in head trauma, prognostication in head injury, prognostic scales in traumatic brain injury.

Introduction

Prognostication in medicine is predicting the future course of an illness based on medical knowledge and evidence. Prediction of outcome in TBI helps preparing the patient's family in case of expected unfavourable outcome,

---

* Corresponding Author's Email: drvgramesh@hotmail.com

In: Rehabilitation in Neurotrauma
Editors: VD Sinha, Amit Chakraborty, Jitin Bajaj et al.
ISBN: 978-1-68507-787-7

triaging the patients in mass casualty and also helps the physician in clinical decision making process in planning better treatment to improve the outcome in patients with possible poor outcome. Prognostic models can also help in: "(a) guiding health-care policy by generating global predictive scenarios, (b) assisting comparative audit among hospitals by (case-mix adjusted) mortality predictions, (c) determining study eligibility of patients for new treatments, (d) defining inclusion criteria for clinical trials to control for variation in prognosis, (e) cost reimbursement programs, and (f) selecting appropriate tests and therapies in individual patient management including supporting decisions on withholding or with-drawing therapy" (Abu-Hanna & Lucas, 2001).Because of the heterogeneous and dynamic nature of TBI, the prediction of outcome following TBI has been a challenge.

Prognostic Models in TBI

There are well established factors affecting the prognosis in TBI. Age, Glasgow Coma Scale (GCS) score, Size of the pupils and their reaction to light, brainstem reflexes like oculocephalic reflex, Hypotension and Computerised Tomographic (CT) Scan features are well established prognostic factors (Jiang, Gao, Li, Yu, & Zhu, 2002). Intracranial pressure (ICP), multimodality evoked potentials, biochemical parameters like creatinine phosphokinase isoenzyme BB (CPK-BB), neuron specific enolase (NSE), myelin basic protein (MBP), S-100 protein, etc., are also other prognostic indicators. (Adams et al., 2017; Herrmann et al., 2001)Prognostic models or scoring systems involve quantification of the severity of disease based on established prognostic factors and predicting possible outcome based on the score.

Various prognostic models for TBI have been developed over the years. Narayan's logistic model (1981) used clinical factors (age, GCS, pupillary response), CT findings, ICP and motor evoked potentials (MEP) and a linear logistic regression model was applied to predict the prognosis in two groups - good outcome or poor outcome. Outcome in 96% patients could be predicted accurately. (Narayan et al., 1981) Choi's model (1988) based on age, motor response of GCS and unilateral or bilateral absent pupillary response and prediction was made by locating the variables in a ready-reference graphs created for this purpose. Outcome in 90% of patients could be predicted accurately (Choi, Narayan, Anderson, & Ward, 1988). In Leed's Scoring system factors such as age, non-reactive pupils, ICP, systolic blood pressure,

GCS score, other extracranial injuries and hyperdense lesions on CT scans. This system predicted outcome in 80% of patients accurately. (Feldman, Contant, Robertson, Narayan, & Grossman, 1991; Myles Gibson & Stephenson, 1989) · Klauber's model (1989) used the GCS motor score, pupillary light reaction, systolic pressure, age, chest injury, abdominal injury with a logistic regression coefficient assigned for each of the factors to calculate the predicted outcome. (Klauber et al., 1989) The mathematical model developed at the Post-Graduate Institute of Medical Education and Research, Chandigarh, India, (Chandigarh mathematical model 2000), is based on the GCS motor score, Reaction Level Scale, and brain stem reflexes, assigning coefficient to each parameter based on linear logistic regression and a formula to calculate the predicted outcome. This model predicted outcome accurately in 84% of patients (Mukherjee, Sharma, Ramanathan, Khandelwal, & Kak, 2000). The National Institute of Mental Health and NeuroSciences, Bangalore, India model (NIMHANS model, 2003), used the GCS motor score, oculo-cephalic response and midline shift on CT scan and developed an equation based on these factors and the outcome was predicted. The model had a sensitivity of 75% in predicting the outcome. (Pillai, Kolluri, & Praharaj, 2003).

Despite having a good predictive value, these prediction models seldom find usage in the routine clinical practice because: 1) some of them involve parameters like ICP, evoked potentials, etc., which are not available in all centers; 2) most of them involve complex equations and mathematical calculations or charts; 3) many of the models have not had cross or external validation, which would have ensured universal validity of these models in predicting outcome in other centers also. Some of the recently developed prognostic models have tried to address these concerns.

Madras Head Injury Prognostic Scale (MHIPS)

The Madras Head Injury Prognostic Scale (MHIPS, 2008) bases prediction on six easily available clinical parameters, namely, age, GCS motor score on admission, reaction of pupils to light, oculo-cephalic reflex, CT scan findings, other major skeletal and systemic injuries. Everyone of these parameters is subdivided into 3 groups, which are assigned a score according to the expected prognosis (Table 1).

Out of the maximum possible score of 18, those patients with MHIPS score of 15 and above have good outcome; those with 13 and 14 are vegetative or have severely disability; those with 12 and less had mortality. Prospective study involving 104 patients showed 87.5% accuracy of prediction. (Ramesh, Thirumaran, & Raja, 2008) MHIPS has validated in other centers also, which predicted an accuracy of prediction of 92.3% to 100% (Ebrahimi et al., 2016; Mendoza Astolingon, 2014). MHIPS is a simple numerical scale like the GCS and can be easily applied at the bedside, using readily available clinical and CT parameters. MHIPS is now available onweb (http://www. medical algorithms.com/madras-head-injury-prognostic-scale-mhips-head-trauma-assessment) and mobile app (Medical calculators -'Medal'- Google playstore) (Ramesh, 2021).

Table 1. Madras Head Injury Prognostic Scale (MHIPS)

Prognostic Factor	**Sub Group**	**Score**
Age	> 45 Years 15 – 45 Years < 15 Years	1 2 3
Best Motor Response (GCS)	1 – 2 3 – 4 5 – 6	1 2 3
Pupillary light reflex	Absent Impaired Normal	1 2 3
Oculo Cephalic Response	Absent Impaired Normal	1 2 3
CT scan findings	Absent basal cisterns/ Midline shift > 5 mm./ Lesion density > 3 cm. Diameter Partly effaced basal cisterns/ Midline shift < 5 mm./ Lesion density < 3 cm. Diameter Normal basal cisterns/ No midline shift/ No lesions	1 2 3
Systemic injuries	Thoracic/Abdominal visceral injuries/ > 2 long bone fractures. One or two long bone fractures No other systemic or long bone injuries	1 2 3

TBI-IMPACT Model

International Mission for Prognosis and Analysis of Clinical Trials in TBI (TBI-IMPACT, 2008) investigators developed prognostic models for predicting outcome at the end of 6 months for moderate and severe TBI (GCS 12 and less). Three models of increasing complexities have been developed (Table 2).

Table 2. TBI-IMPACT (Prediction models for 6 months outcome)

Characteristics	Value	Score	Sum
Age (Years)	< 30	0	
	30-39	1	
	40-49	2	
	50-59	3	
	60-69	4	
	70+	5	
Motor score	None/extension	6	
	Abnormal flexion	4	
	Normal flexion	2	
	Localizes/obeys	0	
	Untestable/ missing	3	
Pupillary reactivity		0	
	Bilateral reactive	2	
	Unilateral reactive	4	
	Bilateral non-reactive		________
Sum Score Core Model			
Hypoxia	Yes/suspected	1	
	No	0	
Hypotension	Yes/suspected	1	
	No	0	
CT classification	I	-2	
	II	0	
	III/IV	2	

Table 2. (Continued)

Characteristics	Value	Score	Sum
	V/VI	2	
Traumatic subarachnoid hemorrhage	Yes No	2	
Epidural hematoma	Yes No	-2 0	________
Sum score extended model	Sub score CT	________	
Glucose (mmol/l)	<6 6-8.9 9-11.9 12-14.9 15+	0 1 2 3 4	
Hb (g/dl)	<9 9-11.9 12-14.9 15+	4 3 2 1	
Sum score lab model	Sub score lab	________	________

Sum scores can be calculated for the core model (age, motor score, pupillary reactivity), the extended model (core + hypoxia + hypotension + CT characteristics), and a lab model (core + hypoxia + hypotension + CT + glucose + Hb). Th e probability of 6 mo outcome is defi ned as 1 / (1 + e-LP), where LP refers to the linear predictor in a logistic regression model. Six LPs were defi ned as follows:

- LPcore, mortality=-2.55 + 0.275 * sum score core
- LPcore, unfavorable=-1.62 + 0.299 * sum score core
- LPextended, mortality=-2.98 + 0.256 * sum score extended
- LPextended, unfavorable=-2.10 + 0.276 * sum score extended
- LPlab, mortality=-3.42 + 0.216 * sum score lab
- LPlab, unfavorable=-2.82 + 0.257 * sum score core lab

(reproduced from Steyerberg et al., PLoS Medicine 5(8):5165)

The predicted outcome is arrived at using complex mathematical calculations where the linear predictor for each model is calculated using logistic regression equations for each of the three models. (Steyerberg et al., 2008) For easy practical application, computer based TBI-IMPACT calculator is available in the internet (http://www.tbi-impact.org/?p=impact/calc). The TBI-IMPACT model is a well validated model internationally. It has the disadvantage of requiring a computer-based app. for prediction of outcome. This model has been recommended by the authors only for studying large group of patients and not for predicting outcome in a single patient.

CRASH Model

Corticosteroid Randomisation After Significant Head Injury Model (CRASH model, 2008) has been advocated for estimating the possibility of death in 14 days and mortality and severe disability at six months in TBI. It uses the parameters like age, GCS, Pupil reaction to light, other major systemic injury, CT scan findings and the economic category of the country (high-, middle- or low-income country). Two prediction models are available as a chart with mutivariate prediction with and without CT findings, shown as odds ratio at 95% confidence interval. (Perel et al., 2008) Like TBI-IMPACT, CRASH model also has a web based calculator for easy application (www.crash2.lshtm.ac.uk/). The CRASH model also has been validated internationally and has been found to be very reliable. The authors also have urged caution while making judgment on individual patients.

GCS-PA Prognostic Charts

In 2018, Murray, Brennan and Teasdale modified the GCS to include the pupillary light reflex to further refine GCS to include brainstem function and called it GCS-P score (Brennan, Murray, & Teasdale, 2018):

Pupils Reactive to Light	Pupil Reactivity Score
Both Pupils	0
One Pupil	1
Neither Pupil	2

GCS-P = GCS - Pupil Reactivity Score

GCS-P has been intended to serve as an index of the severity of the patient's clinical status as well as the prognosis. They have further developed graphic charts for predicting the outcome after TBI, on the basis of Age, GCS, Pupillary reaction to light and CT scan findings (GCS-PA charts) and are able to prognosticate the possibility of death and independent recovery at six months (expressed as % of probability) (Brennan et al., 2018). These charts are also very user-friendly and are finding wide acceptance.

Conclusion

The recently developed prognostic models for TBI like, MHIPS, TBI-IMPACT, CRASH, GCS-PA are highly reliable. MHIPS is very simple and can be easily used like the GCS in the bedside, as it does not involve any complex formulae or equations and web based app is also available for those who need it. TBI-IMPACT and CRASH models are popular, but always require web-based calculator to predict the prognosis. GCS-PA charts are finding wide acceptance, but require the use of graphical charts. The prediction tools in TBI, when used judiciously, can help in better planning of treatment strategies, counseling of the patient's relatives and also for epidemiological studies. The ability to predict the prognosis should not hamper the intensity of treatment of a seriously injured patient with TBI.

References

Abu-Hanna, A., & Lucas, P. J. (2001). Prognostic models in medicine. AI and statistical approaches. *Methods Inf Med, 40*(1), 1-5.

Adams, H., Donnelly, J., Czosnyka, M., Kolias, A. G., Helmy, A., Menon, D. K., . . . Hutchinson, P. J. (2017). Temporal profile of intracranial pressure and cerebrovascular reactivity in severe traumatic brain injury and association with fatal outcome: An observational study. *PLoS Med, 14*(7), e1002353. doi:10.1371/journal.pmed.1002353.

Brennan, P. M., Murray, G. D., & Teasdale, G. M. (2018). Simplifying the use of prognostic information in traumatic brain injury. Part 1: The GCS-Pupils score: an extended index of clinical severity. *J. Neurosurg., 128*(6), 1612-1620. doi:10.3171/2017.12.jns172780.

Choi, S. C., Narayan, R. K., Anderson, R. L., & Ward, J. D. (1988). Enhanced specificity of prognosis in severe head injury. *J. Neurosurg., 69*(3), 381-385. doi:10.3171/jns.1988.69.3.0381.

Ebrahimi, H., Abbasi, A., Hoseini, A., Shamsizadeh, M., Bazghaleah, M., & Hekmtafshar, M. (2016). Comparison of patient's prognostic based on Madras Head Injury Prognostic Scale and Glasgow Outcome Scale in head trauma patients admitted in emergency ward of 5th Azar educative and therapeutic center in Gorgan, 2011. *Journal of Clinical Nursing and Midwifery, 4*, 68-79.

Feldman, Z., Contant, C. F., Robertson, C. S., Narayan, R. K., & Grossman, R. G. (1991). Evaluation of the Leeds prognostic score for severe head injury. *The Lancet, 337*(8755), 1451-1453. doi:10.1016/0140-6736(91)93137-X.

Herrmann, M., Curio, N., Jost, S., Grubich, C., Ebert, A. D., Fork, M. L., & Synowitz, H. (2001). Release of biochemical markers of damage to neuronal and glial brain tissue is associated with short and long term neuropsychological outcome after traumatic brain injury. *J. Neurol. Neurosurg. Psychiatry, 70*(1), 95-100. doi:10.1136/jnnp.70.1.95.

Jiang, J. Y., Gao, G. Y., Li, W. P., Yu, M. K., & Zhu, C. (2002). Early indicators of prognosis in 846 cases of severe traumatic brain injury. *J. Neurotrauma, 19*(7), 869-874. doi:10.1089/08977150260190456.

Klauber, M. R., Marshall, L. F., Luerssen, T. G., Frankowski, R., Tabaddor, K., & Eisenberg, H. M. (1989). Determinants of head injury mortality: importance of the low risk patient. *Neurosurgery, 24*(1), 31-36. doi:10.1227/00006123-198901000-00005.

Mendoza Astolingon, E. P. (2014). Comparación de scores de severidad del trauma en la predicción de mortalidad en pacientes con traumatismo encéfalo craneano. *Universidad Privada Antenor Orrego.*

Mukherjee, K., Sharma, B., Ramanathan, S., Khandelwal, N., & Kak, V. (2000). A mathematical outcome prediction model in severe head injury : a pilot study. *Neurol. India, 48*(1), 43-48.

Myles Gibson, R., & Stephenson, G. C. (1989). Aggressive Management of Severe Closed Head Trauma: Time for Reappraisal. *The Lancet, 334*(8659), 369-371. doi:10.1016/s0140-6736(89)90546-1.

Narayan, R. K., Greenberg, R. P., Miller, J. D., Enas, G. G., Choi, S. C., Kishore, P. R., . . . Becker, D. P. (1981). Improved confidence of outcome prediction in severe head injury. A comparative analysis of the clinical examination, multimodality evoked potentials, CT scanning, and intracranial pressure. *J. Neurosurg., 54*(6), 751-762. doi:10.3171/jns.1981.54.6.0751.

Perel, P., Arango, M., Clayton, T., Edwards, P., Komolafe, E., Poccock, S., . . . Yutthakasemsunt, S. (2008). Predicting outcome after traumatic brain injury: practical prognostic models based on large cohort of international patients. *Bmj, 336*(7641), 425-429. doi:10.1136/bmj.39461.643438.25.

Pillai, S. V., Kolluri, V. R., & Praharaj, S. S. (2003). Outcome prediction model for severe diffuse brain injuries: development and evaluation. *Neurol India, 51*(3), 345-349.

Ramesh, V. G. (2021). Head Trauma Assessment Prognostic Scale | Medical Algorithm | Medicalalgorithms.com. Retrieved from https://www.medicalalgorithms.com/.

Ramesh, V. G., Thirumaran, K. P., & Raja, M. C. (2008). A new scale for prognostication in head injury. *J. Clin. Neurosci., 15*(10), 1110-1113; discussion 1113-1114. doi:10.1016/j.jocn.2007.08.033.

Steyerberg, E. W., Mushkudiani, N., Perel, P., Butcher, I., Lu, J., McHugh, G. S., . . . Maas, A. I. (2008). Predicting outcome after traumatic brain injury: development and international validation of prognostic scores based on admission characteristics. *PLoS Med, 5*(8), e165; discussion e165. doi:10.1371/journal.pmed.0050165.

Chapter 7

Nutrition in Brain Trauma, Cognitive Sequelae and Quality of Life in Mild Head Injury

Shilpi Pandey[1], Ved Prakash Maurya[2,*], Mayank Singh[2] and Kamlesh Singh Bhaisora[2]

[1]Department of Neurology, Sanjay Gandhi Postgraduate Institute of Medical Sciences, Lucknow, India

[2]Department of Neurosurgery, Sanjay Gandhi Postgraduate Institute of Medical Sciences, Lucknow, India

Abstract

The modern developed world has significantly raised the incidence of traumatic brain injury and the individuals living with the sequelae of traumatic brain injury. The global burden of head injury has raised to such an extent that it has become the third leading cause of death. Following a traumatic head injury, there is an immediate injury to an individual in the form of mechanical injury to the brain parenchyma and a hematoma formation in various combinations and locations. The extensive physiological commitment of brain plays a vital role in regulating the metabolic activities of almost all body organs. These metabolic alterations result in increased state of catabolism, leading to enhanced protein degradation resulting in negative protein balance. These abrupt alterations in homeostasis make an individual prone to many physiological stresses leading to infections. The delayed effects of traumatic brain injury (TBI) reflect an increased financial burden on the family and society. Available evidence suggests that mild traumatic brain injury patients require a shorter duration of hospitalization but the

---

* Corresponding Author's Email: vpmsurgery@gmail.com

In: Rehabilitation in Neurotrauma
Editors: VD Sinha, Amit Chakraborty, Jitin Bajaj et al.
ISBN: 978-1-68507-787-7

cognitive and rehabilitative measures are not less crucial than candidates with moderate and severe brain injury. The effect of head trauma reflects impairment of the quality of life, resulting in poor health-related quality of life (HRQoL) and an unfavourable Glasgow outcome scale (GOS). The present chapter will discuss the nutritional demand and change in metabolic needs, cognitive outcome, and aberration in quality of life following mild brain trauma.

Introduction

Brain trauma refers to an injury to the brain parenchyma resulting from various underlying mechanisms, such as road traffic accidents, fall from height, gunshot injury to the head or a sudden blow to the head. Features of traumatic brain injury (TBI) appears following fracture of skull bone, hematoma collection outside (extradural hematoma) or inside the dural covering (subdural hematoma) of the brain, as well as bleed in the brain parenchyma (contusion). For practical purposes, the severity of the head injury is categorized based on the Glasgow Coma Scale (GCS) and the duration of disrupted memory following head trauma (Mahan and Raymond, 2017; Stern et al., 2015). With the advent of industrialization and the availability of modern automobiles, TBI is now the third leading cause of death and disability worldwide. The burden of disability reflects that there are about 200 victims per 100 000 populations and the adolescent and youth between 15 years to 35 years are the most affected age group (Mahan and Raymond, 2017).

The head injury event has been considered a point epidemic of the modern world. Following TBI, there are short term and long term consequences that affect the individual and society to a variable degree. The human brain is the complex organ system that continuously regulates the autonomic, endocrine, metabolic, and external challenges in day-to-day activity. Following a head injury, a complex metabolic alteration occurs, which affects the internal homeostasis of an individual. This alteration initiates a cascade of aberrant inflammatory, cellular, metabolic, and endocrine responses. The available literature supports a significant metabolic alteration that increases catabolism after head trauma. The classic symptoms following head injury are headache, confusion, decreased attention span and blurring of vision- the severity of these symptoms increases in case of moderate to severe head injury. The long-term dysfunction following head injury may include depression, agitation, impaired speech or gait, seizure disorder, and behavioural dysfunction (Shen et al., 2016).

Nutrition in Brain Trauma

Head trauma initiates a state of hypermetabolism which leads to nearly double the amount of energy expenditure. This state of hypermetabolism extends for weeks up to a year following head injury (Lee-anne et al., 2015). This hypermetabolism is followed by a state of increased catabolism wherein an increased loss of muscle tissue, up to 20 gram/ day, and increased urinary excretion of nitrogen up to 25-30 gram/ day are the usual metabolic disturbances. Enhanced mobilization of nitrogen from the muscle tissue, leading to gluconeogenesis, decreased muscle mass, and excessive nitrogen excretion. Excessive urinary depletion of zinc results in decreased serum levels of zinc (Daradkeh et al., 2014; Duraski, Lovell and Roth, 2014). The inflammatory response to head trauma leads to a surge in cytokine production (IL-1, IL-6, 1L-8 and TNF). These inflammatory mediators result in altered amino acid metabolism and increased hepatic acute phase reactants production. Reduction in muscle mass and increased counter-regulatory hormones (cortisol, glucagon and catecholamines) are the by-products. Even though the head-injured patient is bedridden, enhanced systemic and cerebral energy requirements are the rule (Campos and Machado, 2012).

Gut-Brain Axis in the Regulation of Nutrition

As discussed earlier, the brain is the final regulatory centre of food intake, homeostasis of fluid and electrolytes, and activation of feeding and satiety centres.

The hypothalamus and brainstem are directly involved in regulating gut activity via a variety of neuronal pathways. These pathways regulate food intake and the gastrointestinal system's mechanical activities (Dodds, 2017). The lateral nucleus of the hypothalamus serves as the feeding centre, and stimulation of this centre increases the food intake. The paraventricular, dorsomedial, and arcuate nucleus of the hypothalamus has a significant role in regulating food intake. The injury to the dorsomedial nucleus is associated with decreased intake of food and results in weight loss or starvation. These features of the brain-gut axis support a pivotal role of traumatic brain injury in disturbing the internal milieu of an individual and alteration in food habits. Following a head injury, a reduction in body weight and significant weight gain has been reported. A prospective study suggested a nearly 15% increase in body weight of the individuals following head trauma (Crenn et al., 2014).

Physiological functions of appetite and energy metabolism are regulated by Adipokines, which are expressed profusely in the central nervous system. A dysregulation in the level of these Adipokines is associated with several neurological disorders (Parimisetty et al., 2016). Orexin neuron activity is mitigated by tumour necrosis factors (TNF). In most head trauma cases, decreased Orexin level was a frequent physiological derangement. Decreased Orexin, in turn, is responsible for reduced appetite and weight loss (Clark and Vissel, 2014).

Nutritional Support and Clinical Outcomes

The head injury patients who require hospital care undergo significant protein and energy deficits, and these events are associated with unfavourable outcomes (Lee-anne et al., 2016). Irrespective of the degree of injury or severity of head trauma, those patients who receive adequate nutritional care lead to better outcomes.

This clinical improvement reflects decreased hours of mechanical ventilation, reduction in the days of hospitalization, and an overall reduction in the expense of medical care. In order to restore homeostasis and prevent secondary complications by reactivating the immune system, early initiation of nutritional support is mandatory. After trauma, enteral or parenteral nutritional support must be initiated (Aadal, Mortensen and Nielsen, 2015). After 1- 2 days, advanced nutritional planning needs to be initiated following traumatic brain injury. A cohort study conducted at multiple centres advocates the importance of early initiation of enteral feeding following TBI. Those patients with early commencement of enteral nutrition performed much better in the form of early improvement in the GCS on the seventh post-trauma day, improved clinical status at one month following trauma, and better overall survival rates (Chiang et al., 2012). On the contrary, those subjected to delayed initiation of enteral nutrition resulted in significant protein and calorie depletion ($p < 0.001$). This protein-energy malnutrition resulted in a significant increment in the duration of mechanical ventilation and prolonged hospital stay (Dodds, 2017).

Specific Challenges in Nutrition for Brain Trauma Patients

The hypermetabolic state of physiological alteration following head injury not only affects the initial period of hospitalization but equally influences the recovery and rehabilitation as long term sequelae. The continued inflammatory response and inability to walk appropriately lead to hypermetabolism and negative protein balance in the body. After the initial phase of acute crisis, the muscles' resultant tone is also responsible for deciding the extent of daily energy expenditure. Increased calories are required in the spastic conditions of the muscle because of persistent sympathetic neuronal discharges responsible for maintaining the increased tone of the muscles. This hypermetabolic state and decreased nutritional intake results in cachexia, which indirectly increases hospital stay duration, decreased wound healing rate, and complication development such as urinary tract infections and deep vein thrombosis. The oral intake of these patients is significantly below average due to impaired swallowing and depressed level of sensorium. The transition of patients out of intensive care units favours the transition from hypertonic ICU based fluid to isotonic and ample volume of dietary preparations. Initiation of enteral nutrition must be reassessed regularly to look for inadequate intake, which brings the role of parenteral nutrition into the picture. Adequate fluid with electrolyte replacement is paramount if the patient is undergoing supplementation with an enteral diet. Replacement of free water and electrolytes is crucial to maintain a balance between serum sodium, serum creatinine, and blood urea nitrogen.

Renal and hepatic dysfunctions that result in a significant electrolyte, metabolic, and mental status alterations are well avoided once adequate monitoring is performed.

Several case reports and case series report the altered food behaviour and individual's personality following TBI. Most of the literature discusses malnutrition following TBI, but few of these mentions hyperphagia. The disruption in the regular physiological activity of the hypothalamus leads to an alteration in food habits. Several studies advocate no change in nutritional status following head injury. There is a significant disparity in the objective findings of cerebral imaging of individuals with TBI and nutritional status of an individual because the diffuse axonal injury is not readily noticed on conventional CT and MRI scans. There is a lack of robust evidence to correlate head injury and alteration in food habits. In the future, studies should be designed that focus on the alteration in food habits with the category of head injury.

Cognitive Sequelae in Mild Head Injury

Mild traumatic brain injury (mTBI) contributes most common type of head injury and is also labelled as concussion (Alexander, 1992; Barth et al., 1983). According to the mTBI Committee of the American Congress of Rehabilitation Medicine, this event of head trauma results in loss of consciousness for a brief duration, after which there occurs an impairment in cognitive function. mTBI is characterized by a spectrum of symptoms of which headache is the commonest one.

The other notable symptoms include fatigue, anxiety, irritability to a variable extent (Tyerman and King, 2009).

A set of skilled functions known as executive function are involved following head injury, which inhibits the individual in carrying out flexible thinking, planning the organizational activity, and multitasking. This results in a significant amount of stress and inability to carry out their task smoothly at the workplace. The subtle cognitive dysfunctions may not be evident in the early period following trauma. This is because the memory and the educational skills remain pretty intact, and hence the day-to-day activity or conversation goes unnoticed. Once these individuals are subjected to neuropsychological evaluation, the cognitive deficits become apparent and need therapeutic intervention. In the case of mild TBI, there is a significant improvement in cognitive dysfunction during the recovery phase, but this does not happen in moderate or severe head injury. Certain aspects of cognition need to be discussed to emphasize the impact of head trauma on an individual's personality.

Memory Dysfunction

Memory dysfunction is one of the most typical problems nearly all individuals face after trauma, and it takes various forms. The significant problem is regarding the amnesia of the event following the episode. There occurs a significant problem in recalling the events before trauma and registration of new information following head injury. Retrograde amnesia refers to memory loss of events landing up to the injury. The individual finds it difficult to recall the events that resulted in the injury. This period may range from a few seconds, minutes, hours, days, weeks, or even longer. The prolonged duration of amnesia becomes significantly distressing to the individual and family members.

Post-traumatic amnesia: The impairment in memory that arises following trauma is referred to as post-traumatic amnesia. In this situation, the individual is confused about the activities after trauma and finds it challenging to retain the events later on. This duration is also variable and may range from seconds, minutes to months. In this situation, the individual carries on a sensible conversation about the familiar objects or topics but finds it difficult to remember them longer.

Concentration and Attention

The individuals following head trauma find it difficult to concentrate on a topic for a significant amount of time. Some individuals have difficulty conducting multi-tasking, while others have the problem of easy distractibility. Such individuals find it challenging to initiate and complete a task in a single setting and requires repeated sessions to carry out relatively simple and trim work. Such problems carry a far-reaching implication and significantly affect work, social activity, and interpersonal relationships.

Language Dysfunction

After mTBI, the difficulty in language skills is not an uncommon issue. There may be issues related to word-finding, and often experiences the lack of vocabulary. There may be difficulty organizing their thoughts while conversating on a complex issue. There may be problems recognizing the words and speech of a familiar personality. The problem of word selection, as well as fair use of grammar, may be challenging. The task of reading and writing may become challenging and often becomes a topic of distress for the individual and the family.

Executive Function

Executive Function is one of the most familiar and distressing issues noticed after head trauma. The individual experiences difficulty in planning, reasoning and decision making. During the daily conversation, the continuity of the thought process is broken frequently, and they find it difficult to express their opinion in a group discussion. It becomes a difficult task for an individual to identify the problem, make a judgement and think about the possibilities of a solution. Such individuals have compromised planning, monitoring and evaluating their performance.

Awareness and Insight

After head trauma, there occurs a significant impairment in awareness of an individual about self and the surrounding. Such individuals are unaware of their presentation and the problems they have been undergoing. The lack of awareness and insight is noticed in the early stage following trauma and gradually starts regaining awareness over time. The impact of head trauma is such that with time, individuals start regaining awareness and insight into their mobility, speech, and self-awareness but often fail to regain normalcy.

Perceptual Skills

The perceptual skills are impaired following trauma, and individuals who follow head injury finds it difficult in their daily activity. The most common perceptual skills impaired are recognizing and identifying the known objects and individual faces. This problem may often get complicated due to diplopia, decreased visual acuity and impaired ocular movement leading to a restricted field of vision. Similar problems may be noticed in auditory and tactile perception and carry significant hearing and sensation challenges.

Spatial and Constructional Skills

Individuals with head trauma may face difficulty in accurately judging objects in their surroundings, leading to wrong assessment of distance between two objects. There are problems related to correct laterality and difficulty locating a familiar object even with familiar routes. Few individuals face difficulty in constructional skills and feel distressing in carrying out activities such as copying, drawing, cooking in the correct sequence of orders (S. S. Dikmen et al., 2003).

Quality of Life in Mild Head Injury

The majority of the patients who seek medical attention following head injury fall in mild Traumatic Brain Injury (mTBI) category. The majority of the mTBI are categorized based on the crude clinical signs of patients upon hospital admission (GCS score of 13-15). It has been well established that following moderate to severe head injury, there is a significant possibility of permanent disability, but there is an ongoing debate about the clinical recovery and disability following mTBI (Maas, Stocchetti and Bullock, 2008; Nelson et al., 2016). Mild TBI manifests acute symptoms in impaired cognitive function and difficulty executing day-to-day activities (Carroll et al., 2014; Rimel et al., 1981). These findings manifest even after the acute phase has elapsed, and the residual disability persists even for months to a year following injury (S. Dikmen, Machamer and Temkin, 2017).

The consequences arising as a result of TBI can be assessed with the help of a generic and the measures specific to the disease for the measurement of HRQoL (health-related quality of life), which is recommended (Polinder et al., 2015; Attenberger, Amsler and Gross, 2012). Although there seems to be a significant advancement in managing patients with head trauma or polytrauma, the post-trauma outcome and impact on the individual's life is still a less explored area. These alterations in one's daily activity and the level of care involved for an individual from the family and society reflects the quality of life or HRQoL. Several tools or scales have been employed to assess the assessment of QOL (Quality of life) of individuals following trauma or surgery. There is a significant deficit of standardized interpretation tools for the integrated use of available measures. The POLO (Polytrauma outcome) chart represents a combination of scores developed for the patients who sustained polytrauma, including head injury. This POLO chart comprises the GOS (Glasgow outcome scale), the EQ-5D and the SF-36 (Short form- 36) (Pirente et al., 2002). On a day-to-day basis, the practical applicability of these scoring systems appears difficult for individuals. The applicability of trauma-specific TOP addresses both the factors related to the general criteria of HRQoL and the parameters related to trauma for long-term survival and outcome. Von Steinbuchel et al. proposed that the components of QOLIBRI (Quality of life after brain injury) focused mainly on the cognitive, emotional and psychological factors rather than the physical changes noticed in an individual's body following trauma (Von Steinbüchel et al., 2010). There is literature that focuses on the severity of the head injury, which correlated the HRQoL and their recovery pattern. The application of the QOLIBRI scale was postulated that those patients with mild head injury do not have better cognitive functioning than those with a severe head injury (Soberg et al., 2017).

Conclusion

The nutrition requirement of mild traumatic head injury patients' needs to be individualized depending upon one's daily requirement keeping in mind the increased catabolic rate. The cognitive impairment and quality of life are often less discussed but carries a massive impact on the recovery of these patients with a head injury.

References

Aadal Lena, Mortensen Jesper and Feldbæk Nielsen Jørgen 2015 'Weight Reduction after Severe Brain Injury: A Challenge during the Rehabilitation Course'. *Journal of Neuroscience Nursing* 47 (2): 85-90.

Alexander Michael P 1992 'Neuropsychiatric Correlates of Persistent Postconcussive Syndrome'. *The Journal of Head Trauma Rehabilitation* 7 (2): 60-69.

Attenberger Corinna, Amsler Felix and Gross Thomas 2012 'Clinical Evaluation of the Trauma Outcome Profile (TOP) in the Longer-Term Follow-up of Polytrauma Patients'. *Injury* 43 (9): 1566-74.

Barth Jeffrey T, Macciocchi Stephen N, Giordani Bruno, Rimel Rebecca, Jane John A and Boll Thomas J 1983 'Neuropsychological Sequelae of Minor Head Injury'. *Neurosurgery* 13 (5): 529-33.

Campos Brenno Belazi Nery de Souza and Santana Machado Fabio 2012 'Nutrition Therapy in Severe Head Trauma Patients'. *Revista Brasileira de Terapia Intensiva* 24: 97-105.

Carroll Linda J, Cassidy J David, Cancelliere Carol, Côté Pierre, Hincapié Cesar A, Kristman Vicki L, Holm Lena W, Borg Jörgen, Nygren-de Boussard Catharina and Hartvigsen Jan 2014 'Systematic Review of the Prognosis after Mild Traumatic Brain Injury in Adults: Cognitive, Psychiatric, and Mortality Outcomes: Results of the International Collaboration on Mild Traumatic Brain Injury Prognosis'. *Archives of Physical Medicine and Rehabilitation* 95 (3): S152-73.

Chiang Yung-Hsiao, Chao Dan-Ping, Chu Shu-Fen, Lin Hui-Wen, Huang Shih-Yi, Yeh Yi-Shian, Lui Tai-Ngar, Binns Colin W and Chiu Wen-Ta 2012 'Early Enteral Nutrition and Clinical Outcomes of Severe Traumatic Brain Injury Patients in Acute Stage: A Multi-Center Cohort Study'. *Journal of Neurotrauma* 29 (1): 75-80.

Clark Ian A and Vissel Bryce 2014 'Inflammation-Sleep Interface in Brain Disease: TNF, Insulin, Orexin'. *Journal of Neuroinflammation* 11 (1): 1-11.

Crenn Pascal, Hamchaoui Sabrina, Bourget-Massari Aliette, Hanachi Mouna, Melchior Jean-Claude and Azouvi Philippe 2014 'Changes in Weight after Traumatic Brain Injury in Adult Patients: A Longitudinal Study'. *Clinical Nutrition* 33 (2): 348-53.

Daradkeh Ghazi, Mohamed Essa Musthafa, Al-Adawi S Samir, Subash Selvaraju, Mahmood Lubna and Kumar Parvathy R 2014 'Nutritional Status, Assessment, Requirements and Adequacy of Traumatic Brain Injury Patients.' *Pakistan Journal of Biological Sciences: PJBS* 17 (10): 1089-97.

Dikmen Sureyya, Machamer Joan and Temkin Nancy 2017 'Mild Traumatic Brain Injury: Longitudinal Study of Cognition, Functional Status, and Post-Traumatic Symptoms'. *Journal of Neurotrauma* 34 (8): 1524-30.

Dikmen Sureyya S, Machamer Joan E, Powell Janet M and Temkin Nancy R 2003 'Outcome 3 to 5 Years after Moderate to Severe Traumatic Brain Injury'. *Archives of Physical Medicine and Rehabilitation* 84 (10): 1449-57.

Dodds WJ 2017 'Central Nervous System Regulation of Appetite in Humans and Pet Animals'. *Ann Clin Exp Metabol* 2017 2 (1) 1013: 34-35.

Duraski Sylvia A, Lovell Linda and Roth Elliot J 2014 'Nutritional Intake, Body Mass Index, and Activity in Postacute Traumatic Brain Injury: A Preliminary Study'. *Rehabilitation Nursing* 39 (3): 140-46.

Lee-anne S Chapple, Chapman Marianne J, Lange Kylie, Deane Adam M and Heyland Daren K 2015 'Nutrition Support Practices in Critically Ill Head-Injured Patients: A Global Perspective'. *Critical Care* 20 (1): 1-11.

Lee-anne S Chapple, Deane Adam M, Heyland Daren K, Lange Kylie, Kranz Amelia J, Williams Lauren T and Chapman Marianne J 2016 'Energy and Protein Deficits throughout Hospitalization in Patients Admitted with a Traumatic Brain Injury'. *Clinical Nutrition* 35 (6): 1315-22.

Maas Andrew IR, Stocchetti Nino and Bullock Ross 2008 'Moderate and Severe Traumatic Brain Injury in Adults'. *The Lancet Neurology* 7 (8): 728-41.

Mahan LK and Raymond JL 2017 'Krauses Food & The Nutrition Care Process. 14a'. Missouri: Elsevier Inc.

Nelson Lindsay D, LaRoche Ashley A, Pfaller Adam Y, Lerner E Brooke, Hammeke Thomas A, Randolph Christopher, Barr William B, Guskiewicz Kevin and McCrea Michael A 2016 'Prospective, Head-to-Head Study of Three Computerized Neurocognitive Assessment Tools (CNTs): Reliability and Validity for the Assessment of Sport-Related Concussion'. *Journal of the International Neuropsychological Society* 22 (1): 24-37.

Parimisetty Avinash, Dorsemans Anne-Claire, Awada Rana, Ravanan Palaniyandi, Diotel Nicolas and Lefebvre d'Hellencourt Christian 2016 'Secret Talk between Adipose Tissue and Central Nervous System via Secreted Factors—an Emerging Frontier in the Neurodegenerative Research'. *Journal of Neuroinflammation* 13 (1): 1-13.

Pirente N, Bouillon B, Schafer B, Raum M, Helling H-J, Berger E and Neugebauer E 2002 'A Systematically Developed Instrument for the Assessment of Health-Related Quality of Life in Multiple Injured Patients. The Polytrauma Outcome (POLO) Chart'. *Der Unfallchirurg* 105 (5): 413-22.

Polinder Suzanne, Haagsma Juanita A, van Klaveren David, Steyerberg Ewout W and Van Beeck Ed F 2015 'Health-Related Quality of Life after TBI: A Systematic Review of

Study Design, Instruments, Measurement Properties, and Outcome'. *Population Health Metrics* 13 (1): 1-12.

Rimel Rebecca W, Giordani Bruno, Barth Jeffrey T, Boll Thomas J and Jane John A 1981 'Disability Caused by Minor Head Injury'. *Neurosurgery* 9 (3): 221-28.

Shen Qiuhua, Hiebert John B, Hartwell Julie, Thimmesch Amanda R and Pierce Janet D 2016 'Systematic Review of Traumatic Brain Injury and the Impact of Antioxidant Therapy on Clinical Outcomes'. *Worldviews on Evidence-Based Nursing* 13 (5): 380-89.

Soberg Helene Lundgaard, Roe Cecilie, Brunborg Cathrine, von Steinbüchel Nicole and Andelic Nada 2017 'The Norwegian Version of the QOLIBRI–a Study of Metric Properties Based on a 12 Month Follow-up of Persons with Traumatic Brain Injury'. *Health and Quality of Life Outcomes* 15 (1): 1-13.

Stern Theodore A, Fava Maurizio, Wilens Timothy E and Rosenbaum Jerrold F 2015 *Massachusetts General Hospital Comprehensive Clinical Psychiatry*. Elsevier Health Sciences.

Tyerman Andy and King Nigel S 2009 *Psychological Approaches to Rehabilitation after Traumatic Brain Injury*. John Wiley & Sons.

Von Steinbüchel Nicole, Wilson Lindsay, Gibbons Henning, Hawthorne Graeme, Höfer Stefan, Schmidt Silke, Bullinger Monika, Maas Andrew, Neugebauer Edmund and Powell Jane 2010 'Quality of Life after Brain Injury (QOLIBRI): Scale Development and Metric Properties'. *Journal of Neurotrauma* 27 (7): 1167-85.

Chapter 8

Disorders of Memory and Their Rehabilitation

Orlin Pavlov*, MD and Kalina Koleva, MD, PhD
[1]Department of Neurosurgery, Helios Klinikum Krefeld, Germany
[2]Department of Pharmacology and Toxicology, Medical University of Sofia, Bulgaria

Abstract

Traumatic brain injury (TBI) remains one of the most significant public health problems associated with high mortality and morbidity rates. TBI survivors are exposed to a range of TBI-associated deficits, including paresis, epilepsy, memory disturbances, chronic fatigue syndrome, and mood changes. All of these deficits negatively impact quality of life and often require extensive rehabilitation to overcome them.

The simultaneous treatment of all TBI-related disorders has a synergic positive effect. Neurorehabilitation after a TBI is a complex process involving all aspects of post-TBI disturbances, including cognition, memory, seizure control, pain control, muscular rehabilitation, and psychological support.

The therapies for post-TBI memory disorders are divided into three groups: pharmacological, non-pharmacological, and neurophysiological. Many pharmacological agents have been used to treat post-TBI memory disorders; however, only a few, including rivastigmine, methylphenidate, modafinil, and donepezil, have been effective. Non-pharmacological therapy consists of the utilization of new technologies, such as virtual reality (VR), computer-based cognitive retraining (CBCR), and non-invasive brain stimulation. VR could be one of the most important innovations in the rehabilitation of memory disturbances. An enriched environment based on individual experience stimulates episodic and semantic memories, which affect positively the patients with TBI.

* Corresponding Author's Email: orlinpavlov88@gmx.de

In: Rehabilitation in Neurotrauma
Editors: VD Sinha, Amit Chakraborty, Jitin Bajaj et al.
ISBN: 978-1-68507-787-7

Internalized strategy training and external memory compensation techniques (individual or group memory rehabilitation) are simple, cost-effective methods of improving working and episodic memory and, in turn, improving patients' overall quality of life.

Introduction

Traumatic brain injury (TBI) remains one of the most significant public health problems associated with high mortality and morbidity rates. TBI survivors are exposed to a range of TBI-associated deficits, including paresis, epilepsy, memory disturbances, chronic fatigue syndrome, and mood changes. All of these deficits negatively impact quality of life and often require extensive rehabilitation to overcome them.

For a long time, TBIs have been seen as static injuries. However, it is now clear that TBIs can trigger a cascade of processes leading to neurodegeneration and dementia. Memory loss, processing speed problems, and executive dysfunction are common cognitive impairment findings in TBI survivors (Scheid et al., 2006). Memory disturbances and dementia are commonly found together in patients with post-TBI syndrome. A recent meta-analysis of the post-TBI risk of dementia estimated a 1.6–1.8 times higher risk of dementia in post-TBI individuals compared to the general population (Raj et al., 2017, Li et al., 2017).

TBIs alter the brain's anatomical and functional integrity through cellular, structural, and functional changes. From an anatomical perspective, the structural changes include strokes, diffuse axonal injury, and substance defects due to hematoma. Through these mechanisms, TBIs affect the three processes of memory: encoding, maintenance, and retrieval (Tulving 1985). Encoding is a complex process of transforming experience (e.g., sight, touch, and smell) into a neuronal chain, which is also known as a memory engram. The ability to store a memory engram across time is called maintenance. Retrieval is the ability to voluntarily reinstate the engram into the forefront of consciousness (Paterno, Folweiler, and Cohen 2017). The anatomical substrate of memory is located in the hippocampus and frontal neocortex; thus, anatomical alterations in these areas lead to functional memory disturbances.

The current research divides memory into the following categories: working, episodic, and semantic. Working memory is the cognitive ability to transiently hold, process, and manipulate information (Diamond 2013, Paterno, Folweiler, and Cohen 2017). Episodic and semantic memories are based on personal experience. For instance, episodic memory is connected to temporally dated episodes and temporal–spatial relations between those episodes, therefore representing the ability to recollect specific episodic situations concerning time and space. Episodic memory remains short-term compared to semantic memory. Semantic memory describes the meaning applied to objects through personal experience. The three types of memories constantly exchange information. The process of consolidation describes the transformation of episodic memory into semantic memory. Neurocognitive sciences describe this as a process of consolidation in which the memory engram is transferred from the medial temporal lobe to the cerebral cortex (Alvarez and Squire 1994).

Post-TBI neurorehabilitation is a complex process involving all aspects of post-TBI disturbances, including cognition, memory, seizure control, pain control, muscular rehabilitation, and psychological support. A memory disturbance cannot be seen as a separate entity and is thus treated alone. A multimodal approach by an experienced team is thus mandatory for achieving optimal results. The simultaneous treatment of all TBI-related disorders has a synergic positive effect. For instance, individuals who have experienced a mild TBI (mTBI) typically perform worse on tasks requiring advanced cognitive load than they do on easier tasks (McAllister et al., 2006). Semantic and episodic memories are also affected in TBI cases. Auditory verbal episodic memory usually improves over one year in individuals with mTBIs, but in complex TBI cases, it worsens (Halgren et al., 2011). Semantic memory disturbances improve over 30 years, and younger age is associated with a greater chance of recovery and faster recovery (Himanen et al., 2009).

Neurorehabilitation strategies are based on neuroplasticity. The brain's ability to modify and create neuronal connections is the primary objective in compensating for post-TBI memory deficits.

The efficacy of memory rehabilitation programs has been of great interest because of the costs related to neurorehabilitation. Eliott et al., conducted a meta-analysis of 26 studies (from 1985 to2013) in which memory training and recovery were assessed in patients after TBIs and strokes. Surprisingly, in both groups (the treated group versus the non-treated group), an improvement over time was found; however, the improvement among the treatment group was greater. The authors concluded that memory recovery programs are useful and cost-effective for post-TBI and post-stroke patients but that spontaneous recovery also occurs (Elliott and Parente 2014).

Pathoanatomical Findings and Their Effects on Memory

The current understanding of the pathophysiology of memory disturbances in patients with TBI is based on animal models and human pathoanatomical findings.

Table 1. Anatomical regions and types of memory impairment

Anatomical Structure	Type of Memory Disturbance
Hippocampus	Episodic memory, including spatial memory
Dentate gyrus	Episodic memory, including spatial memory
Area CA3	Episodic memory encoding and retrieval
Area CA1	Episodic memory encoding and retrieval
Prefrontal cortex	Working memory

Assessment of Patients with Memory Disorders and Prognosis for Rehabilitation

The assessment of a patient with a post-TBI memory disorder should begin with the patient's personality type. The five-factor model, the predominant dimensional model of general personality structure, consists of the five broad domains of neuroticism (or negative affectivity), extraversion (versus introversion), openness (or unconventionality), agreeableness (versus antagonism), and conscientiousness (or constraint) (Clark 2007, Widiger et al., 2018). Identifying adaptive and maladaptive traits through the five-factor model is one of the main factors of successful neurorehabilitation therapy.

Identifying a patient's previous job and hobbies is also a vital step in creating a patient-based approach for post-TBI neurorehabilitation. Some jobs and hobbies require extensive hand–eye coordination, and these activities could be recreated in virtual reality (VR) to improve one's working memory. Other hobbies (e.g., chess and other board games) require extensive semantic and episodic memory capabilities. A positive approach based on previously known facts would improve patient compliance and overall results.

The family environment is another important aspect of neurorehabilitation. Through a friendly family environment, it is possible to obtain a sufficient intensity of neurorehabilitation to achieve the maximum degree of generalization from formalized training to the patient's daily environment and mobilize cognitive reserves (Mogensen and Wulf-Andersen

2017). Through the family environment, it is possible to move to home-based neurorehabilitation, allowing for a higher intensity of training and the utilization of pre-traumatic cognitive strategies.

To complete an assessment of a patient with a TBI, frequent brain imaging is required. A major complication after a TBI is posttraumatic hydrocephalus (PTH). Incidences of PTH are reported in up to 29% of post-TBI patients (Marmarou et al., 1996). In the majority of cases, PTH develops up to 12 weeks post-TBI. Interestingly the patients with higher Glasgow Coma Scale (GCS) scores had a later onset of PTH symptoms, whereas patients with lower GCS scores showed an earlier onset of symptoms (Yoon et al., 2018). One of the most common clinical features of PTH is arrested neurological improvement, which is one of the main reasons for the referral of post-TBI patients to neurosurgical departments. Its incidence is reported in up to 20% of cases. The treatment of choice remains ventriculoperitoneal shunt (VPS) surgery. Another concern in post-TBI patients is the delayed development of chronic subdural hematoma, which may require surgical decompression for symptom relief. The decompression of the chronic subdural hematoma could lead to hyperperfusion syndrome, which could further worsen the neurological outcome. Consequently, it is recommended to slowly decompress such hematomas slowly (Pavlov 2020).

The following factors significantly impact the memory improvement prognosis of post-TBI patients:

Table 2. Prognostic factors for positive and negative post-TBI outcomes regarding memory function

Positive factors	**Negative factors**
1. Young age (< 40)	1.Old age (> 40)
2. No history of memory impairment diseases	2. History of dementia (e.g., Alzheimer's), previous strokes
3. Personality types: extraversion, openness, and agreeableness	3. Personality types: neuroticism, negative affectivity, unconventionality, and antagonism
4. Challenging memory and motor skills required for pre-traumatic job/hobbies	4. Non-challenging memory and motor skills required for pre-traumatic job/hobbies
5. Friendly family environment	5. Friendly family environment
6. Lack of radiological criteria for PTH/chronic subdural hematoma	6. Radiological criteria for PTH/ chronic subdural hematoma

Pharmacology Agents Used in Treating Post-TBI Memory Disorders

Many pharmacological agents are used in neurorehabilitation to achieve better cognitive, memory, behavioral, and neurological outcomes. In this chapter, only pharmacological agents used in memory disturbances will be reviewed.

Rivastigmine

Silver et al., published one of the first studies on the pharmacological treatment of post-TBI memory deficits with rivastigmine (Silver et al., 2006). In this study, the patients were treated with 3 to 6 mg of rivastigmine daily for 12 weeks. The Cambridge Neuropsychological Test Automated Battery (CANTAB) Rapid Visual Information Processing (RVIP) A' subtest, and the Hopkins Verbal Learning Test (HVLT) were used as the primary efficacy measurement scales. In the group with moderate to severe memory deficits, both the CANTAB RVIP A' subtest and the HVLT indicated statistically significant improvement with rivastigmine treatment. All the subjects showed good tolerance of this pharmacological treatment.

Methylphenidate

Manktelow et al., reported behavioral, functional, and structural MRI data from a group of 15 healthy controls and a group of 15 TBI patients obtained during the execution of an N-back task after the administration of either a placebo or 30 mg of methylphenidate. The authors concluded that methylphenidate improves the cognitive outcomes in working memory tasks (Manktelow et al., 2017).

Donepezil

Donepezil, an acetylcholinesterase inhibitor, was introduced as a memory enhancer for post-TBI patients with memory disturbances. This pharmacological agent demonstrated high selectivity and therefore minimal side effects for neuronal acetylcholinesterase (Taverni, Seliger, and Lichtman

1998). The improvement in working memory is observed as early as three weeks after the beginning of the therapy. After three months of therapy with donepezil, an improvement in processing speed, learning, and divided attention in 80% of patients was observed (Khateb et al., 2005). Therapy with donepezil may also positively impact behavioral deficits (Agarwal, Biswas, and Agarwal 2007).

Modafinil is another off-label pharmacological agent used in the treatment of chronic TBIs with memory disturbances. Its mechanism of action relies on the inhibition of norepinephrine and dopamine transporters, thus improving the extracellular environment and neuronal connectivity. The literature is limited to case reports, with results indicating promising post-TBI memory improvement. A daily augmentation of 300 mg of modafinil is associated with a 50% improvement in everyday activities and working memory (Tcheremissine and Rachal 2017).

Non-Pharmacological Neurorehabilitation

Modern technologies offer new possibilities for brain–machine interaction and conceptualization. Three approaches to patients with post-TBI memory disturbances are based on brain–machine interaction: VR, computer-based cognitive retraining, and non-invasive brain stimulation.

VR is rapidly entering everyday life. In neurorehabilitation, VR plays an important role in retraining and sustaining memory through repetition and various enriched stimuli. VR tools also allow physicians to record various parameters and thus obtain a more in-depth, precise understanding of memory deficits and develop strategies to improve them. VR is also a part of cognitive rehabilitation. One of VR's greatest advantages is that it offers the possibility of extracting information from real-life situations and importing it into VR via fragments. This process of segregation allows patients to concentrate on a specific task. Shin et al., conducted a systematic review of cognitive improvement therapies using VR, which showed that a cognitive improvement in attention positively impacts the recovery of general cognitive function (Shin and Kim 2015).

Computer-based cognitive retraining (CBCR) uses the principles of brain plasticity to improve working memory, cognition, and processing speed. Using CBCR, Olesen et al., found increased brain activity (using functional MRI) in the medial frontal gyrus and superior and inferior parietal cortices. The majority of the available research on CBCR concerns patients with neurodegenerative diseases. The authors concluded that these changes in cortical activity could be evidence of training-induced plasticity in the neural systems that underlie working memory (Olesen, Westerberg, and Klingberg 2004). The improvement of working memory positively impacts attention, reasoning, and problem solving.

Non-invasive brain stimulation uses two main strategies—transcranial magnetic stimulation (TMS) and transcranial direct current stimulation (tDCS)—to increase the activity of the damaged brain region directly or indirectly. Based on the principle of electromagnetic induction, TMS causes depolarization and hyperpolarization in cells. A subtype of TMS is repetitive transcranial magnetic stimulation (rTMS), in which pulses are delivered at constant intervals at the same intensity. It has been shown that rTMS improves interaction with cortical activity and can positively affect short-term cognitive performance and improve the rehabilitation potential of neurological patients (Miniussi et al., 2008). On the other hand, tDCS is a less expensive, easier-to-handle method of changing the resting membrane potential and thus altering the level of spontaneous neuronal excitability and activity (Johansson 2011, Spreij et al., 2014).

Neurophysiological Methods for Improving Post-TBI Memory Disorders

The compensatory strategies in post-TBI memory impairments relies simplicity and repetition. The two most common of these memory aids are internalized strategy training and external memory compensation techniques. Internal strategy training involves re-teaching the brain to retain information using different mental strategies, including counting, face/name associations, and mental visualization (Perna and Perkey 2016). Internal strategy training must focus on daily activities to improve the outcomes of patients with mild to severe TBI. External memory compensation techniques involve assistance from aids outside the patient's brain, such as notebooks, organizers, and to-do lists. The aim of external memory compensation techniques is to improve quality of life.

Group memory rehabilitation programs are another way to improve memory in patients with TBI. The patients are enrolled for ten consecutive weeks, usually three months after an mTBI. These programs are intended to reduce rehabilitation costs and improve outcomes at six and twelve months after they begin. However, no study has compared the benefits of group memory rehabilitation programs to those of the individual approach (das Nair et al., 2019).

Conclusion

Post-TBI memory rehabilitation remains part of the broader process of neurorehabilitation. A pretherapeutic assessment of a patient's neurophysiological status including an identification of the positive and negative factors has a crucial role in determining recovery time and overall outcome. A patient-based approach utilizing the patient's positive traits is essential. In selected cases, new technologies such as VR could have a dramatic positive effect on patients with memory impairment. Group memory rehabilitation has not yet demonstrated superiority over the individual-based approach.

References

Agarwal, Arun Lata, Devdutta Biswas, and Sanjay Agarwal. 2007. "Donepezil in traumatic brain injury: Report of two cases." *The Indian Journal of Neurotrauma* 4 (2):129-131. doi: https://doi.org/10.1016/S0973-0508(07)80030-X.

Alvarez, P., and L. R. Squire. 1994. "Memory consolidation and the medial temporal lobe: a simple network model." *Proc Natl Acad Sci U S A* 91 (15):7041-5. doi: 10.1073/pnas.91.15.7041.

Clark, L. A. 2007. "Assessment and diagnosis of personality disorder: perennial issues and an emerging reconceptualization." *Annu. Rev. Psychol.* 58:227-57. doi: 10.1146/annurev.psych.57.102904.190200.

das Nair, R., L. E. Bradshaw, H. Carpenter, S. Clarke, F. Day, A. Drummond, D. Fitzsimmons, S. Harris, A. A. Montgomery, G. Newby, C. Sackley, and N. B. Lincoln. 2019. "A group memory rehabilitation programme for people with traumatic brain injuries: the ReMemBrIn RCT." *Health Technol. Assess* 23 (16):1-194. doi: 10.3310/hta23160.

Diamond, A. 2013. "Executive functions." *Annu. Rev. Psychol.* 64:135-68. doi: 10.1146/annurev-psych-113011-143750.

Elliott, M., and F. Parente. 2014. "Efficacy of memory rehabilitation therapy: a meta-analysis of TBI and stroke cognitive rehabilitation literature." *Brain Inj.* 28 (12):1610-6. doi: 10.3109/02699052.2014.934921.

Halgren, E., J. Sherfey, A. Irimia, A. M. Dale, and K. Marinkovic. 2011. "Sequential temporo-fronto-temporal activation during monitoring of the auditory environment for temporal patterns." *Hum. Brain Mapp.* 32 (8):1260-76. doi: 10.1002/hbm.21106.

Himanen, L., R. Portin, O. Tenovuo, T. Taiminen, S. Koponen, H. Hiekkanen, and H. Helenius. 2009. "Attention and depressive symptoms in chronic phase after traumatic brain injury." *Brain Inj.* 23 (3):220-7. doi: 10.1080/02699050902748323.

Johansson, B. B. 2011. "Current trends in stroke rehabilitation. A review with focus on brain plasticity." *Acta Neurologica Scandinavica* 123 (3):147-159. doi: https://doi.org/10.1111/j.1600-0404.2010.01417.x.

Khateb, Asaid, Jussara Ammann, Jean-Marie Annoni, and Karin Diserens. 2005. "Cognition-Enhancing Effects of Donepezil in Traumatic Brain Injury." *European neurology* 54:39-45. doi: 10.1159/000087718.

Li, Yanjun, Yongming Li, Xiaotao Li, Shuang Zhang, Jincheng Zhao, Xiaofeng Zhu, and Guozhong Tian. 2017. "Head injury as a risk factor for dementia and Alzheimer's disease: a systematic review and meta-analysis of 32 observational studies." *PloS one* 12 (1):e0169650.

Manktelow, Anne E., David K. Menon, Barbara J. Sahakian, and Emmanuel A. Stamatakis. 2017. "Working Memory after Traumatic Brain Injury: The Neural Basis of Improved Performance with Methylphenidate." *Frontiers in Behavioral Neuroscience* 11 (58). doi: 10.3389/fnbeh.2017.00058.

Marmarou, A., M. A. Foda, K. Bandoh, M. Yoshihara, T. Yamamoto, O. Tsuji, N. Zasler, J. D. Ward, and H. F. Young. 1996. "Posttraumatic ventriculomegaly: hydrocephalus or atrophy? A new approach for diagnosis using CSF dynamics." *J. Neurosurg.* 85 (6):1026-35. doi: 10.3171/jns.1996.85.6.1026.

McAllister, T. W., L. A. Flashman, B. C. McDonald, and A. J. Saykin. 2006. "Mechanisms of working memory dysfunction after mild and moderate TBI: evidence from functional MRI and neurogenetics." *J. Neurotrauma* 23 (10):1450-67. doi: 10.1089/neu.2006.23.1450.

Miniussi, Carlo, Stefano F. Cappa, Leonardo G. Cohen, Agnes Floel, Felipe Fregni, Michael A. Nitsche, Massimiliano Oliveri, Alvaro Pascual-Leone, Walter Paulus, Alberto Priori, and Vincent Walsh. 2008. "Efficacy of repetitive transcranial magnetic stimulation/transcranial direct current stimulation in cognitive neurorehabilitation." *Brain Stimulation: Basic, Translational, and Clinical Research in Neuromodulation* 1 (4):326-336. doi: 10.1016/j.brs.2008.07.002.

Mogensen, J., and C. Wulf-Andersen. 2017. "Home and family in cognitive rehabilitation after brain injury: Implementation of social reserves." *NeuroRehabilitation* 41 (2):513-518. doi: 10.3233/nre-160007.

Olesen, Pernille J., Helena Westerberg, and Torkel Klingberg. 2004. "Increased prefrontal and parietal activity after training of working memory." *Nature Neuroscience* 7 (1):75-79. doi: 10.1038/nn1165.

Paterno, Rosalia, Kaitlin A. Folweiler, and Akiva S. Cohen. 2017. "Pathophysiology and Treatment of Memory Dysfunction After Traumatic Brain Injury." *Current neurology and neuroscience reports* 17 (7):52-52. doi: 10.1007/s11910-017-0762-x.

Pavlov, Orlin. 2020. "Rapid evacuation of chronic subdural hematoma – A possible traumatic brain injury (TBI)." *Medical Hypotheses* 137:109539. doi: https://doi.org/10.1016/j.mehy.2019.109539.

Perna, Robert, and Hana Perkey. 2016. "Internal Memory Rehabilitation Strategies in the Context of Post-acute Brain Injury: A Pilot Study." *International Journal of Neurorehabilitation* 03. doi: 10.4172/2376-0281.1000199.

Raj, Rahul, Jaakko Kaprio, Miikka Korja, Era D Mikkonen, Pekka Jousilahti, and Jari Siironen. 2017. "Risk of hospitalization with neurodegenerative disease after moderate-to-severe traumatic brain injury in the working-age population: A retrospective cohort study using the Finnish national health registries." *PLoS medicine* 14 (7):e1002316.

Scheid, Rainer, Kathrin Walther, Thomas Guthke, Christoph Preul, and D. Yves von Cramon. 2006. "Cognitive Sequelae of Diffuse Axonal Injury." *Archives of Neurology* 63 (3):418-424. doi: 10.1001/archneur.63.3.418.

Shin, HyeonHui, and KyeongMi Kim. 2015. "Virtual reality for cognitive rehabilitation after brain injury: a systematic review." *Journal of physical therapy science* 27 (9):2999-3002. doi: 10.1589/jpts.27.2999.

Silver, J. M., B. Koumaras, M. Chen, D. Mirski, S. G. Potkin, P. Reyes, D. Warden, P. D. Harvey, D. Arciniegas, D. I. Katz, and I. Gunay. 2006. "Effects of rivastigmine on cognitive function in patients with traumatic brain injury." *Neurology* 67 (5):748-55. doi: 10.1212/01.wnl.0000234062.98062.e9.

Spreij, Lauriane A., Johanna M. A. Visser-Meily, Caroline M. van Heugten, and Tanja C. W. Nijboer. 2014. "Novel insights into the rehabilitation of memory post acquired brain injury: a systematic review." *Frontiers in Human Neuroscience* 8 (993). doi: 10.3389/fnhum.2014.00993.

Taverni, J. P., G. Seliger, and S. W. Lichtman. 1998. "Donepezil medicated memory improvement in traumatic brain injury during post acute rehabilitation." *Brain Inj.* 12 (1):77-80. doi: 10.1080/026990598122881.

Tcheremissine, Oleg V., and James C. Rachal. 2017. "Modafinil Augmentation Therapy in Patient with Traumatic Brain Injury." *Innovations in clinical neuroscience* 14 (3-4):11-11.

Tulving, Endel. 1985. "How many memory systems are there?" *American psychologist* 40 (4):385.

Widiger, Thomas A., Cristina Crego, Stephanie L. Rojas, and Joshua R. Oltmanns. 2018. "Basic personality model." *Current opinion in psychology* 21:18-22. doi: 10.1016/j.copsyc.2017.09.007.

Yoon, Jae Eon, Cheol Young Lee, Eui Gyu Sin, Jihye Song, and Hyun Woo Kim. 2018. "Clinical Feature and Outcomes of Secondary Hydrocephalus Caused by Head Trauma." *Korean journal of neurotrauma* 14 (2):86-92. doi: 10.13004/kjnt.2018.14.2.86.

Chapter 9

Motor System, Gait and Balance

Rakesh Mishra[1,*], Bukkambudhi V. Murlimanju[2] and Amit Agrawal[3,†]

[1]Department of Neurosurgery, Institute of Medical Sciences, Banaras Hindu University, Varanasi, Uttar Pradesh, India
[2]Department of Anatomy, Kasturba Medical College, Mangalore, Manipal Academy of Higher Education, Manipal, Karnataka, India
[3]Department of Neurosurgery, All India Institute of Medical Sciences, Bhopal, Madhya Pradesh, India

Abstract

The motor system is crucial for independence and a person quality of life. When an individual loses his ability to use his limbs, it has dramatic consequences. Motor function implies a wide range of functions subserved by the motor system in humans. It includes locomotor, gait, and balance. In the event of motor dysfunction, there is an abnormality in gait that makes a person walk less and sets in the vicious cycle with an impact on other organ systems like the cardiovascular system. The main principle behind motor learning is neuroplasticity. It is based on the findings that repetitive movements induce plasticity in functionally preserved brain areas and neural networks take over repetitive movements. The objective of the present chapter is to present an outline principles of motor learning, neurobiological control of motor rehabilitation and to sensitize physicians and surgeons on the neurorehabilitation aspects of motor gait and balance disorder.

---

* Corresponding Author's Email: rakeshmishra_afmc@yahoo.co.in.
† Corresponding Author's Email: dramitagrawal@gmail.com.

In: Rehabilitation in Neurotrauma
Editors: VD Sinha, Amit Chakraborty, Jitin Bajaj et al.
ISBN: 978-1-68507-787-7

Introduction

Motor function implies a wide range of functions subserved by the motor system in humans. It includes locomotor, gait, and balance. A significant proportion of grey matter and the neural circuitry is dedicated to adequate motor system functioning and compensating when the deficit arises. Readers may refer to the neuroanatomical and physiological texts to further understand the neural architecture of motor functioning. The motor system is crucial for independence and a person quality of life. When an individual loses his ability to use his limbs, it has dramatic consequences. The direct consequence of loss of motor function manifest as monoparesis/monoplegia, hemiparesis/hemiplegia or other combinations. The more disturbing aspects of motor function loss are those which do not manifest directly. These are the indirect consequences. In the event of motor dysfunction, there is an abnormality in gait that makes a person walk less and sets in the vicious cycle with an impact on other organ systems like the cardiovascular system. Balance disorders arise due to motor dysfunction, and the resultant ataxia makes a person prone to fall-related injuries. Therefore, motor dysfunction appearing just as the loss of power is the tip of the iceberg, hiding many grave issues underneath.

Motor dysfunction in neurological disorders may arise acutely or over a long duration of time. Spinal cord injuries were associated with severe motor dysfunction and loss of years spent in disability for ages (Wyndaele and Wyndaele 2006). Most spinal cord injuries were traumatic in past years; however, more non-traumatic spinal cord injuries are witnessed in the last few decades (Wyndaele and Wyndaele 2006). Stroke is a significant neurosurgical disease and one of the most rapidly growing neurological disorders due to increased lifespan and lifestyle changes (Boursin et al. 2018, Feigin et al. 2009). Stroke typically results in hemiparesis, which makes it difficult for an individual to walk. In addition, based on the brain's territory affected by stroke, some patients might have predominantly ataxia and are at risk of secondary injuries due to falls (Boursin et al. 2018). Other major neurological disorders which manifest as motor dysfunction, gait, or balance disorders are Parkinson disease, multiple sclerosis and normal pressure hydrocephalus (Fritsch et al. 2012, Trenkwalder et al. 1995, Tullman 2013). The objective of the present chapter is to present an outline principles of motor learning, neurobiological control of motor rehabilitation and to senitize physicians and surgeons on the neurorehabilitation aspects of motor gait and balance disorder.

Physiology of Walking

Walking has two periods of double stance phase in every gait cycle when both the feet are off the ground. When the leg is on the ground, it is called the stance phase, and when the leg is off the ground, it is called the swing phase. The swing and stance phases are further subdivided. A detailed evaluation of the swing and stance phase and its subsections helps in identifying the gait disorder. Walking is very carefully coordinated and orchestrated by neurons in the cerebral cortex, basal ganglia and spinal cord (Lyon and Day 1997). As humans are bipedal; walking is unstable because the centre of gravity is higher and the support base is narrower (DA 1995). During walking, there is a fall forward of the centre of gravity during the stance phase, and the leg's swing phase halts this fall (Lyon and Day 1997). Any incoordination in these elements of gait can create gait disorder. Essential constituents of neurobiological control for locomotor systems are:

1. CPG: a cluster of neurons for the generation of rhythmic movements. Further described in detail later
2. Sensory inputs: from sensory nerve endings, including Golgi tendon organs, to perform stretch reflex. Other associated sensory inputs are crucial for normal gait, like proprioceptive input and visual input. Vestibular sensory disorders can affect gait adversely, resulting in gait imbalance and a tendency to fall.
3. Subcortical systems: Pedunculopontine nucleus in the midbrain is also known as the mesencephalic locomotor pattern generator, and it triggers walking when stimulated in animals. Similar functions are proposed for humans (Collomb-Clerc and Welter 2015). PPN receives direct inputs from the basal ganglia and send output to the reticulospinal tracts (Mori 1987). Other subcortical nuclei and white matter involved in locomotor function in humans include vestibular nuclei, reticular nuclei and reticulospinal tract to the spinal cord (Mori 1987).

Concepts in the Rehabilitation of Gait Disorders

Two main concepts used in the rehabilitation of gait disorders are compensation and restoration. Compensation refers to how preserved functions or assistive technologies substitute the lost motor function.

Compensation is the preferred approach in severe and complete sensory-motor loss, as seen in complete spinal cord injuries. In contrast, restoration is used when the motor function loss is not complete and can be restored with training exercises. An example of compensation to increase functional independence in individuals with persistent handicap is functional electrical stimulation (FES) of the common peroneal nerve for spastic foot drop due to an upper motor neuron lesion. In a study involving 126 patients, Taylor et al. (Taylor, Humphreys, and Swain 2013) found that FES was a pract6ical, cost-effective, long term and efficacious compensatory strategy to increase walking speed, dorsiflexion and eversion in foot drop patients due to stroke and multiple sclerosis. Critical components of compensatory strategies include:movement strategies to assist gait training, strengthening of the innervated muscles and use of assistive equipments. (Eng and Tang 2007). In contrast, restoration aims to restore normal motor function while minimizing compensatory muscle action. This has gained importance with better scientific evidence on neuroplasticity. Restoration is preferred in patients with a higher potential for recovery of neural function, like an incomplete spinal cord injury. Critical components of restoration include:

1. Body weight-supported step training on a treadmill or overground.
2. Conventional gait training involving the practice of static and dynamic standing balance, stepping and walking
3. Functional electrical stimulation therapy for neuromuscular re-education and functional training emphasizing normal movement patterns.

If we plot the rehabilitation strategy on the y-axis and the injury severity on the x-axis, the graph follows an s-shaped curve. This means that restoration strategies are better than compensatory strategies with increased time from CNS injury and less severe injury. However, the distinction in moderate impairments gets blurred, and restorative strategies support compensatory strategies and vice-versa.

Progressive Resisted Exercise

An upper motor neuron disease usually leads to muscle paresis. Muscle paresis can occur secondary to disuse atrophy. Gait parameters are affected to a different degree based on the muscle involved. For example, studies have shown that paresis of plantar flexors results in the reduction of walking speed (Bohannon 2007). In progressive resisted exercise, repetitive exercises against resistance is performed to induce muscle hypertrophy. This is also likely to induce changes in the descending regulatory pathways. American College of Sports Medicine (ACSM) guidelines advocate 60-80% of the one-repetition maximum: 6-12 repetitions per set and three sets. Progression should occur, and training should last at least 8-12 weeks as this is the minimum time before physiological changes occur. There is fair to strong evidence grade 3B to 1B that resistance training produces increased strength, gait speed, and functional outcomes and improved quality of life without exacerbation of spasticity.

Functional Electrical Stimulation

Functional electrical stimulation is helpful in patients who have damage to the central nervous system but preserved peripheral nervous system. In FES, the peripheral nerve is stimulated to activate the muscle. Any muscles involved in the gait cycle can be targeted; however, the most common peroneal nerve is stimulated for ankle dorsiflexion. This can be achieved by using sensors in the soles to target muscle activation for appropriate timing during the gait cycle.

Stretching and Splinting

Spasticity and atrophy results in the shortening of sarcomeres and connective tissue. Though there is no evidence that stretching increases the length of sarcomeres, studies have found that passive movements at the ankle to 5 degrees improve walking (Katalinic, Harvey, and Herbert 2011). A randomized trial showed a beneficial effect on walking sustained at three months with casting and botulinum injection at the ankle in adult stroke patients (Carda S and 1119-27. 2011).

Bodyweight Supported Treadmill Training

Several protocols are in use for bodyweight supported treadmill training (BWSTT) by rehabilitation therapists. The basic structure of body weight supported treadmill training is that patients steps on the treadmill with partial body weight and manual assistance (Duncan et al. 2011). The individual walks on a treadmill at a pace needed and per individual protocol, usually for 20-30 minutes and at 3 km/hour. This often is supplemented by progressive walking on the ground for 15 minutes. There are robotic bodyweight support systems that provide dynamic support to the patient and ergonomic sitting support to the therapist assisting the patient manually (Duncan et al. 2011). In BWSTT, dtatic support is provided by the harness and counterweights, and dynamic support is provided by the springs. Dynamic support is particularly helpful to coiunter the inertia due to shift of gravity crntre due to counterweights at higher speed.

BWSTT has emerged as standalone effective rehabilitation therapy for motor control in stroke, multiple sclerosis and stroke patients over the years (Duncan et al. 2011, Mehrholz, Thomas, and Elsner 2017, Lo and Triche 2008). In a randomized control trial, six weeks of BWSTT improved the walking distance and balance and reduced fatigue and pain in moderate and severe Parkinson disease (Atan et al. 2019). Another RCT is underway comparing BWSTT with traditional physiotherapy in critically ill patients (Kwakman et al. 2020).

Anatomical Substrates of Motor System Reorganization

For two centuries, it was known that locomotor functions are based on segmental spinal reflexes. However, the therapeutic use of this knowledge gained momentum after Sherrington published his physiological experiments on cats. Sherrington found that when appropriate sensory stimulation was given to the spianlised cats, they generated a pattern of movements similar to the swing and stance phase of gait (Sherrington 1910). What brown and Sherrington termed as intrinsic factors in their experiments came to be known as central pattern generators (CPG) (Sherrington 1910). CPG are a cluster of neurons located in the neuraxis to perform functions involving rhythmic muscle movements like breathing, chewing and walking. Later, animal and human studies found that the lower thoracic and upper lumbar levels of CPG for locomotor function in humans (Grillner and Zangger 1975, Dimitrijevic, Gerasimenko, and Pinter 1998, Harkema et al. 2011). The CPG for locomotor control is not autonomous and is under the regulatory control of supraspinal cortical neurons (Singh et al. 2011). In addition, it needs afferent stimulation of the generation of the gait pattern (Lacquaniti, Ivanenko, and Zago 2012). Therefore, some stimuli are more effective in gait pattern generation than others (Pearson 2000). In a study involving complete spinal cord injury, it was found that movement at the hip joint, particularly extension is the key trigger factor for gait pattern generator based on load-sharing from the soles (Dietz, Müller, and Colombo 2002). Among the set of factors necessary for long term retention of newly acquired skill includes the degree of active participation and motivation of the patient, an appropriate intrinsic and extrinsic feedback, the adaptation of the complexity of the movement task, and contextual interference, in which variability and diversification of the movement tasks are explicit components of the gait training (Krakauer 2006). Other rehabilitative modalities under investigation for improving locomotor function include robotic and electromechanical training (Mehrholz and Pohl 2012), virtual reality (Laver et al. 2015) and deep brain stimulation (Collomb-Clerc and Welter 2015).

Conclusion

The main principle behind motor learning is neuroplasticity. It is based on the findings that repetitive movements induce plasticity in functionally preserved brain areas and neural networks take over repetitive movements. Therefore, repetition is the crucial factor for successful motor learning. Though this can enhance the performance in the short term however is not sufficient for long term performance.

Conflicts of Interest

None.

Disclosure of Funding

None.

References

Atan, T., Ö Özyemişci Taşkıran, A. Bora Tokçaer, G. Kaymak Karataş, A. Karakuş Çalışkan, and B. Karaoğlan. 2019. "Effects of different percentages of body weight-supported treadmill training in Parkinson's disease: a double-blind randomized controlled trial." *Turk J Med Sci* 49 (4):999-1007. doi: https://10.3906/sag-1812-57.

Bohannon, R. W. 2007. "Muscle strength and muscle training after stroke." *J Rehabil Med* 39 (1):14-20. doi: https://10.2340/16501977-0018.

Boursin, P., S. Paternotte, B. Dercy, C. Sabben, and B. Maïer. 2018. "[Semantics, epidemiology and semiology of stroke]." *Soins* 63 (828):24-27. doi: https://10.1016/j.soin.2018.06.008.

Carda, S, Invernizzi M, Baricich A, Cisari C., and 1119-27. 2011. "Casting, taping or stretching after botulinum toxin type A for spastic equinus foot: A single-blind randomized trial on adult stroke patients." *Clin. Rehabil.* 25(12).

Collomb-Clerc, A., and M. L. Welter. 2015. "Effects of deep brain stimulation on balance and gait in patients with Parkinson's disease: A systematic neurophysiological review." *Neurophysiol Clin* 45 (4-5):371-88. doi: https://10.1016/j.neucli.2015.07.001.

DA, Winter. 1995. *Human balance and posture control during standing and walking*. 3rd ed, *Gait and Posture*.

Dietz, V., R. Müller, and G. Colombo. 2002. "Locomotor activity in spinal man: significance of afferent input from joint and load receptors." *Brain* 125 (Pt 12):2626-34. doi: https://10.1093/brain/awf273.

Dimitrijevic, M. R., Y. Gerasimenko, and M. M. Pinter. 1998. "Evidence for a spinal central pattern generator in humans." *Ann N Y Acad Sci* 860:360-76. doi: https://10.1111/j.1749-6632.1998.tb09062.x.

Duncan, P. W., K. J. Sullivan, A. L. Behrman, S. P. Azen, S. S. Wu, S. E. Nadeau, B. H. Dobkin, D. K. Rose, J. K. Tilson, S. Cen, and S. K. Hayden. 2011. "Body-weight-supported treadmill rehabilitation after stroke." *N Engl J Med* 364 (21):2026-36. doi: https://10.1056/NEJMoa1010790.

Eng, J. J., and Pei-Fang Tang. 2007. "Gait training strategies to optimize walking ability in people with stroke: a synthesis of the evidence." *Expert review of neurotherapeutics* 7 (10):1417-1436. doi: https://10.1586/14737175.7.10.1417.

Feigin, V. L., C. M. Lawes, D. A. Bennett, S. L. Barker-Collo, and V. Parag. 2009. "Worldwide stroke incidence and early case fatality reported in 56 population-based studies: a systematic review." *Lancet Neurol* 8 (4):355-69. doi: https://10.1016/s1474-4422(09)70025-0.

Fritsch, T., K. A. Smyth, M. S. Wallendal, T. Hyde, G. Leo, and D. S. Geldmacher. 2012. "Parkinson disease: research update and clinical management." *South Med J* 105 (12):650-6. doi: https://10.1097/SMJ.0b013e318273a60d.

Grillner, S., and P. Zangger. 1975. "How detailed is the central pattern generation for locomotion?" *Brain Res* 88 (2):367-71. doi: https://10.1016/0006-8993(75)90401-1.

Harkema, S., Y. Gerasimenko, J. Hodes, J. Burdick, C. Angeli, Y. Chen, C. Ferreira, A. Willhite, E. Rejc, R. G. Grossman, and V. R. Edgerton. 2011. "Effect of epidural stimulation of the lumbosacral spinal cord on voluntary movement, standing, and assisted stepping after motor complete paraplegia: a case study." *Lancet* 377 (9781):1938-47. doi: https://10.1016/s0140-6736(11)60547-3.

Katalinic, O. M., L. A. Harvey, and R. D. Herbert. 2011. "Effectiveness of stretch for the treatment and prevention of contractures in people with neurological conditions: a systematic review." *Phys Ther* 91 (1):11-24. doi: https://10.2522/ptj.20100265.

Krakauer, J. W. 2006. "Motor learning: its relevance to stroke recovery and neurorehabilitation." *Curr Opin Neurol* 19 (1):84-90. doi: https://10.1097/01.wco.0000200544.29915.cc.

Kwakman, R. C. H., J. Sommers, J. Horn, F. Nollet, R. H. H. Engelbert, and M. van der Schaaf. 2020. "Steps to recovery: body weight-supported treadmill training for critically ill patients: a randomized controlled trial." *Trials* 21 (1):409. doi: https://10.1186/s13063-020-04333-y.

Lacquaniti, F., Y. P. Ivanenko, and M. Zago. 2012. "Patterned control of human locomotion." *J Physiol* 590 (10):2189-99. doi: https://10.1113/jphysiol.2011.215137.

Laver, K. E., S. George, S. Thomas, J. E. Deutsch, and M. Crotty. 2015. "Virtual reality for stroke rehabilitation." *Cochrane Database Syst Rev* 2015 (2):CD008349. doi: https://10.1002/14651858.CD008349.pub3.

Lo, A. C., and E. W. Triche. 2008. "Improving gait in multiple sclerosis using robot-assisted, body weight supported treadmill training." *Neurorehabil Neural Repair* 22 (6):661-71. doi: https://10.1177/1545968308318473.

Lyon, I. N., and B. L. Day. 1997. "Control of frontal plane body motion in human stepping." *Exp Brain Res* 115 (2):345-56. doi: https://10.1007/pl00005703.

Mehrholz, J., and M. Pohl. 2012. "Electromechanical-assisted gait training after stroke: a systematic review comparing end-effector and exoskeleton devices." *J Rehabil Med* 44 (3):193-9. doi: https://10.2340/16501977-0943.

Mehrholz, J., S. Thomas, and B. Elsner. 2017. "Treadmill training and body weight support for walking after stroke." *Cochrane Database Syst Rev* 8 (8):CD002840. doi: https://10.1002/14651858.CD002840.pub4.

Mori, S. 1987. "Integration of posture and locomotion in acute decerebrate cats and in awake, freely moving cats." *Prog Neurobiol* 28 (2):161-95. doi: https://10.1016/0301-0082(87)90010-4.

Pearson, K. G. 2000. "Neural adaptation in the generation of rhythmic behavior." *Annu Rev Physiol* 62:723-53. doi: https://10.1146/annurev.physiol.62.1.723.

Sherrington, C. S. 1910. "Flexion-reflex of the limb, crossed extension-reflex, and reflex stepping and standing." *J Physiol* 40 (1-2):28-121. doi: https://10.1113/jphysiol.1910.sp001362.

Singh, A., S. Balasubramanian, M. Murray, M. Lemay, and J. Houle. 2011. "Role of spared pathways in locomotor recovery after body-weight-supported treadmill training in contused rats." *J Neurotrauma* 28 (12):2405-16. doi: https://10.1089/neu.2010.1660.

Taylor, P., L. Humphreys, and I. Swain. 2013. "The long-term cost-effectiveness of the use of Functional Electrical Stimulation for the correction of dropped foot due to upper motor neuron lesion." *J Rehabil Med* 45 (2):154-60. doi: https://10.2340/16501977-1090.

Trenkwalder, C., J. Schwarz, J. Gebhard, D. Ruland, P. Trenkwalder, H. W. Hense, and W. H. Oertel. 1995. "Starnberg trial on epidemiology of Parkinsonism and hypertension in the elderly. Prevalence of Parkinson's disease and related disorders assessed by a door-to-door survey of inhabitants older than 65 years." *Arch Neurol* 52 (10):1017-22. doi: https://10.1001/archneur.1995.00540340109020.

Tullman, M. J. 2013. "Overview of the epidemiology, diagnosis, and disease progression associated with multiple sclerosis." *Am J Manag Care* 19 (2 Suppl):S15-20.

Wyndaele, M., and J. J. Wyndaele. 2006. "Incidence, prevalence and epidemiology of spinal cord injury: what learns a worldwide literature survey?" *Spinal Cord* 44 (9):523-9. doi: https://10.1038/sj.sc.3101893.

Chapter 10

Chronic Fatigue Syndrome

Brajesh Kumar*, MD
Department of Neurosurgery, IGIMS, Patna, India

Abstract

Chronic fatigue syndrome (CFS) is disease in which the patient is suffering from various debilitating physical and mental symptoms without a definitive diagnosis. They present with severe fatigue without much exertion, muscular pain, pain all over body and multiple aching joints. Their suffering causes a lack of refreshing sleep, depression, lack of concentration and other behavioral abnormalities. The presence of so much physical and mental suffering without clear-cut diagnostic criteria and investigation makes the problem worse for both the clinician and the patient as this can only be diagnosed by clinically excluding other diseases.

There is no definitively identified cause that has been found so far, though many theories have been proposed. Patient education regarding the disease along with psychological, social and pharmacological support is crucial for the management of the disease. A good patient-physician relationship of respect and trust is important to motivate and involve the patient for therapy. Different workouts are planned according to the individual needs of the patient. Drugs have a supportive role in disease management.

We need to change the way patients look at their suffering and divert their attention from symptoms through *Cognitive Behavioral Therapy (CBT)* and *Graded Exercise Therapy (GET)* which has been found to be effective in the management of CFS.

* Corresponding Author's Email: drbrajesh78@gmail.com.

In: Rehabilitation in Neurotrauma
Editors: VD Sinha, Amit Chakraborty, Jitin Bajaj et al.
ISBN: 978-1-68507-787-7

Keywords: chronic fatigue syndrome, depression, cognitive behavioral therapy, graded exercise therapy

Introduction

Chronic fatigue syndrome (CFS) is characterized by debilitating fatigue without much exertion, pain all over the body, muscles and joints. This suffering leads to decreased sleep, chronic headaches and memory disturbances. There is no clear clinical, biochemical and radiological test available to accurately diagnose CFS.

These tests are done to exclude other diseases which present with similar symptoms and are medically treatable. "As per CDC case definition[1] revised in 1994, there should be a minimum 6 months of persistent fatigue which has significantly affected the routine activity of the person. There should be 4 or more symptoms present along with fatigue in last six months to define the disease as CFS. If a person's symptoms fit any of the medical or psychiatric diseases then it is not treated as CFS.

CDC Guideline for Chronic Fatigue Syndrome[1]

(1) Persistent & unexplained fatigue which is of:

- New onset
- Not due to present ongoing exertion
- Not significantly relieved by rest and
- Unable to perform previous levels of activity.

(2) Where four or more of the following symptoms are present for 6 months or more:

- Post exertional malaise (extreme, prolonged exhaustion and exacerbation of symptoms following physical or mental exertion.)
- Memory disturbances
- Disturbed sleep and day time drowsiness
- Muscle pain & multiple joint pain without swelling or redness

- New onset headache (new type or severity)
- Frequent or recurring sore throat
- Presence of tender lymph nodes (cervical or axillary)

Exclusion Criteria as per CDC[1]

- Medical condition which explains fatigue
- Major depressive disorder, bipolar disorder, delusional disorder, dementia and schizophrenia
- Anorexia or bulimia nervosa
- Alcohol and substance abuse

Etiology

As there is no definite identifiable cause has been found for CFS, many theories have been proposed but none of them defines the disease. TNF alpha, IL-1Beta, IL-6, IL-4 may be associated with increased fatigue in CFS, cancer related fatigue and other fatigue states. When the patient is not taken seriously when visiting the physician or confiding in family members causes aggravation in the disease. When patients constantly think about the symptoms, disease and suffering leads to increased disease severity. Other factors which precipitate the disease's severity are pregnancy, stress factors in family or suffering from flu like vial illness or history of sexual abuse in childhood, to name a few.

Differential Diagnosis

Hypothyroidism, obesity, immunological disorder, diabetes mellitus, viral infective diseases, sleep disorders, obstructive sleep apnoea, fibromyalgia, psychiatric (depression, anxiety, substance abuse) and neurological disorder are common diseases which can mimic CFS.

How to Differentiate from CFS from Depression

Table 1. Comparison between CFS and Depression

Domain	CFS	Depression
History	Post exertional malaise	Feeling better after exercise/ activity Insomnia or excessive sleep
	Post exertional malaise Unrefreshing/ Excessive sleep. Fatigue associated with frustration due to feeling of illness. There is less expression of emotional symptoms. Symptoms are more physical in nature. Better with decreasing stress level and decrease in activity. Frequent doctor change and frustration due to non-diagnosis	Fatigue associated with apathy and anhedonia. More likely to be expressed as negative emotional symptoms. Attribute their illness to psychological factors. Better with increasing activities. Doctor patient relationship is well maintained.
Physical and mental status examination	More pain complaints. Frequent and recurring sore throat.	Less pain complaints. Not Present.

Tests

Screening Tests Recommended by CDC (Coutts, Weatherby, and Davie 2001)

Complete blood count (CBC), **u**rine examination (routine and microscopic), fasting and post -prandial blood glucose, liver function test, C-reactive protein (CRP), serum electrolyte, renal function test, antinuclear antibody, RA factor, calcium, phosphorus and thyroid function test (free T4 and TSH)

Supportive and Symptomatic Treatment

- Education of patient regarding CFS and recognizing their illness experience.
- Medical treatment of their most problematic symptoms.
- Encouraging well balanced diet and good nutritional habits.
- Psychological support to patients for achieving normal activities of daily living.

Management of Fatigue

Considering the suffering of the patient without any definitive examination and lab findings, there is need of psychological, social and pharmacological management of the disease. Educating patients about their diagnosis is crucial. The aim of the treatment is to bring change to the patient's approach and perception regarding the disease through behavioral changes. Well-balanced diet with good nutritional habits and fixed bedtime and wake up time are encouraged. Optimum exercise. including aerobic exercises, yoga, meditation, dance, walking and cycling activities are included in the sessions with set goals of maximal heart rate and evenly planned throughout the day to prevent any exhaustion. Exercise should be gradually increased and should neither be too little nor too much activity. Exercise and mood enhancing activities cause a decrease in the stress and an improvement in lowering fatigue (Friedberg, 2002, Natelson et al., 1998, Powell et al., 2004). Motivation of the patient is the only key to fight the disease by bringing the change in the patient's acceptance and tolerance toward fatigue and also divert attention from the symptoms for the sustained effects of therapy.

Drug Therapy in CFS

The most frequently used drugs in these cases are antidepressants. Selegiline is a monoamine oxidase inhibitor which increases the dopamine level in the brain at clinical doses. If doses are increased, it increases serotonin and norepinephrine in the brain. The antidepressant and mood modulating effect is used in the treatment of CFS (Klimas et al., 1993). Fluoxetine is a selective serotonin reuptake inhibitor used in management of depressive and anxiety disorder associated with the disease (Goodnick and Sandoval, 1993). Bupropion was effective for the treatment of fatigue and depression in fluoxetine resistant patients (Lecrubien, 1993). Other drugs used are Paroxetine (White and Cleary, 1997), Venlafaxine, (White and Cleary, 1997) Moclobemide (White and Cleary, 1997) (Hickie et al., 2000) (up to 600mg a day for 6 weeks) and Duloxetine which may have a therapeutic benefit because of its characteristics of targeting pain. Essential fatty acid supplements rich in eicosapentaenoic acid and carnitine supplementation have shown to reduce chronic inflammation and fatigue and improve outcomes. Low dose hydrocortisone therapy has also shown a positive therapeutic response.

Conclusion

Chronic fatigue is disease in which the patient is suffering from various debilitating physical and mental symptoms without a definitive diagnosis. The diagnosis and treatment of chronic fatigue syndrome needs to be carried out individually for each individual patient. We still do not know the exact pathophysiology of the disease. Chronic activation of the immune system may be involved in the pathogenesis of the symptoms. Treatment is based on the presenting symptoms of the patient. Behavior and exercise therapy are more effective in the sustained treatment than drugs. Motivation of the patient and a good doctor patient relationship is key to the successful treatment of the disease.

References

Coutts R, Weatherby R and Davie A. 2001. "The use of a symptom "self-report" inventory to evaluate the acceptability and efficacy of a walking program for patients suffering with chronic fatigue syndrome." *J Psychosom Res,* 51 (2):425-9. doi: 10.1016/s0022-3999(00)00220-8.

Friedberg F. 2002. "Does graded activity increase activity? A case study of chronic fatigue syndrome.. *J Behav Ther Exp Psychiatry,* 33 (3-4):203-15. doi: 10.1016/s0005-7916(02)00038-1.

Goodnick PJ and Sandoval R. 1993. "Psychotropic treatment of chronic fatigue syndrome and related disorders.. *J Clin Psychiatry,* 54 (1):13-20.

Hickie IB, Wilson AJ, Wright JM, Bennett BK, Wakefield D and Lloyd AR. 2000. "A randomized, double-blind placebo-controlled trial of moclobemide in patients with chronic fatigue syndrome." *J Clin Psychiatry,* 61 (9):643-8. doi: 10.4088/jcp.v61n0909.

Klimas Nancy G, Morgan Robert, Van Riel Flavia and Fletcher, Mary Ann. 1993. Observations regarding use of an antidepressant, fluoxetine, in chronic fatigue syndrome. In *chronic fatigue and related immune deficiency syndromes.* Arlington, VA, US: American Psychiatric Association.

Lecrubien Y. 1993. "Antidepressant drugs: similar but different." *New Pharmacological Approaches to the Therapy of Depressive Disorders.* Basel, Switzerland: Karger:83-91.

Natelson BH, Cheu J, Hill N, Bergen M, Korn L, Denny T and Dahl K. 1998. "Single-blind, placebo phase-in trial of two escalating doses of selegiline in the chronic fatigue syndrome." *Neuropsychobiology,* 37 (3):150-4. doi: 10.1159/000026494.

Powell P, Bentall RP, Nye FJ and Edwards RH. 2004. "Patient education to encourage graded exercise in chronic fatigue syndrome. 2-year follow-up of randomised controlled trial." *Br J Psychiatry,* 184:142-6. doi: 10.1192/ bjp.184.2.142.

White PD and Cleary KJ. 1997. "An open study of the efficacy and adverse effects of moclobemide in patients with the chronic fatigue syndrome." *Int Clin Psychopharmacol,* 12 (1):47-52. doi: 10.1097/00004850-199701000-00007.

Chapter 11

Spinal Cord Injuries: Neurological Involvement and Disability Pattern

S. Shashivadhanan[1,*], MCh, MS and Gaurav Mittal[2], MS

[1]Military Hospital Bathinda, Bathinda, Punjab, India

[2]Department of Orthopaedics, MH Kirkee, Pune, India

Abstract

Background: The Spinal Cord Injury Center (SCIC), Kirkee along with Paraplegic rehabilitation center (PRC) and Queen Mary's Technical Institute (QMTI) Kirkee, Pune is one of the largest rehabilitation centers in South East Asia. It provides medical care and extended rehabilitation to the infirm and invalidated soldiers which includes physical, psychological, and financial rehabilitation. It also acts as a nodal agency to impart training to doctors and paramedics of the Armed Forces and civil hospitals for rehabilitation of paraplegics and quadriplegics. Till date, approximately 3000 spinal cord injury patients have been treated here since its inception. On 13 May 2019, the SCIC has completed 51 glorious years. A retrospective study at this center was undertaken to study the injury patterns suffered by soldiers and associated neurological deficits sustained.

Methods: This was a retrospective study conducted from Jan 2019 till Sep 2019. 67 patients in the SCIC were clinically evaluated for the nature of spinal cord injury. They were graded as per the Frankel Grading system. The cervical spinal injury cases were classified as per the Sub axial Cervical Spine Injury Classification (SLIC) system. Observation

* Corresponding Author's Email: drshashivadhanan@gmail.com.

In: Rehabilitation in Neurotrauma

Editors: VD Sinha, Amit Chakraborty, Jitin Bajaj et al.

ISBN: 978-1-68507-787-7

was made regarding the temporal profile of neurological improvement following injury.

Results: Of the total 67 patients studied, 24 had cervical spinal injuries, 33 had dorsal spine injuries and 09 suffered lumbar fractures while 01 suffered a lumbosacral fracture. All individuals with burst cervicodorsal fractures suffered Frankel Grade A injury. 07 out of 13 individuals with dislocation injuries suffered Frankel Grade B injury. Most patients plateaued to a static neurological grade within 45 days of intervention (surgical or nonsurgical).

Conclusion: Outcome from spinal cord injury has not changed much in the past decade but rehabilitation and dedicated involvement by health care providers has helped the disabled soldiers to reintegrate with society. SCIC, Kirkee along with PRC is a validation to this fact.

Keywords: spinal cord injury center (SCIC), paraplegic rehabilitation center (PRC), Kirkee, Frankels Grade

Introduction

Traumatic spinal injury (TSI; injury to spinal column, spinal cord, or both) commonly leads to significant impairment in the quality of life [1]. More than 10% of trauma patients sustain spinal injury and they have a higher mortality rate compared to other traumatic events [2, 3]. The incidence of spinal fractures is reported to vary between 16 and 64 per 100,000, depending on the study area and population concerned [4, 5]. Internationally, most of the injuries are caused by road traffic accidents (RTAs), together with falls from heights. Road traffic and fall accidents are the typical etiologies in young patients, whereas falls and associated osteoporosis causes trauma in the older population. Spinal fractures are often associated with other injuries. Studies have shown that 30 to 55 percent of patients of polytrauma have at least one associated spinal injury [6, 7]. Spinal cord injury (SCI) is one of the most severe consequences coexisting in one-tenth to one-fifth of those with spinal injury [8, 9]. Epidemiological factors of SCI in Indian scenario are different from Western countries, with the major cause being falls in India. The low socioeconomic status and younger age group have a major financial, social, and psychological impact, as majority of the patients are the primary earning members of their families [10].

Previously, combat-related spine injury rates rarely ever exceeded 1% to 2% of all trauma owing to lower survivability; however, multiple studies have now documented a 5% to 8% incidence of spinal wounds during the Iraq and Afghanistan conflicts [11-13].

As per the US Army figures (data accessed from icasualties.org), from 2003 to 2011, a total of 60,288 enlisted personnel sustained mortal injuries during the Iraq & Afghanistan wars. Of these, 38.5% had sustained one or more levels of spinal injury [14].

In the Indian scenario, as in most developing countries, very little is known about the exact incidence of SCIs. Since there is no curative treatment for SCI, prevention of SCI is paramount. Investigating the epidemiological pattern of SCI is the first step in planning for preventive strategies [10].

Spinal Cord Injury Center Kirkee

Origin and establishment: The erstwhile Military Hospital (MH) Kirkee used to be a 600-bed strength hospital during the 1971 war which included a 175 bedded orthopaedic center. Prior to this, there were two paraplegic units in the Armed Forces having 30 beds each in Lucknow and Pune. In 1968, rehabilitation of paraplegics was reorganized by shifting the 30-bedded unit from Military Hospital Poona to Military Hospital Kirkee where facilities for vocational training were available at the adjoining Queen Mary's Technical School. In 1971, it was further reorganized to an 80-bedded spinal cord injury center. By end of December 1971, it had 92 patients who were being provided total medical care and rehabilitation [15]. The center along with the adjoining Paraplegic Rehabilitation center (for rehabilitation of invalidated soldiers) and Queen Mary's Technical institute, forms a unique rehabilitation complex with over 160 beds (SCIC and PRC combined) and 34 family quarters with families living as a community within the center, making it one of the largest centers of its kind in South East Asia.

Management Protocol: Soldiers suffering spinal cord injury are managed in phases in the armed forces. Although there is no defined timeline, it is generally distributed into three phases. *Phase I:* Following acute spinal cord injury the soldiers are treated at the nearest tertiary care hospital. Here surgical intervention and intensive critical care is given to overcome any life-threatening event. (Initially this phase was being provided at the SCIC but has gradually become decentralized). *Phase II:* Most of the patients reach Military Hospital Kirkee during this phase (16 to 18 weeks post trauma), where they are made to undergo passive and active physiotherapy. Interacting with other patients having similar disabilities helps them get over depression and frustration. They are encouraged to undertake sporting activities like basketball, swimming, athletics etc. Occupational therapy is pursued at this stage. *Phase III:* By this time the paraplegic is adequately rehabilitated and requires minimal assistance by the staff. They are voluntarily enrolled into Queen Mary's Technical Institute to subsequently make them self-employed and productive individuals. Subsequently multiple agencies (Government & Non-Government) contribute in providing the disabled ex-servicemen, suitable employment.

Along with being the first center to provide physical, psychological and financial rehabilitation in our country, it is also the first in India to introduce wheelchair sports and also function as a nodal center in training doctors & paramedics in rehabilitation of paraplegics and quadriplegics.

Table1. SLIC Scoring System

Characteristics	**Points**
Morphology	
No abnormality	0
Compression/Burst	1 + 1 = 2
Distraction	3
Rotation/Translation	4
Disco ligamentous Complex	
Intact	0
Indeterminate	1
Disrupted	2
Neurological Status	
Intact	0
Root Injury	1
Complete Cord Injury	2
Incomplete Cord Injury	3

Table 2. Interpretation of SLIC Scoring System

Score	**Interpretation**
< 4	Non-Operative
4	Operative Versus Nonoperative
>/= 5	Operative Treatment

Materials and Methods

This was a retrospective study conducted from Jan 2019 till Sep 2019. Institutional Ethical committee clearance was acquired prior to start of the study. A written, informed consent was also obtained from participating patients. Most of the information regarding the standard of care, history and evolution of Spinal cord injury center were acquired by interacting with inmates and available documents with the staff of Spinal cord injury center. All inmates residing in the SCIC were clinically evaluated for the nature of spinal cord injury. They were graded as per the Frankel Grading system. History of the injury was noted & medical documents including radiological investigations were reviewed. The cervical spinal injury cases were classified as per the Sub axial Cervical Spine Injury Classification (SLIC) system (Tables 1 & 2) [14]. Observation was made regarding the temporal profile of neurological improvement following injury.

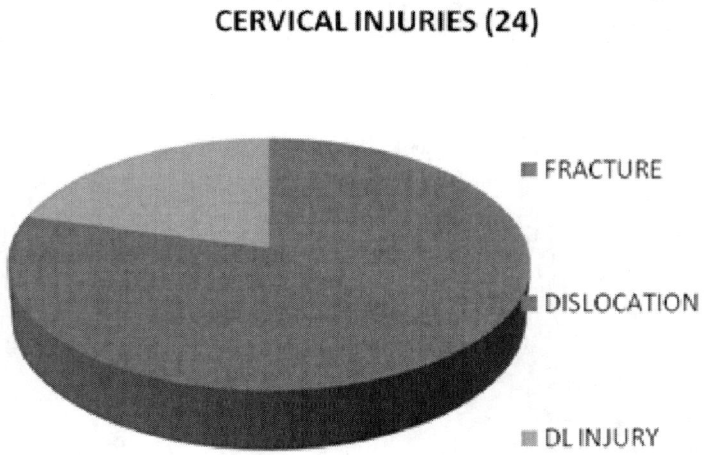

Figure 1. Distribution of cervical injuries as per the SLIC Classification into Fracture, Dislocation and Discoligmantous (DL) injury.

Results

A total of 67 patients were included for analysis in the present study and all were males. The SLIC classification was used for clinical assessment (Tables

1 & 2). The distribution of cervical injuries as per the SLIC Classification into Fracture, Dislocation and Disco ligamentous (DL) injury is as per Figure 1. The distribution of dorsal spine injuries is depicted in Figure 2 and of lumbar spine injuries in Figure 3. The overall distribution of spinal injuries in all 67 patients is as per Figure 4.

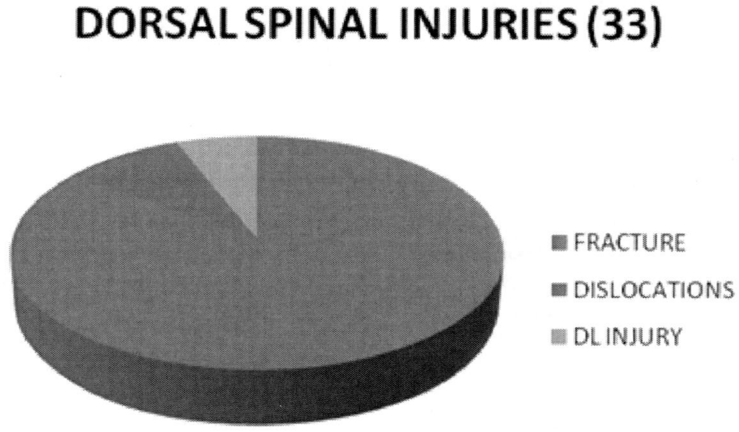

Figure 2. Distribution of dorsal spinal injuries in 33 patients.

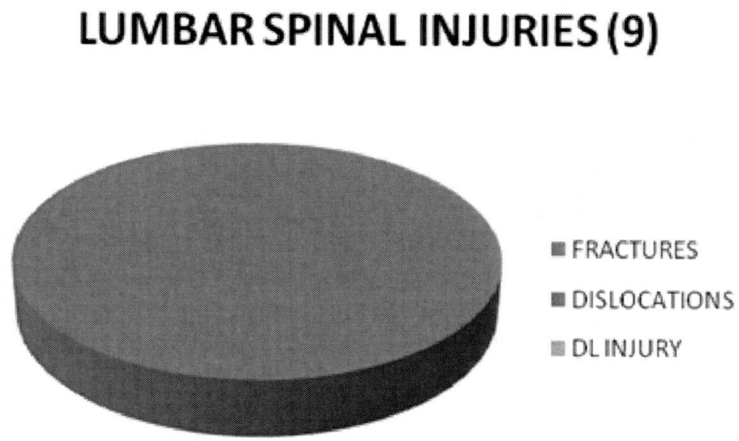

Figure 3. Distribution of Lumbar spine injuries in 9 patients.

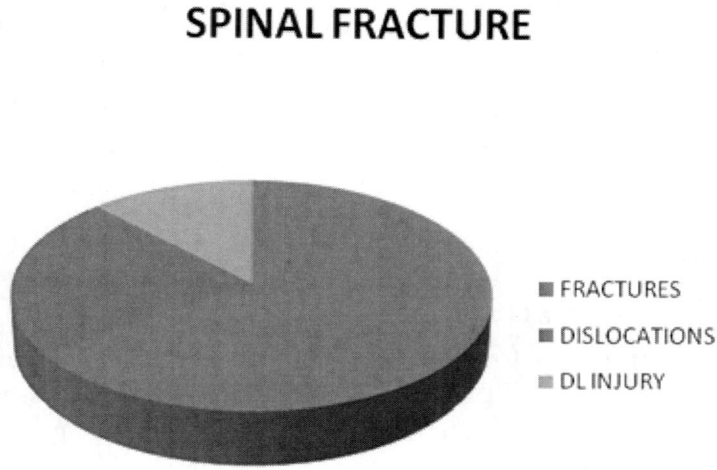

Figure 4. Overall distribution of spinal injuries into Fracture, Dislocations and Disco Ligamentous Injuries.

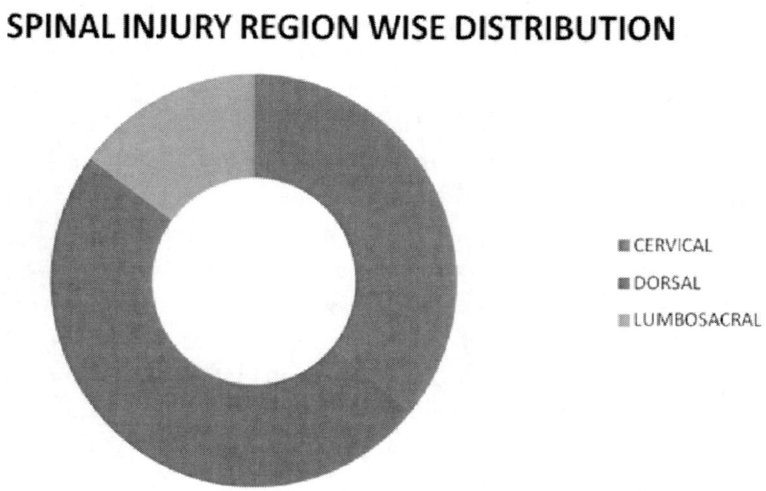

Figure 5. Spine injury by location leading to Frankels Grade A Deficit.

All individuals with burst fractures suffered severe axial compressive pattern of injury making them Frankels Grade A immediately following trauma. Most of the patients plateaued to a static neurological grade within 45 days of intervention (surgical or nonsurgical). Figure 5 shows spine injuries by location leading to a Frankels Grade A Deficit.

Discussion

Spinal Cord injury during the 60s and 70s was primarily sustained by soldiers during war. Later the mode of injury resulted mainly due to road traffic accidents. As the strength of the armed forces increased, so did the incidence of neuro trauma. Right from its inception, the PRC is expanding to meet the requirements of the spinal cord injured patients.

Conclusion

The Spinal Cord Injury Center and Paraplegic Rehabilitation center, Kirkee are doing a yeoman service to the disabled soldier of Indian armed forces for more than 50 years. Not much progress has been made in changing outcome in spinal cord injury, but current research and findings hold immense promise to overcome this disabling and devastating condition. Spinal cord injury as on date is the most devastating trauma afflicting the soldier and his family. Aggressive management in the initial phase of injury helps in reaching a stable neurological state. Subsequent rehabilitation requires intense dedicated and sustained efforts by professionals with a beating heart for these unfortunate soldiers. Interacting with the health care providers and highlighting the importance of this premiere institute will serve not only to focus on its improvement but also reassure our fighting soldiers that the Medical Corps not only provides cure but also world class rehabilitation. Our study proves that nature of injury plays a major role in determining the Neurological status. Morbidity is more in the cervical spinal cord injured patients with burst fracture.

Conflict of Interest

None

Acknowledgments

Dr R. K. Mukherjee, Director PRC and Occupational Therapy staff of MH Kirkee.

References

[1] Bouyer B, Vassal M, Zairi F, Dhenin A, Grelat M, Dubory A, et al. Surgery in vertebral fracture: Epidemiology and functional and radiological results in a prospective series of 518 patients at 1 year's follow-up. *Orthop. Traumatol. Surg. Res.* 2015;101:11-5. Back to cited text no.

[2] Akmal M, Trivedi R, Sutcliffe J. Functional outcome in trauma patients with spinal injury. *Spine* (Phila Pa 1976) 2003;28:180-5. Back to cited text no.

[3] Hasler R M, Exadaktylos A K, Bouamra O, Benneker L M, Clancy M, Sieber R, et al. Epidemiology and predictors of spinal injury in adult major trauma patients: European cohort study. *Eur. Spine J.* 2011;20:2174-80. Back to cited text no.

[4] Moradi-Lakeh M, Rasouli M R, Vaccaro A R, Saadat S, Zarei M R, Rahimi-Movaghar V, et al. Burden of traumatic spine fractures in Tehran, Iran. *BMC Public Health* 2011;11:789. Back to cited text no.

[5] Hu R, Mustard C A, Burns C. Epidemiology of incident spinal fracture in a complete population. *Spine* (Phila Pa 1976) 1996;21:492-9. Back to cited text no.

[6] Wang H, Zhang Y, Xiang Q, Wang X, Li C, Xiong H, et al. Epidemiology of traumatic spinal fractures: Experience from medical university-affiliated hospitals in Chongqing, China, 2001-2010. *J. Neurosurg. Spine* 2012;17:459-68. Back to cited text no.

[7] Leucht P, Fischer K, Muhr G, Mueller E J. Epidemiology of traumatic spine fractures. *Injury* 2009;40:166-72. Back to cited text no.

[8] Oliver M, Inaba K, Tang A, Branco B C, Barmparas G, Schnüriger B, et al. The changing epidemiology of spinal trauma: A 13-year review from a level I trauma center. *Injury* 2012;43:1296-300. Back to cited text no.

[9] Fletcher D J, Taddonio R F, Byrne D W, Wexler L M, Cayten C G, Nealon S M, et al. Incidence of acute care complications in vertebral column fracture patients with and without spinal cord injury. *Spine* (Phila Pa 1976) 1995;20:1136-46.

[10] Mathur N, Jain S, Kumar N, Srivastava A, Purohit N, Patni A, et al. Spinal cord injury: Scenario in an Indian state. *Spinal Cord* 2015;53:349-52.

[11] Blair J A, Patzkowski J C, Schoenfeld A J, et al. Spinal column injuries among Americans in the Global War on Terrorism. *J. Bone Joint Surg. Am.* 2012; 94(1Y9): e135.

[12] Blair J A, Patzkowski J C, Schoenfeld A J, et al. Are spine injuries sustained in battle truly different? *Spine J*. 2012;12:824Y829.

[13] Comstock S, Pannell D, Talbot M, et al. Spinal injuries after improvised explosive device incidents: implications for tactical combat casualty care. *J. Trauma*. 2011;71:S413YS417. [11,12,13]

[14] Vaccaro A R, Hulbert R J, Patel A A, Fisher C, Dvorak M, Lehman R A Jr, et al. The subaxial cervical spine injury classification system: a novel approach to recognize the importance of morphology, neurology, and integrity of the disco-ligamentous complex. *Spine* (Phila Pa 1976). 2007 Oct 1. 32(21):2365-74. [Medline].

[15] Lt Col A S Chahal, *Care of Spinal Cord Injries in the Armed Forces of India*, Paraplegia (1975):13, 25-28.

Chapter 12

Spasticity

Mrinal Joshi*

Rehabilitation Research Centre, Department of Physical Medicine and Rehabilitation, SMS Medical College and Associated Hospitals, Jaipur, India

Abstract

Human muscle tone is maintained by descending excitatory and inhibitory pathways, influencing interneuron pools and motoneurons. Spasticity originated from the word *spasmos* and was used in the 16th century to describe the contraction of muscles around the wound. Spasticity is multifaceted, and its pathophysiology is influenced by two primary mechanisms, spinal mechanisms and supraspinal & suprasegmental mechanisms. Recently, a consensus in 2018 of the IAB-Interdisciplinary Working Group for Movement Disorders, a special interest group promoting multimodal and interdisciplinary therapies in movement disorders, including spasticity, described spasticity as involuntary muscle hyperactivity in the presence of central paresis. Spastic muscles are weak and further weaken post-surgery, so rehabilitation should be planned accordingly with goal setting in consultation with the patient and caregiver.

Keywords: spasticity

Introduction

Spasticity originated from the word *spasmos* and was used in the 16th century to describe the contraction of muscles around the wound. Erb, in 1875 used it

---

* Corresponding Author's Email: dr.m.joshi@gmail.com.

In: Rehabilitation in Neurotrauma
Editors: VD Sinha, Amit Chakraborty, Jitin Bajaj et al.
ISBN: 978-1-68507-787-7

first as a noun in German *Spastizitat* (Erb, W. H. 1875) (Marjoline Boude 2019).

Spasticity results from injury/lesion to the upper motor neuron within the central nervous system (Decq, P. 2003) (Sheean, G. 2002) (M. M. Adams 2005). Tardieu, in 1954 proposed the definition of spasticity as *an increase in a stretch reflex that could be characterised and measured by the speed required to elicit the reflexes* (Tardieu, G. 1954). Lance defined spasticity in 1980 *as a motor disorder characterised by a velocity-dependent increase in tonic stretch reflex as one component of the upper motoneuron syndrome* (Lance, J. W. 1980). Decz, in 2000, modified the definition and categorised it into intrinsic tonic spasticity, intrinsic phasic spasticity and extrinsic spasticity to differentiate between various spasticity-related symptoms (Decq, P. 2003).

Later the Support Program for Assembly of a Database for Spasticity Measurement (SPASM) project reviewed the definition of disordered sensory-motor control resulting from an upper motor neuron lesion, presenting as intermittent or sustained involuntary activation of muscles (Burridge J. 2005).

And recently, a consensus in 2018 of the IAB-Interdisciplinary Working Group for Movement Disorders, a special interest group promoting multimodal and interdisciplinary therapies in movement disorders, including spasticity, described spasticity as involuntary muscle hyperactivity in the presence of central paresis. It consists of spasticity *sensu-strictu* (involuntary muscle hyperactivity triggered by rapid passive joint movement), rigidity (involuntary muscle hyperactivity triggered by slow passive joint motion), dystonia (spontaneous involuntary muscle hyperactivity) and spasms (complex involuntary movements usually triggered by sensory or acoustic stimuli). The committee further distinguished symptoms which are amenable to chemo-denervation by botulinum toxin (Dirk Dressler 2018) (Jacky Ganguly 2021).

Marjoline Baude and colleagues enumerated main features of spastic paresis with the condition of detection, at rest - spastic myopathy, spasticity and spastic dystonia; at a stretch – stretch sensitive paresis, spastic co-contraction, extrapyramidal co-contraction/synkinesis; and nociceptive spasm presenting at both rest and effort (Marjoline Boude 2019). Recently in 2019, a revised taxonomy was proposed for spastic paresis syndrome. The syndrome is defined in two parts, (a) muscle disorder called spastic myopathy, which combines muscle shortening and loss of extensibility, and (b) neurologic disorder comprising of spastic dystonia, spastic co-contraction, spasticity, and stretch sensitive paresis (Gracies, J. M. 2015) (Marjoline Boude 2019). And the authors conclude that *it is probably time that we cease to use the easy term spasticity to encompass all the various pathophysiological features of complexities of deforming spastic paresis.*

Spasticity can have a disabling effect on a patient through pain and reduced mobility, limiting the potential success of rehabilitation. Spasticity can also affect the quality of life and can be both diverse and highly detrimental to daily functioning. Spasticity can result in urinary incontinence, limit sexual intimacy, interfere with walking, sitting, standing, and generally reduce a person's ability to undertake activities of daily living. The physical limitations associated with spasticity confer risk of falls and consequent fractures (Ward 2012).

Extrinsic factors or *noxious triggers* identified by physician's observations that can increase spasticity can be temperature, time of the day, mental stress, physical touch, loud noises, anxiety, tight clothing, poor orthosis fit, poor wheelchair prescription, pain, fever, urinary tract infection, bladder stones, bladder distension, blocked catheter, chronic cystitis, bowel impaction, constipation, peri-rectal abscess, anal fissure, intra-abdominal pathology, muscle strains, muscle fatigue, joint contracture, ingrown toenails, menstrual cycle, labour, delivery, pregnancy, pressure ulcer, lack of sleep etc. (Chetan P. Phadke 2013).

Pathophysiology

Spasticity is multifaceted, and its pathophysiology is influenced by two primary mechanisms, spinal mechanisms and supraspinal & suprasegmental mechanisms.

Spinal influence can be following.

(a) Increased Fusimotor Drive

In the past, it was hypothesised that increased fusimotor activity leads to increased muscle spindle sensitivity, resulting in an exaggerated stretch reflex activity. But various experiments failed to demonstrate it; thus, it was dropped as a possible cause of spasticity (Hagbarth 1981).

(b) Hypersensitivity of Alpha Motor Neurons

Descending monoaminergic pathways have a facilitatory effect on alpha motor neurons at the ventral horn and an inhibitory effect on the dorsal horn. In acute spinal injury, alpha motor neurons have hyperexcitability, but in a chronic spinal state, the plateau potentials (voltage-dependent, persistent Ca+ and Na+ currents result in prolonged depolarization, i.e., plateau potentials) can be induced without an agonistic activity leading to the development of spasticity (C. H. Heckmann 2005) (Angshuman Mukherjee 2010).

(c) Hyperexcitability of Cutaneous Reflexes

Hyperresponsive withdrawal reflexes are observed in spasticity due to failure of presynaptic inhibition and hyperexcitability of propriospinal interneurons system, e.g., mass withdrawal reflex, Babinski sign.

(d) Reduction of Presynaptic Inhibition

There is a reduction of presynaptic inhibition in the presence of spasticity in some cases (Angshuman Mukherjee 2010).

(e) Recurrent Inhibition of Renshaw Cells

Previously it was believed to be a precursor of spasticity, but various observations and experiments have failed to demonstrate its role (Angshuman Mukherjee 2010).

(f) Reciprocal Ia Inhibition

Disynaptic inhibition of antagonist muscle activity during a stretch reflex is reciprocal inhibition. But the damage to descending pathways results in a lack of inhibitory signals from the interneuron, co-contraction of antagonist muscles, an essential accompaniment of spasticity (C. Crone 2006) (Angshuman Mukherjee 2010).

(g) Decreased Ib Inhibition

Alteration of Ib inhibition may play a role in the occurrence of spasticity.

Supraspinal and Suprasegmental Mechanisms

Human muscle tone is maintained by descending excitatory and inhibitory pathways, influencing interneuron pools and motoneurons.

Isolated corticospinal/pyramidal pathways do not cause spasticity but produce weakness, hyporeflexia and hypotonia. Spasticity results when lesions involve tracts from the premotor cortex, Broadman area *6* (Sheean 2008) (Segal 2018). They run with pyramidal tracts and are called parapyramidal tracts.

Medullary reticular formation produces inhibitory influence; dorsal reticulospinal tract inhibits stretch reflex arc and flexor reflex afferents (creating flexor spasms and clasp knife phenomenon).

The facilitatory or excitatory drive is mediated by ventral reticulospinal and, to some extent, by vestibulospinal tracts. Vestibulospinal pathways help maintain postural and anti-gravity (extensor) muscles, but their role in spasticity is doubtful. The ventral reticulospinal tract facilitates muscle stretch reflex & tone and is an inhibitor of flexor reflexes and spasms (W. Fries 1993) (B. T. Shahani 1973) (C. Trompetto 2014) (Brown 1994).

Complete spinal lesions have less spasticity than incomplete lesions. Incomplete lesions involving the dorsal reticulospinal tract have unopposed medial reticulospinal tract activity results in spasticity and hyperreflexia, marked extensor activity. Complete lesions lack the facilitatory influence of medial reticulospinal and vestibulospinal tracts resulting in less hypertonia than incomplete; the release of flexor reflex afferents results in paraplegia in flexion and exaggerated flexor spasms.

In spinal cord injury/lesion, neural reorganisation happens after a period of spinal shock. It results in hypertonicity due to hypersensitivity of neurons and axonal sprouting.

Rheological changes or changes in viscoelastic properties of muscle can also result in hypertonia (V. Dietz 1981) (Angshuman Mukherjee 2010) (A. F. Thilmann 1991). Contractures are extreme effects of these changes, which can be prevented by timely intervention with botulinum toxin.

So, multifactorial influences are responsible for increased muscle tone and associated reactions.

Assessment Scales for Spasticity

Modified Tardieu Scale

The Tardieu scale was developed by Tardieu et al., in 1954 and modified a couple of times by Held et al., and Boyd et al., The last modification is the modified Tardieu scale (Tardieu, G 1954) (Boyd, R. 1999).

It measures spasticity angle; the distal end of a joint is moved with three stretching velocities V1, V2 and V3.

It measures the passive range of movement at different velocities while measuring *the angle of catch.* A limb is moved in three different velocities: as slow as possible (V1), speed equivalent to freefall due to gravity (V2), and as fast as possible (V3). Goniometric measurement of the angle of catch at V1 velocity is called R2, and V3 is called R1. The angle R2-R1 is called the angle of dynamic spasticity. A significant difference means a sizeable dynamic component of spasticity, and a slight difference points to static influence (rheological changes) of the muscle (Roslyn N. Boyd 1999) (Love, S. C. 2001)

Modified Ashworth Scale

It is commonly used for assessing spasticity and quantifying spasticity. Ashworth scale was first proposed by Bryan Ashworth in 1964 and was later modified by Bohannon et al., (Bohannon, R. W. 1987) (Ansari, N. N. 2008).

0: No increase in muscle tone
1: Slight increase in muscle tone, manifested as a catch and release at the end of the range of movement
1+: Slight increase in muscle tone manifested by a catch, followed by minimal resistance throughout the remainder (less than ½) of the range of movement
2: More marked increase in tone, through most of the range of movement, but joint quickly moves
3: Considerable increase in muscle tone, passive movement is difficult
4: Affected part rigid in flexion or extension.

Treatment Options

Treatment depends on the rehabilitation goals directed by the patient and caregiver. The rehabilitation team sets a rehab goal with an objective outcome scale, e.g., goal setting with the Goal Attainment Scale, with discussion among the interdisciplinary team. The patient and caregiver then choose various therapeutic options or pathways to achieve it.

Oral Medications

Baclofen

It is an agonist at the beta subunit of gamma-aminobutyric acid on mono and polysynaptic neurons at the spinal cord level and brain (Albright 1996). It blocks neurotransmitter release, inhibiting motor neuron activity to muscle spindle intrafusal fibres (Christopher F. Terrence 1981). It also has an affinity for voltage-gated calcium channels (Ann Felicia Ambrose 2018). It is available as oral, transdermal and intrathecal administration (Ghanavatian S. Baclofen. 2021).

Tizanidine

Tizanidine is a centrally acting alpha-2 receptor agonist. It inhibits the release of excitatory neurotransmitters from spinal interneurons, enhances presynaptic inhibition, affects spinal polysynaptic pathways (Fuchigami T., 2011). Drug comparison studies show no difference in efficacy compared with baclofen or diazepam (Wallace J. D. 1994) (Shakespeare D. T. 2003). Periodic monitoring of creatinine and liver functions is required in patients on long-term management with tizanidine (Ghanavatian S. Tizanidine 2021).

Dantrolene Sodium

Dantrolene sodium is a directly acting muscle relaxant that decreases the calcium release from the sarcoplasmic reticulum in skeletal muscles, thereby reducing the force of contraction. It causes weakness; thus, it may interfere in ambulation, limiting its use primarily in non-ambulatory patients (Jay M.

Meythaler 2011). Hepatic functions should be evaluated before initiating, and regular monitoring is required during long term use.

Intrathecal Baclofen

In patients with severe spasticity, oral baclofen might not give the desired effect as it does not cross the blood-brain barrier. The intrathecal implantable baclofen pump is used to overcome the limitation. The baclofen dose required for intrathecal administration is much lower than the oral dose. Due to its high cost, risk of complications and maintenance, patient selection and education is of utmost necessity. Generally, patients with poor spasticity control despite a maximal trial of non-invasive modalities are the most appropriate candidates. The delivery system consists of a programmable pump with a reservoir and a catheter to deliver the drug to CSF. Adverse effects include catheter kinks, pump failure, catheter migration, hygroma, infection etc.; also, abrupt withdrawal due to pump failure can lead to seizure, coma and death (Sacelino M. 2016) (Coffey R. J. 2002).

Chemo-Neurolysis

Chemical neurolysis involves the application of chemicals that interfere with the conduction of nerve, alcohol and, more commonly, phenol is used for regional/focal spasticity management. It converts an upper motor neuron syndrome to a partial lower motor neuron syndrome (Lawrence H. Horn 2011). Phenol, also known as carbolic acid, is a benzene derivative; when applied to any tissue at a concentration of 5% or more, it causes tissue necrosis. When applied to nerves, it destroys axons, and recovery depends on the concentration of phenol used (Halpern, D. 1977).

Neurolysis is preferable in motor nerves or mixed motor nerves with limited sensory supply to prevent complications secondary to sensory loss. Its intrathecal use to treat spasticity was described first (Nathan, P. W., 1959) (Kelly R. E. 1959), and later Khalili and associates established its clinical use and published injection techniques for various peripheral nerve blocks using phenol (Khalili A. A. 1964). Diagnostic ultrasound combined with a nerve locator is used for the precise location of neurolysis. It precludes complications by visualising the vascular structure and minimising the effective dose of phenol.

Side-effects of phenol neurolysis can be due to chemical effects (overcorrection/atrophy, sensory loss, dysesthesia, tender nodules, skin sloughing). Even though botulinum toxin has emerged as an effective alternative for managing focal spasticity, phenol neurolysis remains the mainstay in regional/focal spasticity management in the middle- and low-income countries due to the vast disparity in cost between phenol and botulinum toxin.

Chemo-Denervation

Botulinum toxin has become an effective and safer option for managing focal spasticity. So far, only type A and B of botulinum toxin are available for clinical use.

Botulinum toxin inhibits the vesical dependent release of acetylcholine from the presynaptic nerve terminal; as a result, there is no input from the nerve to the muscle resulting in *chemo-denervation.*

Injections are performed using a landmark-based approach, electromyographic stimulation/localisation but now more so by direct visualisation using diagnostic ultrasound. It is usually combined with therapy, orthosis and/or neuromuscular electric stimulation for optimal goal achievement (Bhakta B. B., 2000) (Sheen, G. L., 2001). Motor functions improve in patients where some focal spasticity is causing hindrance with some preserved meaningful functions and voluntary control. The dose of botulinum toxin depends on the patient's weight, the severity of spasticity, functional goal, type of botulinum toxin, and injector experience.

Non-Pharmacological Intervention

Non-pharmacological interventions remain the first-line treatment of spasticity, and then pharmacological and invasive treatments are provided if needed. Various types of interventions are used, which includes shock wave, transcutaneous electric nerve stimulation (TENS), vibratory stimulation, electromyography feedback, therapeutic ultrasound, repetitive transcranial magnetic stimulation, acupuncture, orthosis and more importantly, physical intervention, heat/cold therapy, e.g., stretching and passive movement, serial casts, saeboflex, lycra garments, body weight supported ambulation, functional electric stimulation etc. (Khan F. 2019).

Although there is a paucity of literature for large randomised, double-blind trials, solid scientific evidence supports their use (Stuyvenberg Corri L n.d.). Physical therapy in the form of therapeutic exercises is beneficial as a single and early modality or in combination with other approaches to improve function and outcome (Antonio Naro 2017) (Thamer J. Bovend'Eerdt 2008) (Harvey L. A. 2017) (Singer B. 2001).

Surgical Intervention

Surgical intervention includes orthopaedic and neurosurgical intervention. Surgical intervention must be considered when spasticity and functional improvement cannot be achieved despite a multidisciplinary pharmacologic and non-pharmacologic intervention. Spastic muscles are weak and further weaken post-surgery, so rehabilitation should be planned accordingly with goal setting in consultation with the patient and caregiver. Surgical planning includes clinical examination, functional examination, grading various scales for outcome assessment, evaluating co-morbidities, gait evaluation, dynamic EMG, video analysis and long-term plan post-surgery.

References

Adams, M. M., A. C. Hicks. 2005. "Spasticity after spinal cord injury." *Spinal Cord* 43: 577-586.

Albright, A. Lenland. 1996. "Topical review: Baclofen in the treatment of cerebral palsy." *Journal of child neurology* 11 (2): 77-83.

Ambrose, A. F., Tanya Verghese, Caroline Dohle, Jennifer Russo. 2018. *Physical Medicine and Rehabilitation Clinics of North America* 29: 483-500.

Ansari, N. N., Nagheli S., Arab T. K., Jalaie S. 2008. "The interrater and intrarater reliability of the modified Ashworth scale in the assessment of muscle spasticity: limb and muscle group efferents." *Neurorehabilitation* 23 (3): 231-7.

Bhakta, B. B., Cozens J. A., Chamberlain M. A., Bramford J. M. 2000. "Impact of botulinum toxin type A on disability and carer burden due to arm spasticity after stroke: a randomized, double-blind placebo-controlled trial." *J Neurol Neurosurg Psychiatry* 69: 217-21.

Bohannon, R. W., Smith, M. B. 1987. "Interrater reliability of a modified Ashworth scale of muscle spasticity." *Physical Therapy* 67 (2): 206-7.

Boude, M., Jens Bo Nielson, Jean Michel Gracies. 2019. "The neurophysiology of deforming spastic paresis: A revised taxonomy." *Annals of Physical & Rehabilitation Medicine* 62: 426-430.

Bovend'Eerdt, T. J., Meridith Newman, Karen Barker et al., 2008. "The effect of stretching in spasticity: a systemic review." *Arch Phys Med Rehabil* 89 (7): 1395-406.

Boyd, R. N., H Kerr Graham. 1999. "Objective measurement of clinical findings in the use of botulinum toxin type A for the management of children with cerebral palsy." *European journal of neurology* 6: S 23-35.

Brown, P. 1994. "Pathophysiology of spasticity." *Journal of neurology, neurosurgery & psychiatry* 57 (7): 773-7.

Burridge, J., Wood D., Hermens H. J., Voorman G., Johnson G., Van Wijck F., Platz T., Gregorie M., Hitchcock R., Pandyan A. 2005. "Theoretical and methodological considerations in the measurement of spasticity." *Disability and Rehabilitation* 27: 69-80.

Coffey, R. J., Edgar T. S., Francisco G. E. et al., 2002. "Abrupt withdrawal from intrathecal baclofen: recognition and management of a potentially life-threatening syndrome." *Archives of Physical Medicine Rehabilitation* 83: 735-41.

Crone, C., L. L. Johnsen, F. Bieringsorensen, J. B. Nielsen. 2006. "Appearance of reciprocal facilitation of ankle extensors from ankle flexors in patients with stroke or spinal cord injury." *Brain* 126: 495-507.

Decq, P. 2003. "Pathophysiology of spasticity." *Neurochirurgie* 49: 163-184.

Dietz, V., J. Quimern, W. Berger. 1981. "Electrophysiological studies of gait in spasticity and rigidity. Evidence that altered mechanical properties of muscle contribute to hypertonia ." *Brain* 104: 431-449.

Dressler, D., Roongraj Bhidayasiri, Saeed Bohlega, Pedro Chans, Hsin Fen Chien, Tae Mo Chung, Carlo Colosimo, Markus Ebke, Klemens Fedoroff, Bernd Frank, Ryuji Kaji, Petr Kanovsky, Serdar Kocer, Federico Micheli, Olga Orlova, Sebastian Paus et al., 2018. "Defining spasticity: a new approach considering current movement disorders terminology and botulinum toxin therapy." *Journal of neurology* 265: 856-862.

Erb, W. H. 1875. "Spinaler symptomenkomplex." *Berliner Zeitschrift Psych* 32.

Fries, W., A. Danek, K. Schidumann, C. Hamburg. 1993. "Motor recovery following capsular stroke. Role of descending pathways from multiple motor areas." *Brain* 116: 369-382.

Fuchigami, T., Kakinohana O., Heffran M. P., Marsala S. et al., 2011. "Potent suppression of stretch reflex activity after systemic or spinal delivery of tizanidine in rats with spinal ischemia-induced chronic spastic paraplegia." *Neuroscience* 194: 160-9.

Ganguly, J., Dinkar Kulshreshtha, Mohammad Almotiri, Mandar Jog. 2021. "Muscle tone physiology and abnormalities." *Toxins* 13 (4): 282.

Ghanavatian, S., Derian A. 2021. "Baclofen." *StatPearls.* May 15. https://:www.ncbi.nlm.nih.gov/books/NBK526037/.

Ghanavatian, S., Derian, A. 2021. "*Tizanidine.*" Aug 13. https://www.ncbi.nlm.nih.gov/books/NBK519505/.

Gracies, J. M., 2015. "Coefficients of impairment in deforming spastic paresis." *Annals of Physical and Rehabilitation Medicine* 58: 173-8.

Hagbarth, K. E. 1981. *Fusimotor and stretch reflex function studied in recordings from muscle spindle afferents in man.* Vol. 13, by A Prochazka A Taylor, 109-115. New York: Oxford University Press.

Halpern, D. 1977. "Histological studies in animals after intramuscular neurolysis with phenol." *Arch Phys Med Rehabil* 58 (10): 438-443.

Harvey L. A., Katalinic O. M., Herbert R. D. et al., 2017. "Stretch for the treatment and prevention of contracture: an abridged republication of a Cochrane Systematic Review." *Journal of physical therapy* 63 (2): 67-75.

Heckmann, C. H., M. Gorassini M. A., D. J. Bennette. 2005. "Persistent inward currents in motoneuron dendrites: implications for motor output." *Muscle Nerve* 31: 135-156.

Horn, L. H., Gurtej Singh, Edward R. Dabrowski. 2011. "Chemoneurolysis with phenol and alcohol: a dying art that merits revival." In *Spasticity: diagnosis and management*, by Elie Elovic Allison Brachear. Demos Medical.

Kelly, R. E., Gauthier Smith P. L. 1959. "Intrathecal phenol in the treatment of reflex spasms and spasticity." *Lancet* 274 (7112): 1102-5.

Khalili, A. A., Harmel H. H., Forester S., Benton J. 1964. "Management of spasticity by selective peripheral nerve block with dilute phenol solution in clinical rehabilitation." *Arch Phys Med Rehabil* 45: 513-9.

Khan, F., Amatya B., Bensmail D., Yelnik A. 2019. "Non-pharmacological interventions for spasticity in adults: an overview of systemic reviews." *Annals of physical medicine & rehabilitation medicine* 62 (4): 265-273.

Lance, J. W., 1980. "The control of muscle tone, reflexes, and movement: Robert Wartenberg Lecture." *Neurology* 30: 1303-1313.

Love, S. C., Valentine J. P., Blaur E. M., Price C. J., Cole J. H., Chauvel P. J. 2001. "The effect of botulinum toxin type A on the functional ability of the child with spastic hemiplegia a randomised controlled trial." *Journal of Neurology* 8: 50-8.

Meythaler, J. M., Scott Kowalski. 2011. *Spasticity: diagnosis and management.* Edited by Elli Elovic Allison Brashear. Demos Medical.

Mukherjee, A., Ambar Chakravarty. 2010. "Spasticity mechanism - for the clinician." *Frontiers of neurology* 1: 1-10.

Naro, A., Antonio Leo, Margherita Russo et al., 2017. "Breakthrough in the spasticity management: are non-pharmacological treatment the future?" *Journal of clinical neuroscience* 39: 16-27.

Nathan, P. W., 1959. "Intrathecal phenol to relieve spasticity in paraplegia." *Lancet* 274 (7112): 1099-102.

Phadke, C. P., Chitralakshmi K. Balasubramanian, Farooq Ismail, Chris Boulias. 2013. "Revisiting physiologic and psychologic triggers that increase spasticity." *American journal of physical medicine and rehabilitation* 92 (4): 357-369.

Sacelino, M., Ivanhoe C. B., McGuire J. R. et al., 2016. "Best practices for intrathecal baclofen therapy: patient selection." *Neuromodulation* 19: 607-15.

Segal, M. 2018. "Muscle overactivity in the upper motor neuron syndrome: pathophysiology." *Physical medicine and rehabilitation clinics of North America* 29: 427-436.

Shahani, B. T., R. R. Young. 1973. Human flexor spasm. Vol. 3, in *New developments in electromyography and clinical neurophysiology.*

Shakespeare, D. T., Boggild M., Young C. 2003. "Anti-spasticity agents for multiple sclerosis." *Cochrane database syst. rev.* (2003(4):CD001332).

Sheean, G. 2008. "Neurophysiology of spasticity." In *Upper motor neuron syndrome and spasticity clinical management and neurophysiology*, G. R. Johnson, M. P. Barnes. New York: Cambridge university press.

Sheean, G., 2002. "The pathophysiology of spasticity." *European journal of neurology* 9 (S-1): 3-9.

Sheen, G. L. 2001. "Botulinum treatment of spasticity: why is it so difficult to show a functional benefit?" *Curr Opin Neurol* 14: 771-6.

Singer, B., Singer K. B., Allison G. 2001. "Serial plaster casting to correct equino varus deformity of the ankle following acquired brain injury in adults." *Disabil Rehabil* 23 (18): 829-36.

Stuyvenberg Corri, L., Shaaron E. Brown, Ketaki Inamdar, Megan Evans et al., n.d. "Targeted physical therapy combined with spasticity management changes motor development trajectory for a two-year-old with cerebral palsy." *Journal of personalized medicine* 11 (3): 163.

Tardieu, G., Shentoub S., Delarue R. 1954. "A la recherehe d'une technique de measure de la spasticite." *Rev Neurol* 91: 143-4.

Terrence, C. F., Gerhard H. Fromm. 1981. "Complications of baclofen withdrawal." *Archives of neurology* 38: 588-89.

Thilmann, A. F., S. J. Fellows, E. Grams. 1991. "The mechanism of spastic muscle hypertonus: variations in reflex gain over the time course of spasticity." *Brain* 114: 233-244.

Trompetto, C., L. Marinelli, E. Peosin E. et al., 2014. "Pathophysiology of spasticity: implications to neurorehabilitation." *Biomed research international* 354906.

Wallace, J. D. 1994. "Summary of combined clinical analysis of controlled clinical trials with tizanidine." *Neurology* 44 (11(S-9)): 60-8.

Ward, A. B. 2012. "A literature review of the pathophysiology and onset of post-stroke spasticity." *European journal of neurology,* 19: 21-27.

Chapter 13

Surgery for Spasticity

Vasundhara S Rangan and Suchanda Bhattacharjee*
Department of Neurosurgery, Nizam's Institute of Medical Sciences, Hyderabad, Telangana, India

Abstract

Spasticity, in a simplified view of things, is the unmasking of the tendency of muscles to resist stretch. It has been described as velocity-dependent resistance to movement and is generally accompanied by weakness of the affected muscle groups. It is a common sign noted in a wide range of neurological conditions and is also a common sign observed in clinical practice. It is a major complicating factor in most severe cases of brain and spinal cord injuries and other chronic CNS pathologies. While spastic diplegia forms the most frequent variant of cerebral palsy, spasticity has been noted in up to 97% of chronic stroke survivors with moderate to severe motor impairments. The high incidence and prevalence of this feature in clinical practice, especially in those with chronic illnesses that cause lasting impairment in the quality of life, mandates a thorough knowledge of available management options.

Introduction

A clear-cut comprehensive definition of the phenomenon of spasticity remains elusive but its defining features have known to include: "disordered sensorimotor control of muscles arising from an upper motor neuron (UMN)

---

* Corresponding Author's Email: suchandab2010@gmail.com

In: Rehabilitation in Neurotrauma
Editors: VD Sinha, Amit Chakraborty, Jitin Bajaj et al.
ISBN: 978-1-68507-787-7

lesion," "presentation as intermittent or sustained involuntary contraction of muscles" and "velocity-dependant increase in tonic stretch reflexes" [1, 2]. Being part of the UMN syndrome, it is accompanied by the other consequences of the causative disorders. Incoordination and weakness are common associations, and the formation of contractures is a common complication. In conditions like cerebral palsy where the neurological damage is complex, a variety of motor symptoms besides spasticity may be found. In such cases, thorough evaluation of the positive and negative symptoms and signs of the patient precedes treatment to address predominant motor disturbance which may be weakness, spasticity, rigidity, dystonia, dyskinesia, or incoordination.

Overview

The complete and exact neural mechanism for the development of this state of hypertonia and hyperreflexia remains unclear. The hyperactivity of gamma motor neurons is thought to play a significant role. With the loss of upper motor neuron control (inhibition) of the gamma motor neurons, the muscle spindle mediated stretch reflex becomes prominent. Increased alpha motor neuron excitability is also a feature observed [3]. Such loss of higher control may originate from pathologies involving the neural axis anywhere from the cerebral cortex to the spinal segment supplying the musculature in question. A resultant imbalance of neurotransmitters at the spinal level, especially the lack of the inhibitory gamma aminobutyric acid (GABA), results in the loss of the physiological reciprocal inhibition of antagonistic muscle groups. Imbalance between the inputs from the corticospinal, reticulospinal and possibly the vestibulospinal tracts cumulatively leads to the final clinical picture. Most common examples of cerebral pathology leading to spasticity include cerebral palsy in the pediatric age group and trauma as well as stroke in the adult population [4]. Cerebral causes are thought to result in increased excitability of monosynaptic pathways and tend to present with spasticity predominantly in the antigravity muscles leading to typical postures involving lower limb extension and upper limb flexion. Spinal cord pathology resulting from a variety of causes including trauma, tumors, vascular lesions, or medical conditions including multiple sclerosis, which also manifests as spasticity of the muscles supplied by segments below the affected cord level. Increased polysynaptic responses and activation of multiple spinal segments in response to one peripheral input are notable associated features in these conditions.

Spasticity hampers usage of residual motor function, generates pain, development of contractures and joint deformities, non-aesthetic appearance, difficult nursing care / care taker exhaustion. However, spasticity may help the child in locomotion also.

Evaluation and Treatment Considerations

Muscle tone is vital for muscle function. Since spasticity results from dysregulation of this essential parameter, its management is far from simple. Abolishing spasticity must not result in abolishing of the muscle tone which is needed for posture and normal functioning of the trunk and extremities. In many cases, the increased tone of the spastic musculature masks their weakness and lack of voluntary control and aids overall function. Management of spasticity alone is therefore hardly a solution in most affected patients. The most clinically prominent signs such as exaggerated reflexes may not be the biggest causes of the patient's disability. Clear insight into the most disabling or troublesome components of the illness, which may be cramping, spasms, fatigue, etc., guides the management plan. Keeping a functional end point to be reached through training or rehabilitation in mind, such treatments are mainly undertaken to facilitate its achievement. In many cases, treatment needs to be supplemented by occupational therapy, speech therapy and even orthopedic or plastic surgical procedure. Spasticity itself is only treated when:

a) it prevents normal functioning or movements,
b) it causes harmful effects like involuntary spasms and pain, or,
c) it impedes necessary nursing / care of the individual.

Clinical Evaluation

1) *Posture and Function:* Although specific measures of the degree of muscle spasticity or hyperreflexia are useful, the final effect is noted in the attitude or posture of the limbs and trunk as well as the impairment it produces in the actual functioning of the patient. A record of the patient performing basic activities using the limbs (such as gait) and change demonstrated in a similar record following intervention is the single most useful clinical measure. A comprehensive disability score is a better indicator than most individual tests.

The Gross Motor Function Classification Scale is a useful categorizing tool [5].

Besides active spasticity itself, complications such as shortening, and contractures must be noted as they prevent significant improvement even after addressing the spasticity. Range of motion across joints is assessed. Fixed deformities prevent any meaningful assessment or treatment of the spastic muscles. In such cases the attitude or posture of the limb itself may be a cause of disfigurement and may need to be addressed.

2) *Tone:* Quantification of tone is most done using the Modified Ashworth Scale. Clinical assessment may be confounded by the varying intensity of spasticity at different times and with rest or activity. The Tardieu Scale is another means of evaluating spasticity and focuses on the velocity dependence of this sign. Spasticity at the knee joint may be assessed by the pendulum test.

3) *Power:* Muscle power assessment is often impaired by the presence of significant hypertonia / spasticity. The presence of some degree of weakness is implied when a muscle group is spastic. It must be taken into consideration that relief of the hypertonia and hyperreflexia may unmask the muscle weakness and leave a worse functional situation after intervention.

4) *Reflex activity:* Hyperreflexia is graded, and clonus is noted.

5) *Coordination and control:* Normal movements are a result of complex control of neuromuscular activity and reflect on more than muscle power. Evaluation of all these aspects are complicated by the presence of spasticity.

6) *Abnormal movements:* Spasms when present must be scored in terms of frequency on the Spasm Frequency Scale. Subjective pain and severity are noted. Dyskinesias, dystonia, tremors, other abnormal movements like chorea, athetosis, etc are noted. These added movement disorders may require specific focus in treatment and may cloud significant improvement even after spasticity has been addressed.

Investigations

Imaging for treatable causes is undertaken in all cases. When the nature of the cause and its relative permanency has been established, investigations pertaining to identifying and characterizing the spastic muscles are performed.

Electromyography is a valuable tool in identifying spastic muscles. Further assessment may be done using local anesthetic agents to block individual muscle groups. This aids in understanding the effect that more permanent treatments will have.

Management Options

Spasticity may be a clinical feature of a variety of pathologies which are amenable to surgical management. In these cases, treatment of the cause may lead to significant relief in the spasticity. Cervical or dorsal compressive myelopathy resulting from congenital, degenerative, inflammatory, or neoplastic conditions can be surgically addressed. Decompression with or without fixation of affected spinal segments constitutes the mainstay of treatment. Other spinal causative conditions amenable to surgical management include tethering of the spinal cord and vascular malformations. Some intracranial causes of spasticity like hydrocephalus and intracranial mass lesions may also be surgically cured.

Here we discuss the management options for spasticity arising from predominantly irreversible causes. More permanent (surgical) treatments for spasticity per se are undertaken once there is non-progression of the disease, and hence the spasticity, is ascertained. Lesser invasive methods are tried initially, and invasive surgical options are resorted to when results from the former have been found wanting [6].

Treatments are focused at one or many sites in the neural pathway leading from the brain up to the effector muscle. Methods often aim to address one of the three perceived contributing problems: dysregulated (abnormal) central (supraspinal) control pathways, unmasked (overly excitable) spinal reflex pathways, consequently altered muscle properties. Targets higher in the chain are more useful in cases of widespread spasticity and more distal targets like the motor fascicle effectively address localized involvement [7].

Non Invasive Non- Pharmacological/Physical Treatments

Physiotherapy is key in rehabilitation or training of patients with motor disabilities. Use of affected muscles to perform essential activities cannot be achieved without motivated training and practice. Pharmacological and/ or invasive measures are best viewed as adjuncts to physical therapy. Stretching of involved muscles and prolonged positioning of the limbs in the desired attitude with the aid of casts / orthotics when needed are the basic methods used. These are complemented by exercises to train the patient to strengthen weak muscle groups and for performance of specific functions [6]. Identification of noxious stimuli and their elimination is a vital aspect of management.

Various adjuncts to physiotherapy training and rehabilitation have been studied and found to be of some use. Non-Invasive Neuromodulation by means of repetitive transcranial magnetic stimulation (rTMS) and transcranial direct current stimulation (tDCS) have been found useful when added to physiotherapy in stroke patients. Transcutaneous electrical nerve stimulation (TENS) is used as an adjunct in limb spasticity. Shock wave therapy, ultrasound, thermotherapy, cryotherapy, vibration and even acupuncture have been studied and found useful in addressing this chronic complex disorder [8].

Deformities caused by the spasticity may be dealt with mechanically resisting their establishment by use of various methods. POP casts and various corrective or preventive orthotics may be used. Fixed deformities are best corrected by surgical release.

Medical Treatments

Orally administered drug therapy forms the first line of treatment of spasticity. As the exact chemical basis of the disorder is unclear, drugs acting by various mechanisms are used in the management. Medication may function through central neural or peripheral muscular action. Baclofen, the most used oral medication, has GABA agonist action by acting on GABA-B receptors. Benzodiazepines may be beneficial via their action on GABA-A receptors. Diazepam is especially useful in cases where rapid relief is needed such as in case of painful spasms. Central alpha 2 adrenergic agonists like Tizanidine have also often been commonly used. Most of these medications have a sedating effect in varying degrees and hence are best prescribed at night. Dantrolene sodium is used for its muscle relaxant action by preventing calcium release from the muscle sarcoplasmic reticulum. Drugs therapy is initiated with individual drugs and gradual stepping up of dosages in recommended. Combinations may be required in case of insufficient response. GABAergic drugs must be gradually withdrawn when stopping therapy. Drug use is limited by eventually diminishing responses, higher dose required and the incidence of adverse effects. Most medication for spasticity treatment has a sedating effect. When high and poorly tolerated doses of baclofen are required, delivery of the drug via an intrathecal pump must be considered [6, 8].

Invasive Treatments

Insertion of a baclofen pump into the thecal sac is a viable alternative for patients responding to baclofen therapy. It is useful in patients with widespread spasticity. This mode uses a hundredth of the dose of the drug required orally and avoids the challenge of crossing the blood brain barrier. Sedation, muscular weakness and other implant and surgery related complications must be looked out for. The pump is usually considered too large for use in extremely young children and in such cases, the use of botulinum toxin may be advisable as a short-term measure.

Local anesthetic blocks help assess the efficacy and the overall usefulness of abolishing spasticity of individual muscles depending on the site injected. They aid evaluation by helping differentiate severe spasticity from bony ankylosis or contracture formation as the cause of restricted mobility in certain cases. They aid treatment planning by providing a picture of the outcome to be expected. Once assessed satisfactorily, more lasting methods including injection of neurolytic agents are employed. The short-lasting nature of local blocks using agents like Bupivacaine understandably prevent them from being considered a treatment modality.

Botulinum toxin is widely used for localised effects that are reversible but last a long duration (months). Injections cause blockade of transmission at the neuromuscular junction and are therefore best used in cases of spasticity pertaining to smaller muscle groups. Cases of widespread spasticity involving multiple limbs would require forbiddingly high doses of the toxin. Adverse effects include the rare incidences of widespread muscle paralysis, respiratory compromise, allergies, etc. Resistance to the toxin also develops with time besides the development of antibodies and requires adoption of other treatment methods eventually. Nevertheless, it is a well-tolerated adjunctive treatment useful in both adults and children with upper or lower limb spasticity [9].

Permanent neurolysis has been achieved by chemical injections or other mechanical means of lesioning including surgical sectioning. Phenol (3 to 12%) or ethyl alcohol (65%) injections were performed and now the indication for such methods seems to not extend beyond cases with severe spasticity who are unfit for open surgery. Percutaneous stimulation and injection may be performed under fluoroscopic guidance. Chemical neurolysis takes immediate effect and is performed on motor nerves alone. Sensory involvement may lead to unwanted dysesthesias.

Surgical Treatments

The ability of the patient to cooperate with the rehabilitation plan is vital in decision making for undertaking surgery. For instance, in children with significant intellectual impairment resulting from cerebral palsy or in adults in a vegetative state following massive strokes or trauma, surgical management of spasticity is only undertaken when the hypertonia causes gross difficulty in caring for the patient. Medical and mechanical management is invariably the first line of treatment. Once that fails, local less invasive therapies are tried before invasive surgery is undertaken [10].

Surgical methods target in two ways:

1) to modulate the intra-axial neural circuits thought to contribute spasticity, and
2) those that section peripheral neural pathways.

The first (central) type includes:

1) Stereotactic procedures including stimulation or lesioning of central targets including cortical areas and deep nuclei
2) Spinal cord stimulation
3) Myelotomy

The second (peripheral) type includes:

1) Rhizotomy
2) Neurotomy

Intimate anatomical knowledge of the operative site, an operating microscope, an electrical stimulator (bipolar or tripolar), EMG facility (if deemed necessary), local anesthetic agents for administration of a nerve block, micro instruments including atraumatic suction, microsurgical knife which can be substituted with a thin bored needle knife using an insulin needle, micro scissors, fine micro tipped bipolar electrocautery and essential implantable hardware are basic surgical requirements depending on the procedure chosen.

Anesthesia and medication allowing for intraoperative electrophysiological monitoring is advised. Effect of muscle relaxation during surgery is avoided to allow for response to motor stimulation and agents like nitrous oxide and propofol are also avoided as they alter excitability.

Intracranial Targeted Treatments

Stimulation as well as lesioning of various intracranial targets has been attempted as treatment for spasticity. Direct stimulation of the cerebral cortex at motor area, sensory areas and the cerebellar cortex has been studied in the past. Deep nuclear targets that gained some importance in addressing spasticity included areas of the thalamus and the dentate nucleus of the cerebellum. Dentatotomy has been found to be an effective treatment measure. However, these methods did not gain popularity. Lack of clarity in mechanism, superior outcomes and greater experience with more peripheral procedures, the financial burden of stereotaxic procedure and complications of intracranial surgery may all be the contributing factors [11].

Myelotomy

Lateral division within the spinal cord matter with the aim of interrupting the spinal reflex arc was first performed using a coronal cut. This was employed to address severe spasticity of lower limbs in patients with severe impairment of voluntary motor and sphincter function (typically those confined to the bed). Extending across the lumbar and sacral segments through a laminectomy exposing the conus and the epiconus, this procedure was called a Longitudinal Myelotomy. In cases where paraplegia is not absolute, myelotomy attempting to spare the corticospinal fibers is done by making right angled cuts after a posterior midline myelotomy is done. This divides the connection between the ventral and dorsal horns.

Peripheral Neurotomy

The procedure for sectioning of selected motor fibres supplying the spastic muscle has been termed selective peripheral neurotomy, selective motor fasciculotomy, etc. The spastic muscle or muscular compartment to be addressed is defined and surgical exposure tracing the peripheral nerve supplying the muscles is performed. Using intraoperative mapping, the motor fibres are identified by electrical stimulation and observation of the motor response. Sensory fibers are religiously avoided in order to avoid post-operative complications such as regional pain syndromes, hypoesthesia and dysesthesia. Motor weakness is usually not an outcome to worry about unless sectioning has been particularly excessive. 50 to 80 percent of the motor branches contributing to the spastic muscle are generally sectioned. Electrical monitoring and selectivity in the nerve fibres / motor fascicles targeted has led to the procedure being variously called selective or functional neurotomy and Selective Motor Fasciculotomy (SMF) [12].

The neural lesion is formed using sharp dissection and a segmental resection of few millimetres is performed followed by bipolar cauterisation of the stumps. This procedure generally yields immediate and lasting positive results. However, renervation may lead to long term surgical failure. Local surgical complications including hematoma and infections may occur as with any surgery. Negative functional outcomes are best avoided by thorough preoperative ascertainment using local anesthetic block or botox injections well before surgery and optimal physiotherapy of the muscles in question.

Neurotomies performed for specific targets are listed here in the format of: (Anatomical unit: abnormal spastic posture addressed, predominant involved muscles, targeted nerves).

Upper Limb

Shoulder

- Adduction and internal rotation, Pectoralis major and teres major,
- Ansa pectoralis and branches of lower and middle subscapular nerves.

Elbow

- Flexion, Biceps brachii and brachialis, Musculocutaneous nerve.

Forearm

- Pronation, Pronator teres and quadratus, Median nerve

Wrist

- Flexion, Flexor carpi radialis and palmaris longus, Median nerve
- Flexion with ulnar deviation, Flexor carpi ulnaris, Ulnar nerve

Fingers

- Proximal interphalangeal joint and metacarpophalangeal joints:
- Flexion, Flexor digitorum superficialis, Median nerve

Distal Interphalangeal Joint

- Flexion, Flexor digitorum profundus, Median and Ulnar nerves

Swan Neck Deformity / Clawing

- Lumbricals and Interossei, Median and Ulnar nerves

Thumb

- Adduction and flexion, Adductor policis and flexor policis longus, Ulnar and Median nerves

Lower Limb

Hip

- Adduction, Adductor longus, Obturator nerve (anterior branch)

Knee

- Flexion, Hamstring muscles (primarily semitendinosus), Sciatic nerve branches
- Extension, Quadriceps femoris (primarily vastus intermedius and rectus femoris), Femoral nerve branches

Foot

- Equinus (plantar flexion), Gastrocnemius and soleus (primarily soleus), Tibial nerve branches
- Varus, Tibialis posterior, Tibial nerve branch

Toes

- Hallux extension, Extensor hallucis longus, Anterior tibial nerve branch
- Claw toes (flexion), Flexor hallucis longus and flexor digitorum longus, tibial nerve branches

Rhizotomy and Drez Lesioning

Neurotomies are best performed to manage segmental or focal spasticity, the management of spasticity involving entire limbs is better treated by more proximally acting procedures. Reduction in spasticity by sectioning dorsal roots was observed in experiments performed on cats over a century ago. While ventral root sectioning that has also been historically performed, understandably translates to reduction in muscular activity, the mechanism of action of dorsal root lesions is less clear. Nevertheless, the observed efficacy of these procedures by multiple pioneers demonstrates a sensory cause to spasticity of the muscles [11, 13].

The dorsal roots have been targeted by multiple methods at various anatomical points including portions of the dorsal horn and the root entry zone.

Selective Dorsal Rhizotomy (SDR)

SDR has been the most widely practiced and reported successful despite recent sources assessing the overall evidence available as being inconclusive about the long-term functional outcomes [14, 15]. Patients with spastic paraparesis were the ones favored to receive the Selective Doral Rhizotomy (SDR) as described by Peacock who modified and revived the use of this procedure [16]. L2 to S1 lesions (sparing L4 root which is considered important for knee extension and therefore standing posture) are performed. Further, targeting the lower sacral roots while monitoring sphincter activity may help relieve a spastic urethral and/or anal sphincter. The individual rootlets are visualized under the microscope and tested for supply and excitability by electrical bipolar stimulation. 30 to 80% of the rootlets at the levels charted in the preoperative plan are then sectioned. Intraoperative use of electrical stimulation testing with relative sparing of muscle groups vital to normal antigravity posture and targeting the rootlets which elicit a motor response on stimulation constitutes the selectivity in SDR. Rootlets are divided sharply as in the case of neurotomy. A secondary effect causing improvement in upper limb spasticity has been observed following lumbar rhizotomies in children with spastic cerebral palsy. The reason is not clear but the role of internuncial neurons has been said to be involved in the process.

DREZotomy

Targeting the dorsal root fibres as they enter the dorsolateral sulcus is done in the form of DREZotomy and has been advocated in cases with painful spasticity of limbs and hyperactive bladder besides other indications [17]. Dorsal rootlets carrying nerve fibres to the posterior columns are spared in such procedures and lesioning targets the more ventrolaterally placed fibres. The dorsal roots at the target segments are retracted dorsomedially, the dorsolateral sulcus is exposed and DREZ is entered. A 2 to 3 mm deep cut is performed directed at a 35-degree angle in the cervical cord and a 45-degree angle in the lumbar segments, directing the microblade ventromedially. Low coagulation is then applied. Cuts carried to a greater depth in the dorsal horn are said to have beneficial effects in patients with associated dystonia. Intraoperative ultrasonography may be used to delineate the white-grey junction and guide the procedure. Microsurgical DREZotomy (MDT) has also been practiced with success in cervical levels [18].

All the lesioning mentioned above may also be performed using radiofrequency. All surgeries performed on the spinal cord or proximal portions of the roots require multisegmented exposure of the spinal canal by laminectomy / laminotomy / laminoplasty and durotomy. Contraindications for these approaches form contraindications for this surgery. Sensory disturbances, worsening of dystonic features, weakness, bowel, and bladder disturbances, are all well documented complications of these procedures. The use of intraoperative neuromonitoring and stimulation coupled with EMG helps reduce the complication incidence. Possible future deformities of the spine may be a risk in younger children with such laminectomies [19]. Therefore, lesser invasive approaches like single level / shorter segment laminectomies (exposing the conus region alone), keyhole laminotomies, etc have been increasingly adopted over time [13].

Summary

Spasticity is a difficult to manage condition. It requires a multispecialty approach. Neurosurgeon, orthopaedician, physiotherapist is primarily involved in the management on a long-term basis. Neurologists and other specialties like ophthalmologists, dentists and plastic surgeons are also called often. Surgery is one of the facets of management and it helps the child with a better activity of daily living and makes the caretakers job little easier. Early consultation and dynamic evaluation and optimal surgery at the optimal time is the key to a better outcome post-surgery. The table below (Table 1) simplifies the neurosurgical procedures done for a patient with spasticity [20].

Table 1. Neurosurgical procedure for a patient of spasticity

	Non ablative	**Ablative**
Peripheral	Peripheral nerve blocks temporarily[Bupivacaine]	Peripheral nerve blocks temporarily[phenol, alcohol]]
Central		
Spinal	Intrathecal baclofen Spinal cord stimulation	Drezotomy Myotomy Stereotactic myelotomy
Central	Cerebellar stimulation Cerebral stimulation Thalamic stimulation	Cerebellar dentetectomy Fastigii lesioning Thalamotomy Pulvinotomy

References

[1] Pandyan A D, Gregoric M, Barnes M P, Wood D, Van Wijck F, Burridge J, Hermens H, Johnson GR. Spasticity: clinical perceptions, neurological realities, and meaningful measurement. *Disabil. Rehabil.* 2005 Jan 7-21;27(1-2):2-6.

[2] Lance, J. W. (1980) Pathophysiology of Spasticity and Clinical Experience with Baclofen. In: Lance, J. W., Feldman, R. G., Young, R. R. and Koella, W. P., Eds., *Spasticity: Disordered Motor Control*, Yearbook, Chicago, 185-204.

[3] Nielsen J B, Crone C, Hultborn H. The spinal pathophysiology of spasticity--from a basic science point of view. *Acta Physiol.* (Oxf). 2007 Feb;189(2):171-80.

[4] Martin A, Abogunrin S, Kurth H, Dinet J. Epidemiological, humanistic, and economic burden of illness of lower limb spasticity in adults: a systematic review. *Neuropsychiatr. Dis. Treat.* 2014 Jan 23; 10:111-22.

[5] Palisano R, Rosenbaum P, Walter S, Russell D, Wood E, Galuppi B. Development, and reliability of a system to classify gross motor function in children with cerebral palsy. *Dev. Med. Child Neurol.* 1997 Apr;39(4):214-23.

[6] Mugglestone M A, Eunson P, Murphy M S; Guideline Development Group. Spasticity in children and young people with non-progressive brain disorders: summary of NICE guidance. *BMJ.* 2012 Jul 26;345: e4845.

[7] Sitthinamsuwan B, Nunta-Aree S. Ablative neurosurgery for movement disorders related to cerebral palsy. *J. Neurosurg. Sci.* 2015 Dec;59(4):393-404.

[8] Naro A, Leo A, Russo M, Casella C, Buda A, Crespantini A, Porcari B, Carioti L, Billeri L, Bramanti A, Bramanti P, Calabrò RS. Breakthroughs in the spasticity management: Are non-pharmacological treatments the future? *J. Clin. Neurosci.* 2017 May; 39:16-27.

[9] Barnes M. Botulinum toxin--mechanisms of action and clinical use in spasticity. *J. Rehabil. Med.* 2003 May;(41 Suppl):56-9.

[10] Lazorthes Y, Sol J C, Sallerin B, Verdié J C. The surgical management of spasticity. *Eur. J. Neurol.* 2002 May;9 Suppl 1:35-41; dicussion 53-61.

[11] Smyth M D, Peacock W J. The surgical treatment of spasticity. *Muscle Nerve.* 2000 Feb;23(2):153-63.

[12] Puligopu A K, Purohit A K. Outcome of selective motor fasciculotomy in the treatment of upper limb spasticity. *J. Pediatr. Neurosci.* 2011 Oct;6(Suppl 1): S118-25.

[13] Enslin J M N, Langerak N G, Fieggen A G. The Evolution of Selective Dorsal Rhizotomy for the Management of Spasticity. *Neurotherapeutics.* 2019 Jan;16(1):3-8.

[14] Park T S, Dobbs M B, Cho J. Evidence Supporting Selective Dorsal Rhizotomy for Treatment of Spastic Cerebral Palsy. *Cureus.* 2018 Oct 19;10(10): e3466.

[15] Tedroff K, Hägglund G, Miller F. Long-term effects of selective dorsal rhizotomy in children with cerebral palsy: a systematic review. *Dev. Med. Child Neurol.* 2020 May;62(5):554-562. Epub 2019 Jul 24.

[16] Peacock W J, Staudt L A. Spasticity in cerebral palsy and the selective posterior rhizotomy procedure. *J. Child Neurol.* 1990 Jul;5(3):179-85.

[17] Sindou M. Microsurgical DREZotomy (MDT) for pain, spasticity, and hyperactive bladder: a 20-year experience. *Acta Neurochir.* (Wien). 1995;137(1-2):1-5.

[18] Mertens P, Sindou M. La drezotomie microchirurgicale pour le traitement de la spasticité des membres [Microsurgical drezotomy for spastic limbs]. *Neurochirurgie.* 2003 May;49(2-3 Pt 2):325-38. French.

[19] Abbott R. The selective dorsal rhizotomy technique for spasticity in 2020: a review. *Childs Nerv. Syst.* 2020 Sep;36(9):1895-1905.

[20] Purohit A. K. (1996). Neurosurgery in spasticity. In:, B Ramamurthi, P.N. Tandon, Eds., *Textbook of Neurosurgery*,Vol.2;B.I Churchill Livingstone Pvt. Ltd, New Delhi, 1258 – 1267.

Chapter 14

Bowel and Bladder Dysfunction

Rakesh Mishra[1,*], Bukkambudhi V. Murlimanju[2] and Amit Agrawal[3,†]

[1]Department of Neurosurgery, Institute of Medical Sciences, Banaras Hindu University, Uttar Pradesh, India
[2]Department of Anatomy, Kasturba Medical College, Manipal Academy of Higher Education, Manipal, Karnataka, India
[3]Department of Neurosurgery, All India Institute of Medical Sciences, Madhya Pradesh, India

Abstract

The function of bladder and bowel continence is the first priority in patients with fracture of dorsolumbar spine and subsequent spinal cord injury. Adequate management of bowel and bladder dysfunction in neurological diseases is often the primary goal of neurorehabilitation A knowledge of bowel and bladder dysfunction can be very useful while managing patients with neurodegenerative disorders and neurotrauma. Inadequate treatment of bowel and bladder dysfunction is detrimental to health and interferes with other rehabilitation measures. This chapter aims to sensitize neurologists, neurosurgeons, psychiatrists and other caregivers to patients suffering from neurological diseases and is not meant to deal with the subject exhaustively.

* Corresponding Author's Email: rakeshmishra_afmc@yahoo.co.in.
† Corresponding Author's Email: dramitagrawal@gmail.com.

In: Rehabilitation in Neurotrauma
Editors: VD Sinha, Amit Chakraborty, Jitin Bajaj et al.
ISBN: 978-1-68507-787-7

Introduction

Bowel and bladder dysfunction is common in patients with neurodegenerative disorders and neurotrauma. Its adds to the significant emotional, physical and financial burden on the individual, family, caregivers and society. Adequate management of bowel and bladder dysfunction in neurological diseases is often the primary goal of neurorehabilitation (Anderson, 2004). Inadequate treatment of bowel and bladder dysfunction is detrimental to health and interferes with other rehabilitation measures. In this chapter, we present the pathophysiology of bowel and bladder dysfunction in neurological diseases and provide a comprehensive overview of the rehabilitation aspects in the management. The chapter concludes with recent advances and therapeutic modalities under investigation. This chapter aims to sensitize neurologists, neurosurgeons, psychiatrists and other caregivers to patients suffering from neurological diseases and is not meant to deal with the subject exhaustively. For a detailed understanding of this chapter's sections, readers are suggested to refer to the recommended references.

Physiological Control of the Urinary System

The bowel and bladder are the main components of the excretory system. The urinary tract is divided into the upper urinary tract (UUT), comprising of ureters and kidneys and the lower ureter tract (LUT), comprising of the urinary bladder (including detrusor), bladder neck, urethra and external urethral sphincter. Adequate functioning requires a complex interaction of UUT and LUT and a more complex interaction among different parts of LUT. The bladder and LUT primarily have two functions: one to store urine at low pressure and the other to intermittently, self-determined, more or less complete urine removal from the system. Spinal reflexes from different spinal levels regulate these functions of LUT. These spinal reflexes are under supraspinal control.(Fowler, Griffiths, & de Groat, 2008) Supraspinal control is exerted by many brain areas, including periaqueductal grey matter, pons, thalamus, hypothalamus, insula, cerebellum, frontal subcortical regions, cingulate gyrus and prefrontal cortex.(Fowler et al., 2008) This supraspinal control is essential for voluntary regulation of LUT and is essential for social continence. Many neurological diseases disrupt this complex neural interaction.

Neural Circuitry for Storage Function

The storage function of the bladder occupies 98% of the daytime. For storage function, it is required that the bladder remains relaxed and the external urethral sphincter remains closed. A sympathetic input from lumbar intermediate-lateral grey matter is achieved, which maintains the bladder and neck tone. The sympathetic input has an adrenergic effect via beta receptors on the bladder and alpha receptors on the bladder neck. The tone of the external urethral sphincter is regulated by the somatic input from the Onuf's nucleus located in the frontal horn of the sacral spinal cord. Because of this sustained tone, filling happens. As a result of filling, bladder sensations are carried by pelvic nerves via Aď and C fibres. These fibres enter the dorsal horn of the sacral spinal cord. From here, the afferent signals reach periaqueductal grey matter and pons; however, it does not reach thalamus and consciousness at low intravesical pressures. When intravesical pressures increase further, the afferents reach consciousness, and a desire to void is generated. The region of Pons, Pons-L, lateral to Pons-M or Barrington nucleus, plays a role in storage function. When bladder afferents reach periaqueductal grey matter and pons from the sacral spinal cord's dorsal horn but do not reach consciousness, PONS-L sends excitatory inputs to the lumbar level to maintain the balder tone and continue storage. Barrington nucleus and dorsal horn send excitatory inputs to the Onuf's nucleus, which has somatic input to the external urethral sphincter and maintains its tone. This complex neural arrangement for storage function is as shown in Figure 1.

Neural Circuitry for Voiding Function

When the desire to void, peri-aqueductal grey region activates the pontine micturition centre, pontine micturition centre is located between Pons-L and M and acts as a kind of switch such that at a time only one can be activated. The pontine micturition centre inhibits sympathetic neurons in lumbar levels and activates parasympathetic neurons in the sacral spinal cord, which cause detrusor contraction via the muscarinic receptors. These parasympathetic neurons and inhibitory collaterals from the pontine micturition centre inhibit Onuf's nucleus, resulting in the relaxation of the external urethral sphincter. This maintains detrusor-sphincter dyssynergia and results in voiding. The neural circuitry is shown in Figure 2.

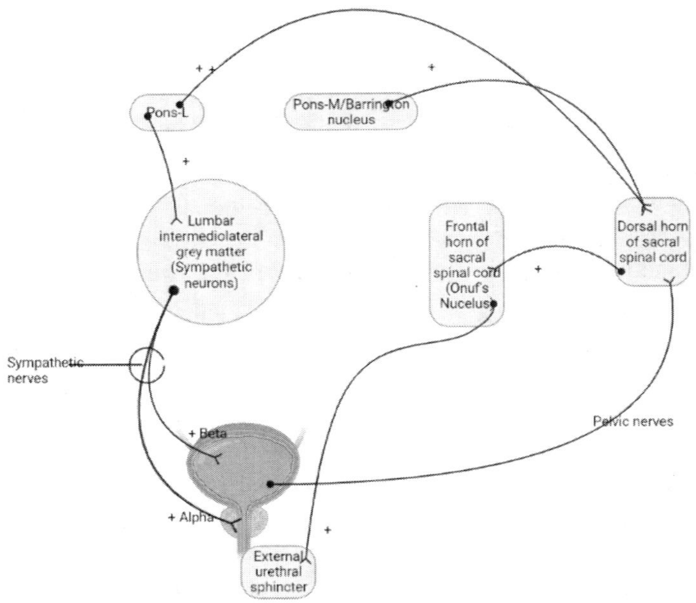

Figure 1. Neural circuitry of storage function of lower urinary tract.

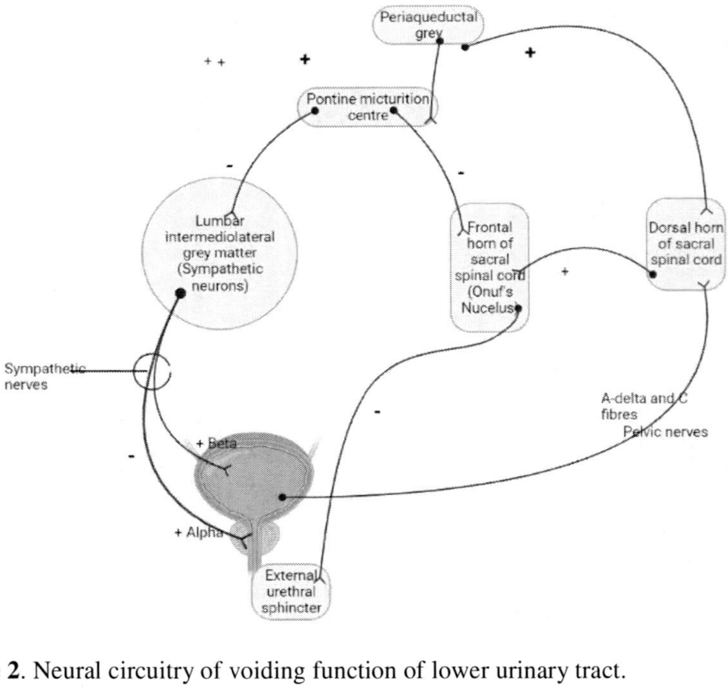

Figure 2. Neural circuitry of voiding function of lower urinary tract.

Epidemiology and Symptoms of Bladder Dysfunction

The prevalence of LUT dysfunction is 91-99% in spinal cord injury patients and 98% in congenital neural tube defects like meningomyelocoele.(Jeong, Cho, & Oh, 2010; Torre, Buffa, Jasonni, & Cama, 2008) When neurological diseases affect the neural networks involved in voiding, it can affect the sensory afferents, motor efferents to detrusor or sphincter function. Accordingly, the symptoms evident are either overacting or underacting of the LUT components. Generally, LUT dysfunction is classified as either dysfunction of storage or that of voiding. Spinal cord injury has provided valuable insights on bladder function, and different types of the bladder are described based on the level of the lesion.

Subsacral Lesions

The sacral micturition centre is in the sacral spinal cord from S2-S3. This centre contains parasympathetic neurons for bladder contraction and motor neurons in Onuf's nucleus for sphincter contraction. Therefore, the connection to the sacral micturition centre is lost in lesions to the subsacral spinal cord or the peripheral nerves (pelvic or pudendal nerves). This loss of connection with the sacral micturition centre results in hypocontractile or non-contractile bladder or sphincter. This neural disconnection translates clinically as incontinence. Some authors also refer to this type of bladder dysfunction as an areflexic bladder. Bladder sensation is reduced.

Suprasacral Spinal Lesions

A suprasacral spinal lesion disrupts the supraspinal control from the pons to the LUT, while spinal reflexes are preserved. This results in an upper motor neuron picture with detrusor overactivity and is termed detrusor hyperreflexia (Abrams et al., 2003). The extent of detrusor overactivity depends on the extent of the lesion. For example, a complete spinal cord injury at the thoracic level will produce a greater degree of detrusor hyperreflexia, while a small frontal subcortical lesion may not have any detrusor overactivity. Under healthy conditions, when an individual micturates, the detrusor contraction while the external urethral sphincter relaxes. This results in the voiding of urine. When there is a lesion in the suprasacral spinal cord, there is detrusor-sphincter dyssynergia. Neurons in the dorsolateral pons are responsible for the synergistic detrusor and external urethral sphincter action, which are lost in these lesions. (Blok, 2002) As a result, there is detrusor hyperreflexia resulting in increased intravesical pressure against the spastic external urethral sphincter. This dyssynergia results in damage to both UUT and LUT.(Karsenty, Reitz, Wefer, Boy, & Schurch, 2005) Autonomic dysreflexia is a typical, and hazardous clinical syndrome see n in spinal cord injury above T5-T6.(Blackmer, 2003) The sympathetic splanchnic nerves to splanchnic blood vessels emanate below T5. Therefore in the lesion above T5, there is disconnection of the central control. As a result, noxious stimuli of bladder dysfunction results in uncontrolled activation of sympathetic splanchnic nerves and uncontrolled hypertension.(Blackmer, 2003) The baroreceptors at the higher level may counter regulate this by decreasing the heart rate, headache, and flushing in the head and neck region.(Blackmer, 2003) Sensation may be impaired or increased with supraspinal lesions. The level of the lesion based on bladder parts involvement is as shown in Table 1.

Table 1. The various types of neurogenic bladder dysfunction

S. No.	Detrusor	External urethral sphincter	Level
1.	Overactive	Normoactive	Suprapontine
2.	Overactive	Overactive	Spinal/suprasacral
3.	Overactive	Underactive	Lumbosacral
4.	Underactive	Overactive	Lumbosacral
5.	Underactive	Normoactive	Lumbosacral
6.	Underactive	Underactive	Subsacral
7.	Normoactive	Overactive	Sphincter only
8.	Normoactive	Underactive	Sphincter only

Pathophysiology of Bowel Dysfunction in Neurological Disorders

The digestive system mainly performs three functions: breaking down food into smaller absorbable molecules, absorption, and excretion of waste products. The intrinsic and extrinsic nervous system mediates neurogenic control of the gastrointestinal system. The intrinsic nervous system comprises the myenteric plexus and submucosal plexus containing 100 million neurons.

The myenteric plexus regulates circular and longitudinal muscles, whereas the submucosal plexus has secretomotor and sensory function and innervates muscularis mucosa and submucosal vessels (Gershon, 1999). External nervous system has sympathetic neurons from T5-L3, which slow gastric motility, and parasympathetic nerves from S2-4 increasing gastric motility. The external anal sphincter innervated by Onuf's nucleus via the pudendal nerve is the only region to have voluntary control. Traditionally neurogenic bowel dysfunction is divided into supra and infraconal lesions depending on sympathetic and parasympathetic involvement.

Principles of management of bowel and bladder dysfunction:

1. *Prevention of damage to UUT*

   Increased intravesical pressure is hazardous and results in detrusor hypertrophy, reflux, calculi, hydronephrosis and increased risk of infection.(McGuire, Woodside, Borden, & Weiss, 1981; Müller, Arbeiter, & Aufricht, 2002; Shingleton & Bodner, 1993; Steinhardt, Goodgold, & Samuels, 1988; van den Berg, Castellote, de Pedro-Cuesta, & Mahillo-Fernandez, 2010) There is minimal evidence which states that intravesical pressure of more than 40 cm of water increases the detrimental effects of vesicoureteral reflex.(McGuire et al., 1981)
2. *Independency in LUT functions to improve self-esteem and social network*

   These include rehabilitation therapies like clean intermittent self-catheterization (CISC), continent catheterize abdominal stoma, sacral anterior root stimulator (SARS), and ileum conduit.
3. *Regular and timely bowel evacuation*
4. *Preventing faecal incontinence*
5. *Improvement in quality of life*

Therapies directed at reducing painful stimuli, achieving continence, achieving independence in managing LUT function and preventing complications and recurrent infection improve quality of life.

Treatment and Rehabilitation of Bladder Dysfunction

All physicians and caregivers should be aware of the treatment modalities and rehabilitation programs for bladder dysfunction. Some valuable, practical points in the management of these patients are:

1. A high index of suspicion in patients suffering from neurological disorders.
2. Rule out non-neurological and treatable causes of LUT dysfunction like prostate hypertrophy.
3. Search for latent neurological disease if the patient presents with LUT without any neurological signs or symptoms.
4. Detailed evaluation to identify the site and level of lesion

If the patient has a peripheral or subsacral lesion and presents with stress urinary incontinence without significant postvoid residue, the diagnosis of an external sphincter is likely. Therapy in these cases constitutes continence products, pelvic floor exercises, behavioural therapy, biofeedback. Surgical therapies constitute the creation of artificial urinary sphincter, bladder neck closure, and bladder neck sling. In contrast, if the patient has significant postvoid residue and stress incontinence following peripheral/subsacral lesion, conservative therapy includes clean intermittent catheterization, intravesical electrotherapy and intravesical bethanechol. Medications used to reduce detrusor overactivity are anti-muscarinic drugs taken orally like oxybutynin, trospium chloride, tolterodine, solifenacin, darifenacin, propiverine, fesoterodine), transdermally (oxybutynin), or intravesically (oxybutynin, propiverine) (Pannek et al., 2009). Other conservative treatment methods include pelvic floor muscle exercises and intravesical electrostimulation. However, these therapies are unlikely to be responsive if there is complete sensory and motor denervation (De Ridder, Vermeulen, Ketelaer, Van Poppel, & Baert, 1999; Decter, Snyder, & Rosvanis, 1992).

Temporary peripheral external neuromodulation affects the peripheral and central nervous sytem by modulating the afferent and efferent nerves in close vicinity of the stimulation site (Blok, Groen, Bosch, Veltman, & Lammertsma, 2006; Kavia, Dasgupta, Critchley, Fowler, & Griffiths, 2010; Mehnert et al., 2008). The exact mechanism is not yet known. However, it is believed that the bladder efferents get blocked at the dorsal horn of the sacral spinal cord due to activation of somatic interneurons with sensations from genitalia, lower limb, perineum and pelvic floor via the pudendal or tibial nerve (Craggs & McFarlane, 1999; Staskin, Peters, MacDiarmid, Shore, & de Groat, 2012). These effects could be similar to the gate theory of pain. Dorsal genital nerve and percutaneous tibial nerve stimulation are currently the most investigated temporary peripheral external neuromodulation. Other interventions and surgical treatment options to address storage function and voiding function are:

1. Botulinum Toxin injection in the detrusor
2. Sacral neuromodulation
3. Sacral deafferentation (with or without sacral anterior root stimulator)
4. Augmentation cystoplasty
5. Cystectomy with urinary diversion
6. Sacral anterior root stimulation
7. Clean self intermittent catheterization
8. Behavioural therapy

Treatment and Rehabilitation of Bowel Dysfunction

Conservative treatment includes patient education, training, and counselling to the patient with caregivers. Stool consistency can be optimized with stool softeners, dietary measures, or laxatives. Incontinence and watery stools can be managed to some extent with anti-diarrheal medications (Ehrenpreis, Chang, & Eichenwald, 2007). When these therapies fail, one can resort to manual stool evacuation or reflex evacuation with suppositories. Anal stimulation with pulsed water irrigation was beneficial in evacuation stool by reflex peristalsis and fragmenting stool (Krassioukov, Eng, Claxton, Sakakibara, & Shum, 2010). Other conservative methods include pelvic floor exercises with biofeedback and continence products such as diapers, pads and anal plugs (Bond et al., 2007). Surgical treatment modalities include perianal injection of bulking agents (for example, dextranomer in stabilized hyaluronic acid) (Maeda, Laurberg, & Norton, 2013), post anal repair involving separating puborectalis from rectum and creating a lattice across the pelvic floor (Mackey et al., 2010), sacral neuromodulation, sacral anterior root stimulator, Malone antegrade continence enema, and artificial anal sphincter.

Conclusion

The function of bladder and bowel continence is the first priority in patients with fracture of dorsolumbar spine and subsequent spinal cord injury. There may be requirement of catheterization to avoid the bladder over distention and bed-wetting, this is a concern to the patients and caregivers (Ward & Hubscher, 2012). Nocturia can be observed in spinal cord injury, which substantially impacts the quality of life. But unfortunately this has been poorly studied (Van Kerrebroeck, 2011). In the animal model research, there was substantial recovery of locomotor function in the mild injury groups, the polyuria was not recovered and it was same as in severe spinal cord injured groups (Ward & Hubscher, 2012). But the residual volume of urine was decreased in the mild injury groups eventually. The patients of nocturnal polyuria can be treated with a synthetic analog of antidiuretic hormone, desmopressin. But this may increase the risk of hyponatremia as the spinal cord injury patients are prone for it (Weiss, Zinner, Klein, & Nørgaard, 2012).

Conflicts of Interest

None.

Disclosure of Funding

None.

References

Abrams, P., Cardozo, L., Fall, M., Griffiths, D., Rosier, P., Ulmsten, U., ... Wein, A. (2003). The standardisation of terminology in lower urinary tract function: report from the standardisation sub-committee of the International Continence Society. *Urology, 61*(1), 37-49. doi:10.1016/s0090-4295(02)02243-4.

Anderson, K. D. (2004). Targeting recovery: priorities of the spinal cord-injured population. *J Neurotrauma, 21*(10), 1371-1383. doi:10.1089/neu.2004.21.1371.

Blackmer, J. (2003). Rehabilitation medicine: 1. Autonomic dysreflexia. *CMAJ, 169*(9), 931-935.

Blok, B. F. (2002). Central pathways controlling micturition and urinary continence. *Urology, 59*(5 Suppl 1), 13-17. doi:10.1016/s0090-4295(01)01633-8.

Blok, B. F., Groen, J., Bosch, J. L., Veltman, D. J., & Lammertsma, A. A. (2006). Different brain effects during chronic and acute sacral neuromodulation in urge incontinent patients with implanted neurostimulators. *BJU Int, 98*(6), 1238-1243. doi:10.1111/j.1464-410X.2006.06521.x.

Bond, C., Youngson, G., MacPherson, I., Garrett, A., Bain, N., Donald, S., & Macfarlane, T. V. (2007). Anal plugs for the management of fecal incontinence in children and adults: a randomized control trial. *J Clin Gastroenterol, 41*(1), 45-53. doi:10.1097/MCG.0b013e31802dcba5.

Craggs, M., & McFarlane, J. (1999). Neuromodulation of the lower urinary tract. *Exp Physiol, 84*(1), 149-160. doi:10.1111/j.1469-445x.1999.tb00080.x.

De Ridder, D., Vermeulen, C., Ketelaer, P., Van Poppel, H., & Baert, L. (1999). Pelvic floor rehabilitation in multiple sclerosis. *Acta Neurol Belg, 99*(1), 61-64.

Decter, R. M., Snyder, P., & Rosvanis, T. K. (1992). Transurethral electrical bladder stimulation: initial results. *J Urol, 148*(2 Pt 2), 651-653; discussion 654. doi:10.1016/s0022-5347(17)36682-x.

Ehrenpreis, E. D., Chang, D., & Eichenwald, E. (2007). Pharmacotherapy for fecal incontinence: a review. *Dis Colon Rectum, 50*(5), 641-649. doi:10.1007/s10350-006-0778-9.

Fowler, C. J., Griffiths, D., & de Groat, W. C. (2008). The neural control of micturition. *Nat Rev Neurosci, 9*(6), 453-466. doi:10.1038/nrn2401.

Gershon, M. D. (1999). The enteric nervous system: a second brain. *Hosp Pract (1995), 34*(7), 31-32, 35-38, 41-32 passim. doi:10.3810/hp.1999.07.153.

Jeong, S. J., Cho, S. Y., & Oh, S. J. (2010). Spinal cord/brain injury and the neurogenic bladder. *Urol Clin North Am, 37*(4), 537-546. doi:10.1016/j.ucl.2010.06.005.

Karsenty, G., Reitz, A., Wefer, B., Boy, S., & Schurch, B. (2005). Understanding detrusor sphincter dyssynergia--significance of chronology. *Urology, 66*(4), 763-768. doi:10.1016/j.urology.2005.04.061.

Kavia, R., Dasgupta, R., Critchley, H., Fowler, C., & Griffiths, D. (2010). A functional magnetic resonance imaging study of the effect of sacral neuromodulation on brain responses in women with Fowler's syndrome. *BJU Int, 105*(3), 366-372. doi:10.1111/j.1464-410X.2009.08819.x.

Krassioukov, A., Eng, J. J., Claxton, G., Sakakibara, B. M., & Shum, S. (2010). Neurogenic bowel management after spinal cord injury: a systematic review of the evidence. *Spinal Cord, 48*(10), 718-733. doi:10.1038/sc.2010.14.

Mackey, P., Mackey, L., Kennedy, M. L., King, D. W., Newstead, G. L., Douglas, P. R., & Lubowski, D. Z. (2010). Postanal repair--do the long-term results justify the procedure? *Colorectal Dis, 12*(4), 367-372. doi:10.1111/j.1463-1318.2009.01800.x.

Maeda, Y., Laurberg, S., & Norton, C. (2013). Perianal injectable bulking agents as treatment for faecal incontinence in adults. *Cochrane Database Syst Rev*(2), CD007959. doi:10.1002/14651858.CD007959.pub3.

McGuire, E. J., Woodside, J. R., Borden, T. A., & Weiss, R. M. (1981). Prognostic value of urodynamic testing in myelodysplastic patients. *J Urol, 126*(2), 205-209. doi:10.1016/s0022-5347(17)54449-3.

Mehnert, U., Boy, S., Svensson, J., Michels, L., Reitz, A., Candia, V., ... Schurch, B. (2008). Brain activation in response to bladder filling and simultaneous stimulation of the dorsal clitoral nerve--an fMRI study in healthy women. *Neuroimage, 41*(3), 682-689. doi:10.1016/j.neuroimage.2008.03.006.

Müller, T., Arbeiter, K., & Aufricht, C. (2002). Renal function in meningomyelocele: risk factors, chronic renal failure, renal replacement therapy and transplantation. *Curr Opin Urol, 12*(6), 479-484. doi:10.1097/00042307-200211000-00006.

Pannek, J., Stöhrer, M., Blok, B., Castro-Diaz, D., Del Popolo, G., Kramer, G., ... Wyndaele, J. (2009). Guidelines on neurogenic lower urinary tract dysfunction. *Eur Assoc Urol, 56*, 81-88.

Shingleton, W. B., & Bodner, D. R. (1993). The development of urologic complications in relationship to bladder pressure in spinal cord injured patients. *J Am Paraplegia Soc, 16*(1), 14-17. doi:10.1080/01952307.1993.11735878.

Staskin, D. R., Peters, K. M., MacDiarmid, S., Shore, N., & de Groat, W. C. (2012). Percutaneous tibial nerve stimulation: a clinically and cost effective addition to the overactive bladder algorithm of care. *Curr Urol Rep, 13*(5), 327-334. doi:10.1007/s11934-012-0274-9.

Steinhardt, G. F., Goodgold, H. M., & Samuels, L. D. (1988). The effect of intravesical pressure on glomerular filtration rate in patients with myelomeningocele. *J Urol, 140*(5 Pt 2), 1293-1295. doi:10.1016/s0022-5347(17)42028-3.

Torre, M., Buffa, P., Jasonni, V., & Cama, A. (2008). Long-term urologic outcome in patients with caudal regression syndrome, compared with meningomyelocele and spinal cord lipoma. *J Pediatr Surg, 43*(3), 530-533. doi:10.1016/j.jpedsurg.2007.10.036.

van den Berg, M. E., Castellote, J. M., de Pedro-Cuesta, J., & Mahillo-Fernandez, I. (2010). Survival after spinal cord injury: a systematic review. *J Neurotrauma, 27*(8), 1517-1528. doi:10.1089/neu.2009.1138.

Van Kerrebroeck, P. (2011). Nocturia: current status and future perspectives. *Curr Opin Obstet Gynecol, 23*(5), 376-385. doi:10.1097/GCO.0b013e32834ac78c.

Ward, P. J., & Hubscher, C. H. (2012). Persistent polyuria in a rat spinal contusion model. *J Neurotrauma, 29*(15), 2490-2498. doi:10.1089/neu.2012.2402.

Weiss, J. P., Zinner, N. R., Klein, B. M., & Nørgaard, J. P. (2012). Desmopressin orally disintegrating tablet effectively reduces nocturia: results of a randomized, double-blind, placebo-controlled trial. *Neurourol Urodyn, 31*(4), 441-447. doi:10.1002/nau.22243.

Chapter 15

Sexual and Reproductive Dysfunction

Rakesh Mishra[1], Bukkambudhi V. Murlimanju[2] and Amit Agrawal[3,*]

[1]Department of Neurosurgery, Institute of Medical Sciences, Banaras Hindu University, Varanasi, Uttar Pradesh, India
[2]Department of Anatomy, Kasturba Medical College, Mangalore, Manipal Academy of Higher Education, Manipal, Karnataka, India
[3]Department of Neurosurgery, All India Institute of Medical Sciences, Bhopal, Madhya Pradesh, India

Abstract

Sexual dysfunction is often ignored in the clinical setting of neurology, neurosurgery, and psychiatry. The caregivers and the patients are not very comfortable discussing sexual problems. Human sexual activity is a complex mechanism that requires interaction with or endocrine and nervous system. Plexus of nerves somatic and autonomic innervate the genitalia. Unlike other mammals, the psychogenic component plays a significant role in human sexual activity. Persons suffering from brain disorders often have sexual dysfunction. Particularly for young men, it can be devastating. With an increase in the incidence of neurotrauma, the prevalence of sexual dysfunction has also increased. There is a requirement of enhanced awareness on options of management available for sexual dysfunction. Such awareness among treating physicians, surgeons, and patients will significantly reduce the emotional burden and stress of sexual dysfunction. As other symptoms of neurological disorders like mood changes, anxiety, and memory issues can impact sexual activity, there are no uniform guidelines for assessing and

* Corresponding Author's Email: dramitagrawal@gmail.com, dramitagrawal@hotmail.com.

In: Rehabilitation in Neurotrauma
Editors: VD Sinha, Amit Chakraborty, Jitin Bajaj et al.
ISBN: 978-1-68507-787-7

managing sexual dysfunction. In this chapter, we present an outline of sexual dysfunction in neurological disorders, physiology, pathogenesis, and management options. We summarize the neurorehabilitation aspects and diagnosis of sexual dysfunction in brain disorders. By no means is the intention to provide an exhaustive list of references to the readers, and for further details, they are suggested for articles on individual neurological disorders.

Keywords: sexual dysfunction, neurorehabilitation, neurological disorders, ejaculatory dysfunction, erectile dysfunction, psychotherapy and counselling

Introduction

The definition of sexual dysfunction is not uniform, with multiple signs and symptoms describing this condition. In everyday language, a patient has sexual dysfunction when he/she cannot engage in satisfactory sexual activity and has issues with desire, arousal, orgasm, or discomfort. Due to issues with the neurological system, nerve pathologies, behavioural or mental disabilities, people with acquired brain disorders frequently develop sexual dysfunction. Sexual performance may be adversely affected further with the hormonal imbalances or drugs used to address other symptoms in these patients.

Physicians treating neurological disorders often ignore sexual dysfunction as part of the illness. It is more devastating, particularly for young and male patients (Calabro, Polimeni, and Bramanti 2014, Anderson 2004). Patient also delays the treatment and often do not open up about their sexual problems due to social taboo. It is often perceived that sexuality is not as important as the illness when a physical or neurological disability patient visits rehabilitation. As a result of the combination of patient hiding and physician not addressing, these problems are kept at bay unaddressed. Sexual dysfunction has a considerable impact on interpersonal relationships, quality of life, social network and self-esteem. Therefore physicians, surgeons and neurorehabilitation service providers should be proactive and aware of the sexual dysfunction in patients with neurological disabilities.

Anatomy of Sexual Function

Sex begins in the brain. Regions of the brain involved in sexual activity are as shown in Figure 1. The limbic and paralimbic regions initiate sexual motivation, whereas parietal areas modulate emotional and motor responses (Rees, Fowler, and Maas 2007). Penis receives innervation from spinal somatic afferents, sympathetic and parasympathetic nerves. Erection and ejaculation occurred as an interaction of the somatic and anatomic stimuli of the penis and mediated by the sympathetic and parasympathetic innervation. Somatic afferents from the penis enter the sacral cord at S2-S4; however, some fibres ascend upwards and synapse with the sympathetic neurons at the thoracic level.

Parasympathetic efferents to the penis cause vasodilation and penile engorgement. Pudendal somatic motor nerves and sympathetic nerves cause propulsion of semen by contraction in the pelvic floor muscles while the bladder neck is closed. This complex interplay of the somatic and autonomic nervous systems is regulated by endocrine, somatic, and psychological changes in physiological states. A pictorial representation of the general outline of neural regulation in the male reproductive system is shown in Figure 2.

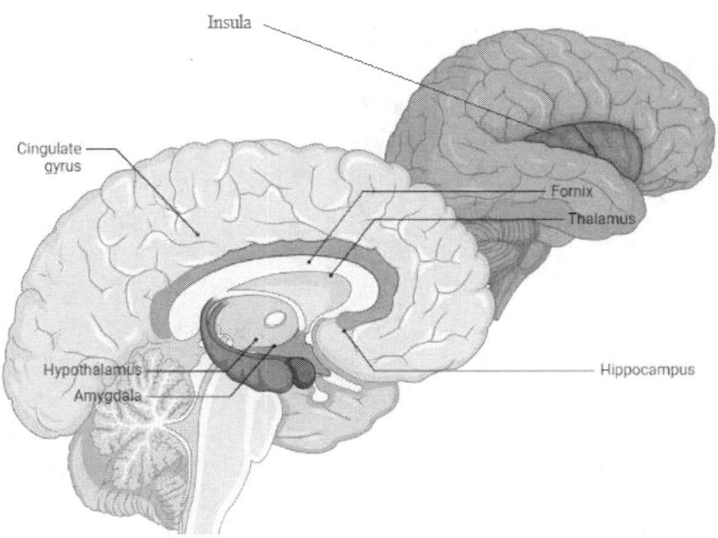

Figure 1. Brain region involved in sexual activity.

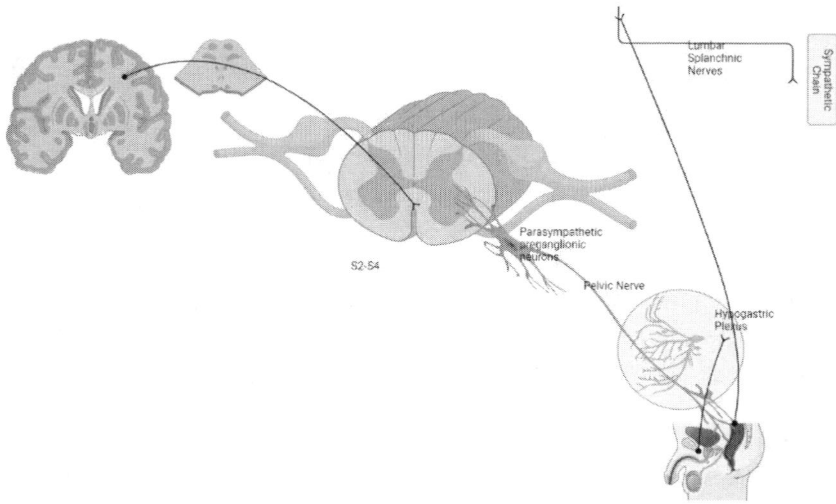

Figure 2. Neural correlates in reproductive function of man.

Sexual Dysfunction in Neurological Disorders

Disruption in the neural connection from the cortex to the sacral cord or the pelvic autonomic nerves results in genital engorgement, erection, ejaculation, or orgasm abnormalities (Rees, Fowler, and Maas 2007). In addition, sensory and motor deficits, cognitive disturbance, personality changes, and bowel and bladder dysfunction affects the ability to embrace and engage in sexual activity (Calabro, Polimeni, and Bramanti 2014). Prevalence of sexual dysfunction varies in studies, population and pathologies. The prevalence of disorders in sexual arousal, desire, erection and ejaculation may be as high as 80% in young men with neurotrauma and individuals with demyelinating and neurodegeneration (Calabro, Polimeni, and Bramanti 2014, Rees, Fowler, and Maas 2007, Calabrò et al. 2011). Erectile dysfunction affects 30% of males after a traumatic brain injury, while orgasm issues affect 40% of men. (Anderson 2004). More than half of the people with a stroke report sexual problems (Boldrini, Basaglia, and Calanca 1991, Korpelainen et al. 1998, Korpelainen, Nieminen, and Myllylä 1999). Medications, reduced functional capacity and quality of life, stress, and dependency further complicate the issue. Spinal cord injury is a preventable disease adding to the social, economic and disability burden. Sexual dysfunction in spinal cord injury varies with the level of the injury and completeness of the injury. Additional motor abnormalities like spasticity and lack of coordination add to the burden. In a high level complete spinal cord injury, there is loss of psychogenic sexual arousal and lubrication, whereas sexual reflexes are preserved. In low level complete spinal cord injury involving cauda equina, there is a complete loss of sexual reflexes, ejaculation and orgasm (Courtois and Charvier 2015).

Sexual dysfunction in neurological disorders can be due to primary, secondary or tertiary effects (Calabrò et al. 2014). Primary effects are the adverse effect of neuropathology on the sexual functional areas of the brain and its connections with the spinal cord. For example, demyelinating plaque lesions of multiple sclerosis in the subcortical frontal white matter, corpus callosum and other areas can directly affect the sexual response and desire (Calabrò et al. 2014). Secondary effects are due to the adverse effects of functional deficits and result in sexual dysfunction indirectly. For example, a patient with spinal cord injury has sexual dysfunction because of limb weakness, spasticity, or bowel/bladder dysfunction, whereas the pathways concerned with sexual arousal and activity are not affected. Tertiary effects are due to social concerns and cognitive dysfunction.

Clinical Evaluation of a Patient with Sexual Dysfunction

The ideal approach in the assessment of a patient with sexual dysfunction should be multidisciplinary, involving neurologists, general physicians, psychologists, psychotherapists, nurses, social workers, and rehabilitation personnel Enquiry about general medical history and history of medical comorbidities like diabetes mellitus and medications is essential in diagnosing sexual dysfunction. The physician should extract maximum information on the problem as the proper understanding of the symptoms will make it easier to diagnose. Specific queries concerning desire, sexual orientation, experiences, abuse, pain, sexual response, orgasm, menstrual cycle (women), libido, or the need to shave facial hair (men) can provide crucial information. A semi-structured clinical interview is the first and mandatory tool for a complete and comprehensive evaluation of sexual dysfunction. The clinical interview should be conducted in the presence and absence of the patient's spouse. These should include but not be restricted to:

1. Nature of the sexual problem in detail.
2. Onset, duration, severity, and frequency of sexual dysfunction symptoms

3. Details on the sexual orientation of individuals, religious beliefs, social and cultural issues
4. Alcohol, smoking, drug abuse, work habits and exercise
5. Details on medical and surgical comorbidity
6. Additional medical details like spasticity and bowel/bladder dysfunction
7. Psychological evaluation with details on past relationships, presence of psychological stressors, mood and anxiety disorders
8. History of previous sexual dysfunction and treatment sought for same
9. Caregivers should try to understand patients and spouses expectations. There is a need for counselling to address the expectations appropriately

This scheme of structured clinical interview provides an initial step of evaluation in patients with sexual dysfunction; however, it should be modified and personalized based on the Patient's characteristics

Standardized Questionnaire for Sexual Dysfunction

Different groups design multiple questionnaires and surveys to evaluate sexual dysfunction. However, the practical and validated instrument is lacking. Available questionnaires include Sasaz's Sexual Health Assessment Framework (Szasz 1989), Sexual Functional Scale of the Minimal Record of Disability (Lottman et al. 1998). These tools provide information on sexual knowledge, sexual activity, sexual response, interest and behaviour (Szasz 1989, Lottman et al. 1998). However, these tools do not categorize the sexual symptoms based on severity and their impact on sexual functioning (Lottman et al. 1998).

Neurological Examination

Physical examination includes assessing communication ability, range of motion, muscle strength and control, sensation, pelvic floor, genitals, and rectum. Neurological examination should include genital sensitive function, search for allodynia, muscle tone, power, reflexes, anal wink, cremasteric and bulbocavernosus reflexes. A decline in facial hair, gynecomastia and testicular atrophy may be indicative of hypoandrogenism. A surgical scar on the abdomen and bruit at the femoral artery may be indicative of neurovascular dysfunction. Autonomic function tests, including heart rate variability and orthostatic hypotension, will provide valuable information. Imaging needs to be done based on neural pathology. For example, an MRI scan of the brain and whole spine is required to identify multiple sclerosis and demyelination lesions. MRI brain may reveal communicating or normal pressure hydrocephalus or other features of neurodegenerative diseases. Electrophysiological evaluation of bulbocavernosus reflex will offer insight into the integrity of the sacral reflex centre or the penile/pudendal nerves. Evoked somatosensory reflex of the pudendal plexus will further enhance the functional status of neural correlates in sexual dysfunction.

Rehabilitation Management

Rehabilitation therapies in the management of sexual dysfunction are multidisciplinary. Essential rehabilitation methods used are:

1. Psychoeducational and counselling intervention
2. Rehabilitation on marital satisfaction and communication
3. Structural cognitive-behavioural psychotherapy
4. Pharmacological approaches
5. Addressing additional medical issues resulting in secondary sexual dysfunction
6. Planning of daily activities
7. Choosing energy-saving techniques or positions which are less strenuous for the sexual activity
8. Therapies to address psychiatric issues of mood disorders and anxiety

Pharmacological Treatment

Drugs used in pharmacological treatment include sildenafil, papaverine and alprostadil (Prostaglandin E1). A double-blind, randomized trial showed significant improvement of erections with sildenafil when compared with placebo (Fowler et al. 2005). More recently, other phosphodiesterase types 5 inhibitors, such as vardenafil and tadalafil with a longer half-life, have been introduced in clinical practice. Injections of vasodilator agents (papaverine and alprostadil) in bulbous cavernosa has also been tried. Discomfort is the most commonly reported side effect. There are automated systems available for drug delivery at the base of the penis in each process more straightforward. Local scar formation, priapism, and penile deformity are the significant adverse effects noticed with vasodilator agents. Stimulatory drugs like amantadine and pemoline have shown potential in reducing sexual dysfunction symptoms. Medications to reduce spasticity are necessary for patients with spinal cord injury and other brain lesions.

Non-Surgical and Surgical Management Options

Non-surgical management options include vacuum devices or pumps in the treatment of erectile dysfunction. Surgical alternatives include inflatable and non-inflatable penile implants. Vibrational stimuli to the glans penis or through the rectal probe are beneficial in patients who could not have sustained erection due to sensory deficits.

Conclusion

The recovery of erectile and sexual function is among the priorities in patients with spinal cord injury (Park et al. 2017). Previous studies focus on the male patients and there is only very little data available about the sexual dysfunction in females (Sipski and Arenas 2006). It was reported that, there will be lower level of testosterone in male patients of spinal cord injury (Barbonetti et al. 2014). Future studies should focus on the blood testosterone levels in the male patients. They can be asked about the lack of interest in the sexual activity and the quality of life (Park et al. 2017). Recent therapeutic advances in managing sexual dysfunction in neurological disorders include transanal electrical stimulation to the pelvic plexus (Kayigil et al. 2007) and percutaneous perineal electrostimulation (Shafik et al. 2008). Virtual reality can speed up the therapeutic psychodynamic process to alleviate premature and delayed ejaculation (Wise ME 2000). Pulsed radiofrequency neuromodulation has been used to treat premature ejaculation by the desensitization of the dorsal penile nerves (Basal et al. 2010).

References

Anderson, K. D. 2004. "Targeting recovery: priorities of the spinal cord-injured population." *J. Neurotrauma* 21 (10):1371-83. doi: 10.1089/neu.2004.21.1371.

Barbonetti, A., M. R. Vassallo, F. Pacca, F. Cavallo, M. Costanzo, G. Felzani, S. Francavilla, and F. Francavilla. 2014. "Correlates of low testosterone in men with chronic spinal cord injury." *Andrology* 2 (5):721-8. doi: 10.1111/j.2047-2927.2014.00235.x.

Basal, S., S. Goktas, A. Ergin, I. Yildirim, A. Atim, L. Tahmaz, and M. Dayanc. 2010. "A novel treatment modality in patients with premature ejaculation resistant to conventional methods: the neuromodulation of dorsal penile nerves by pulsed radiofrequency." *J. Androl.* 31 (2):126-30. doi: 10.2164/jandrol.108.007344.

Boldrini, P., N. Basaglia, and M. C. Calanca. 1991. "Sexual changes in hemiparetic patients." *Arch. Phys. Med. Rehabil.* 72 (3):202-7.

Calabrò, R. S., R. De Luca, V. Conti-Nibali, S. Reitano, A. Leo, and P. Bramanti. 2014. "Sexual dysfunction in male patients with multiple sclerosis: a need for counseling!" *Int. J. Neurosci.* 124 (8):547-57. doi: 10.3109/00207454.2013.865183.

Calabro, R. S., G. Polimeni, and P. Bramanti. 2014. "Recent advances in the treatment of neurogenic erectile dysfunction." *Recent. Pat. CNS Drug Discov.* 9 (1):41-53. doi: 10.2174/2212798406666140131122641.

Calabrò, R. S., G. Polimeni, R. Ciurleo, C. Casella, and P. Bramanti. 2011. "Neurogenic ejaculatory disorders: focus on current and future treatments." *Recent Pat. CNS Drug Discov.* 6 (3):205-21. doi: 10.2174/157488911796958011.

Courtois, F., and K. Charvier. 2015. "Sexual dysfunction in patients with spinal cord lesions." *Handb. Clin. Neurol.* 130:225-45. doi: 10.1016/b978-0-444-63247-0.00013-4.

Fowler, C. J., J. R. Miller, M. K. Sharief, I. F. Hussain, V. J. Stecher, and M. Sweeney. 2005. "A double blind, randomised study of sildenafil citrate for erectile dysfunction in men with multiple sclerosis." *J. Neurol. Neurosurg. Psychiatry* 76 (5):700-5. doi: 10.1136/jnnp.2004.038695.

Kayigil, O., K. Agras, M. Gurdal, E. C. Serefoglu, E. Okulu, and Y. Ucgul. 2007. "Effects of transanal pelvic plexus stimulation on penile erection: clinical implications." *Int. Urol. Nephrol.* 39 (4):1195-201. doi: 10.1007/s11255-007-9205-y.

Korpelainen, J. T., M. L. Kauhanen, H. Kemola, U. Malinen, and V. V. Myllylä. 1998. "Sexual dysfunction in stroke patients." *Acta Neurol. Scand.* 98 (6):400-5. doi: 10.1111/j.1600-0404.1998.tb07321.x.

Korpelainen, J. T., P. Nieminen, and V. V. Myllylä. 1999. "Sexual functioning among stroke patients and their spouses." *Stroke* 30 (4):715-9. doi: 10.1161/01.str.30.4.715.

Lottman, P. E., P. J. Jongen, P. F. Rosier, and E. J. Meuleman. 1998. "Sexual dysfunction in men with multiple sclerosis - a comprehensive pilot-study into etiology." *Int. J. Impot. Res.* 10 (4):233-7. doi: 10.1038/sj.ijir.3900366.

Park, S. E., S. Elliott, V. K. Noonan, N. P. Thorogood, N. Fallah, A. Aludino, and M. F. Dvorak. 2017. "Impact of bladder, bowel and sexual dysfunction on health status of people with thoracolumbar spinal cord injuries living in the community." *J. Spinal Cord. Med.* 40 (5):548-559. doi: 10.1080/10790268.2016.1213554.

Rees, P. M., C. J. Fowler, and C. P. Maas. 2007. "Sexual function in men and women with neurological disorders." *Lancet* 369 (9560):512-25. doi: 10.1016/s0140-6736(07) 60238-4.

Shafik, A., A. A. Shafik, I. A. Shafik, and O. El Sibai. 2008. "Percutaneous perineal electrostimulation induces erection: clinical significance in patients with spinal cord injury and erectile dysfunction." *J. Spinal Cord. Med.* 31 (1):40-3. doi: 10.1080/ 10790268.2008.11753979.

Sipski, M. L., and A. Arenas. 2006. "Female sexual function after spinal cord injury." *Prog. Brain Res.* 152:441-7. doi: 10.1016/s0079-6123(05)52030-2.

Szasz, G. 1989. "Sexuality in persons with severe physical disability: a guide to the physician." *Can Fam. Physician* 35:345-51.

Wise, M. E., Watson, J. P. 2000. "A new treatment for premature ejaculation: a case series for a desensitizing band. *Sexual Relationship Therapy* 15:293-320.

Chapter 16

Stem Cell Application in Neurorehabilitation

Orlin Pavlov[1,*], MD and Kalina Koleva[2], MD, PhD

[1]Department of Neurosurgery, Helios Klinikum Krefeld, Krefeld, Germany
[2]Department of Pharmacology and Toxicology, Medical University of Sofia, Sofia, Bulgaria

Abstract

Many neurological diseases cause irreversible cell death in the spinal cord and brain. Alongside the traditional neurorehabilitation, scientists have been interested in inducing the dormant functional plasticity of nerve cells and cell repair. The application of stem cells in neurorehabilitation has been a topic of significant interest; however, despite promising preclinical results, much work has to be done before establishing strict protocols for neurorehabilitation with stem cells. The complexity of intrinsic factors (neuronal stem cells [NSCs]) and extrinsic factors (the microenvironment of NSCs) and the interactions between them in inducing the differentiation of NSCs lay the foundation for stem cell therapy in neurorehabilitation. Hematopoietic stem cells (HSCs), NSCs, and mesenchymal stem cells (MSCs) have been established as the latest, most commonly used standards for stem cell therapy treatment. There are three ways to apply stem cells: intravenously, intra-arterially and intrathecally. Intravenous application has the significant drawback of first-pass pulmonary sequestration. Intra-arterial application has the drawback of inducing cortical ischemia when applied in the carotid artery. The intrathecal (e.g., the lumbar puncture) application of stem cells lead to maximum loading on the injury site, thus avoiding the drawbacks of the other two methods.

---

* Corresponding Author's Email: orlinpavlov88@gmx.de

In: Rehabilitation in Neurotrauma
Editors: VD Sinha, Amit Chakraborty, Jitin Bajaj et al.
ISBN: 978-1-68507-787-7

The application of stem cell therapy in patients undergoing neurorehabilitation after traumatic brain injury or spinal cord injury (SCI) is gaining momentum. Ongoing clinical trials must reveal the potential for neuroregeneration after the application of stem cells. Neurorehabilitation alone addresses muscle atrophy and the prophylaxis of contractures. When combined with stem cell therapy, a greater neurological improvement in motor and sensory functions could be achieved.

Introduction

Many neurological diseases cause irreversible cell death in the spinal cord and brain. Alongside the traditional neurorehabilitation, scientists have been interested in inducing the dormant functional plasticity of nerve cells and cell repair. The application of stem cells in neurorehabilitation has been a topic of significant interest; however, despite promising preclinical results, much work has to be done before establishing strict protocols for neurorehabilitation with stem cells.

The concept of stem cell application is based on Dr. James Thomson's discovery of human pluripotent embryonic stem cells. The idea of an immature stem cell with self-awareness and the ability to differentiate into other cell types has been an interesting concept for neuroscientists due to its potential to fully repair damaged organs, including nerve cells. The growing number of adult stem cell application reports contradict the generally accepted idea that damage to the brain and spinal nerves tissue is irreversible. The novel works of Park et al. and Yang et al. have shown that adult stem cells, such as neuronal stem cells (NSC), possess the ability to stimulate the generation of three major cell types: new neurons, oligodendrocytes, and astrocytes (D. H. Park 2010, Yang et al. 2013, Kamelska-Sadowska, Wojtkiewicz, and Kowalski 2019). The increased proliferation of NSCs comes from endogenous neural progenitor cells.

Molecular Biology and the Signaling of Neuronal Stem Cells

Neurogenesis, the process of creating new functional neurons, is regulated by dynamic interactions among genomes, epigenetic mechanisms, and extrinsic signals (Shi et al. 2008). The neurogenesis process involves several translation pathways, including Sonic Hedgehog (Shh), Notch, Wnt, and bone morphogenetic proteins, and the activation of transcription factors: Nanog, Oct4, and Sox2 (Chae et al. 2004, Navarro Quiroz et al. 2018a). In this way, pluripotentiality in NSCs is regulated. Of the transcription regulators, the Tlx orphan nuclear receptor is the most important for the maintenance and self-renewal of NSCs in adult brain (Shi et al. 2004). Tlx gene expression is found in postsynaptic neurons and somatosensory neurons. From an anatomical point of view, the Tlx gene is found in regions of the retina, telencephalon, nasal placode, diencephalon, and cortex, showing a strong but dispersed expression in the subgranular zone (SGZ) of the dentate gyrus (GD) and grouped expression in the subventricular zone (SVZ) of the lateral ventricle (Sobhan and Funa 2017, Islam and Zhang 2015). The main function of the Tlx is to keep NSCs in an undifferentiated, self-renewing state. The activation of estrogen receptors by 17-beta estradiol (E2) modulates the proliferation of NSCs by the overexpression of the cyclin-dependent kinase inhibitor p21Cip (Vargas et al. 2016), which thus promotes the proliferation and differentiation of the glial cells of NSCs. Neurogenesis is induced by the interaction of estrogen receptors and insulin-like growth factors because of their synergetic effects. Other transcription factors, such as cAMP response element binding proteins, Pax6, Dlx2, Emx2, and Tbr2, are involved in the proliferation, migration, and differentiation of NSCs.

The Sox protein family belongs to the Sry family of genes and is responsible for maintaining the pool of NSCs in an undifferentiated state. In this family, the Sox 2 gene is responsible for maintaining neural stem cells in neurogenic areas in adults, while the Sox 10 gene maintains the multipotency of stem cells from the neural crest in the peripheral nervous system (Kim et al. 2003).

Neurotransmitters, such as glutamate, dopamine, and GABA, also play a vital role in the process of the proliferation, differentiation, and synaptic integration of adult progenitor cells (Navarro Quiroz et al. 2018b). Multiple electrophysiological and immunohistochemical studies have shown the expression of glutamate receptors in neural progenitor cells in the subventricular adult and SGZ. The activation of these glutamate receptors leads to migration (the olfactory bulb), proliferation, and neurogenesis in the hippocampus. However, GABA released from neuroblasts as the main inhibitory neurotransmitter in the adult brain leads to a reduced rate of proliferation of NSCs. GABA is also responsible for the migration of neuroblasts in the adult SVZ to the olfactory bulb. Dopamine is involved in the ontogenesis and embryonic proliferation of the germinal zone. The application of dopamine agonists increases the proliferation of precursor cells in the adult SVZ and the proliferation of neural precursors in the SGZ (Van Kampen, Hagg, and Robertson 2004, Höglinger et al. 2004).

The complexity of intrinsic (NSCs) and extrinsic (the microenvironment of NSCs) factors and the interactions between them in inducing the differentiation of NSCs lay the foundation for stem cell therapy in neurorehabilitation.

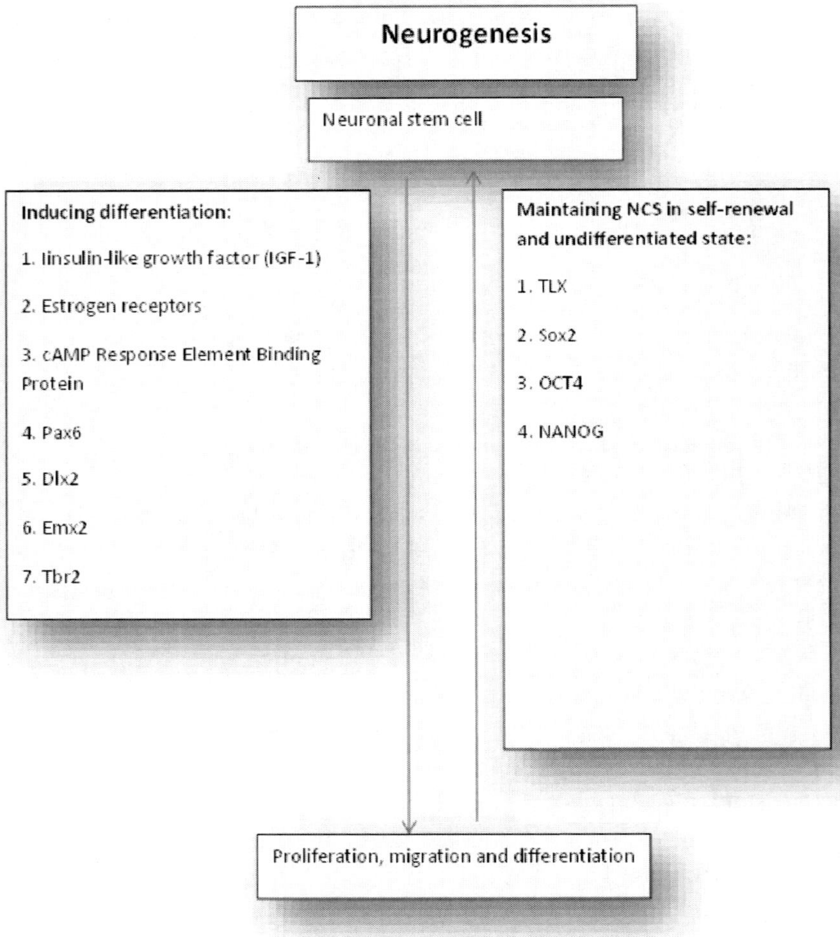

Figure 1. Schematic of neurogenesis.

Stem Cells Used to Promote Neurogenesis and Application Methods

Located deep in the brain parenchyma in the SVZ of the hippocampus, NSCs are unavailable for harvesting and are thus not used for autologous therapeutic application. These cells are harvested from aborted fetuses, disregarding the indication (medical or non-medical), and are prepared for allogeneic transplantation. Due to ethical challenges, the tumorigenic capacity of these cells, and the possibility of the immunological rejection of the transplanted cells, an alternative source of NSCs had to be found. As a result of recent advances in molecular biology, it is now possible to differentiate pluripotent stem cells, including embryonic stem cells and induced pluripotent stem cells, into neural progenitor or NSC-like cells. Nevertheless, it is significant that, until now, no NSC-based therapy has been approved for routine clinical applications. The use of NSCs and NSC-like cells was identified in a review of 27 ongoing clinical trials (Alessandrini et al. 2019b). The majority of these clinical trials are for strokes (5 clinical trials), multiple sclerosis (4 clinical trials) and spinal cord injuries (3 clinical trials).

Hematopoietic Stem Cells

Hematopoietic stem cells (HSCs) are multipotent stem cells used for the treatment of malignant and non-malignant blood diseases and immune system diseases. They are directly harvested from bone marrow, peripheral blood (following the protocol for the stimulation of bone marrow), and umbilical cord blood (Alessandrini et al. 2019b). Depending on the type of disease being treated, HSCs can be harvested from the patient or a donor. Of course, when an allogenic transplantation is necessary, the donor and the patient must have a genetic match to avoid graft versus donor disease or the rejection of the graft. The patient will require lifetime immunosuppressive therapy. In more than 90% of HSC transplantations, a blood or immunological disorder is the indication for therapy. In the last decade, HSCs harvested from umbilical cord blood have been used for neuroregenerative purposes to treat neurological diseases (Dessels, Alessandrini, and Pepper 2018). Currently, 54 clinical trials use HSCs to treat neurological diseases, 40 of which use umbilical cord blood as a source. After umbilical cord blood is harvested, it undergoes a process of separation from mononuclear cells (red blood cells and plasma). The result comprises a high portion of HSCs and, to a lesser extent, mesenchymal stem cells (MSCs), endothelial progenitor cells, and immunosuppressive cells, such as regulatory T-cells and monocyte-derived suppressor cells (Alessandrini et al. 2019a). Due to the paracrine effect after transplantation, these cells 1) promote cell survival, 2) stimulate proliferation and the migration of NSCs, 3) induce the neuroregeneration of damaged brain cells, and 4) promote angiogenesis and reduce inflammation (McDonald et al. 2018). This strategy has mainly been used for the treatment of cerebral palsy and multiple sclerosis. The data on traumatic brain injury (TBI) and spinal cord injury using HSGs remains limited to case reports and case studies. A recent meta-analysis by Novak et al. compared cell therapies used to treat cerebral palsy (olfactory ensheathing cells, NSCs, neural progenitor cells, and allogeneic umbilical cord blood) and found that the use of umbilical cord blood HSGs was superior to the other modalities.

Mesenchymal Stem Cells

MSCs are a unique pool of cells possessing attractive properties for scientists, including the ability to travel to the site of injury, immune privilege, and the possibility of being harvested from many sources, including bone marrow, adipose tissue, and the umbilical cord. The immune privilege of MSCs excludes the necessity for immunosuppressive therapy after transplantation. One of the main disadvantages of MSC therapy is that MSCs harvested from a specific tissue, such as bone marrow (BM-MSCs), are committed to differentiating back to the cells specifically to the harvested tissue. There are numerous indications for preclinical and clinical trials with MSCs, including osteoarthritis, emphysema, bone fractures, and wounds. Only three MSC-derived products have been approved for clinical use in human subjects, while only one, stemirac (autologous bone marrow-derived MSCs), is used for the treatment of spinal cord injuries (Alessandrini et al. 2019a). From the 53 currently registered clinical trials with MSCs for neurological diseases, 27 involve patients with strokes and 26 involve patients with spinal cord injuries.

There are three ways to apply stem cells: intravenously, intra-arterially, and intrathecally. Intravenous application has the significant drawback of first-pass pulmonary sequestration. Intra-arterial application has the drawback of inducing cortical ischemia when applied in the carotid artery. The intrathecal (e.g., the lumbar puncture) application of stem cells leads to maximum loading on the injury site, thus avoiding the drawbacks of the other two methods (Tolar et al. 2006, Walczak et al. 2008).

Outcomes of Neurorehabilitation after Stem Cell Therapy

Currently, there are nine human clinical trials - five completed, two enrolling, and two withdrawn - involving stem cell therapy for TBI. None of these studies have officially published results. The data in the literature is mainly based on preclinical trials, animal models, and clinical trials approved by local ethics committees. Wang et al. (Wang et al. 2013) conducted a study to evaluate the efficacy and safety of UC-MSC transplantation in subjects with TBI. A total of 40 participants were enrolled, 20 of whom underwent stem cell therapy with 2 ml of stem cell suspension containing 1×10^7 SCs via lumbar puncture. The baseline parameters of both groups were matched. The authors concluded that compared to the non-treatment group, there was a statistically significant improvement in sensation, motor, and walking function in the stem cell treatment group six months after beginning the therapy. The patients in the treatment group also showed better mobility, locomotion, and communication and an increased ability to live independently. Four of the patients in the treatment group exhibited mild adverse reactions, such as dizziness and headaches, 48 hours after the initial treatment. Another clinical trial, conducted by C. Tian et al. (Tian et al. 2013) examined the efficacy and safety of autologous BM-MSCs in patients with TBI. A total of 97 patients were enrolled, 24 of whom were in a vegetative state and 73 of whom had severe motor deficits. At least one month after trauma, 100 ml of bone marrow was harvested from each patient. BM-MSCs were administrated intrathecally at a dosage of 1×10^6 cells/ml. At the follow-up, 14 days after the therapy ended, the participants underwent a secondary neurological examination. A total of 38 of the 97 participants showed improvement in their neurological states. The most astonishing results were observed in the group of vegetative state patients: 11 out of 24 of these patients showed improvement in consciousness. A total of 27 of the 73 patients showed improvement in motor function. Age was also a factor in improving outcomes. A younger age, which was not specified in the current study, was associated with greater and quicker improvement after stem cell therapy.

The timing of stem cell therapy is essential. This therapy typically has to be initiated as soon as possible for several reasons. The chemokines released at the injury site could attract stem cells. In acute TBI, the blood-brain barrier is disrupted, which could allow the stem cells to pass through more easily. Advocates for beginning stem cell therapy late apply the theory of a hostile microenvironment following acute TBI and thus recommend waiting a week before initiating it.

Of the 26 registered clinical trials for MSCS therapy in patients with spinal cord injuries, the majority (16) have used MSCs expanded from bone marrow, six from adipose tissue, and only four from umbilical cords. In a recent review of 11 published clinical trials in which the outcomes have already been published, it was found that the application of MSCs is a safe, well-tolerated therapy (Xu and Yang 2019). Patients with spinal cord injuries were treated with MSCs extracted from bone marrow (6) or from umbilical cords (5). The cells were applied intrathecally, intravenously, or in combination in various therapeutic doses. The review indicated that patients treated with MSCs rather than rehabilitation alone showed an improvement in neurological functions (e.g., light touch, pinprick sensation and bladder control) but no improvement in motor function.

Another clinical trial (NCT01909154) aimed to determine the efficacy and feasibility of local autologous BM-MSC transplantation in lesion areas. A total of 12 non-randomized patients aged 18-60 years with SCI (ASIA A) were enrolled. BM-MSC transplantation in the lesion area was carried out in each patient via intrathecal microinjection. Three months after the initial treatment, each patient received a second dose of lumbar subarachnoid transplantation. At the 12-month follow-up, seven of the patients experienced recovery in sensory function, which was also recorded in sensory-evoked potentials. Urodynamic studies also revealed a decrease in detrusor pressure, which correlates with patients' clinical improvement (Silvestro et al. 2020).

Conclusion

The application of stem cell therapy for patients undergoing neurorehabilitation after traumatic brain injury or spinal cord injury is gaining momentum as a treatment. Ongoing clinical trials have revealed the potential for neuroregeneration after the application of stem cells. The preliminary results from clinical trials approved by local ethics committees and many case reports and case series show the safety and feasibility of stem cell therapy. Neurorehabilitation alone addresses muscle atrophy and the prophylaxis of contractures. When combined with stem cell therapy, the aim is neurological improvement of motor and sensory functions. The combination of different treatment modalities is best way to achieve successful neurorehabilitation.

References

Alessandrini, M., O Preynat-Seauve, K. de Bruin, and M. S. Pepper. 2019a. *Stem Cell Therapy for Neurological Disorders*. Vol. 109, 2019.

Alessandrini, M., O. Preynat-Seauve, K. De Bruin, and M. S. Pepper. 2019b. "Stem cell therapy for neurological disorders." *S. Afr. Med. J.* 109 (8b):70-77. doi: 10.7196/SAMJ.2019.v109i8b.14009.

Chae, T. H., S. Kim, K. E. Marz, P. I. Hanson, and C. A. Walsh. 2004. "The hyh mutation uncovers roles for alpha Snap in apical protein localization and control of neural cell fate." *Nat. Genet.* 36 (3):264-70. doi: 10.1038/ ng1302.

D. H. Park, D. J. Eve, P. R. Sanbergetal. 2010. "Increased neuronal proliferation in the dentate gyrus of aged rats following neural stem cell implantation," *Stem Cells and Development*, (vol. 19, no. 2): pp. 175-180.

Dessels, Carla, Marco Alessandrini, and Michael Sean Pepper. 2018. "Factors Influencing the Umbilical Cord Blood Stem Cell Industry: An Evolving Treatment Landscape." *STEM CELLS Translational Medicine* 7 (9):643-650. doi: https://doi.org/10.1002/sctm.17-0244.

Höglinger, G. U., P. Rizk, M. P. Muriel, C. Duyckaerts, W. H. Oertel, I. Caille, and E. C. Hirsch. 2004. "Dopamine depletion impairs precursor cell proliferation in Parkinson disease." *Nat. Neurosci.* 7 (7):726-35. doi: 10. 1038/nn1265.

Islam, M. M., and C. L. Zhang. 2015. "TLX: A master regulator for neural stem cell maintenance and neurogenesis." *Biochim. Biophys. Acta* 1849 (2):210-6. doi: 10.1016/j.bbagrm.2014.06.001.

Kamelska-Sadowska, A. M., J. Wojtkiewicz, and I. M. Kowalski. 2019. "Review of the Current Knowledge on the Role of Stem Cell Transplantation in Neurorehabilitation." *Biomed. Res. Int.* 2019:3290894. doi: 10.1155/2019/3290894.

Kim, J., L. Lo, E. Dormand, and D. J. Anderson. 2003. "SOX10 maintains multipotency and inhibits neuronal differentiation of neural crest stem cells." *Neuron* 38 (1):17-31. doi: 10.1016/s0896-6273(03)00163-6.

McDonald, Courtney A., Michael C. Fahey, Graham Jenkin, and Suzanne L. Miller. 2018. "Umbilical cord blood cells for treatment of cerebral palsy; timing and treatment options." *Pediatric Research* 83 (1):333-344. doi: 10.1038/pr.2017.236.

Navarro Quiroz, E., R. Navarro Quiroz, M. Ahmad, L. Gomez Escorcia, J. L. Villarreal, C. Fernandez Ponce, and G. Aroca Martinez. 2018a. "Cell Signaling in Neuronal Stem Cells." *Cells* 7 (7). doi: 10.3390/cells 7070075.

Navarro Quiroz, Elkin, Roberto Navarro Quiroz, Mostapha Ahmad, Lorena Gomez Escorcia, Jose Luis Villarreal, Cecilia Fernandez Ponce, and Gustavo Aroca Martinez. 2018b. "Cell Signaling in Neuronal Stem Cells." *Cells* 7 (7):75. doi: 10.3390/cells7070075.

Shi, Y., D. Chichung Lie, P. Taupin, K. Nakashima, J. Ray, R. T. Yu, F. H. Gage, and R. M. Evans. 2004. "Expression and function of orphan nuclear receptor TLX in adult neural stem cells." *Nature* 427 (6969):78-83. doi: 10.1038/nature02211.

Shi, Y., G. Sun, C. Zhao, and R. Stewart. 2008. "Neural stem cell self-renewal." *Crit. Rev. Oncol. Hematol.* 65 (1):43-53. doi: 10.1016/j. critrevonc.2007.06.004.

Silvestro, Serena, Placido Bramanti, Oriana Trubiani, and Emanuela Mazzon. 2020. "Stem Cells Therapy for Spinal Cord Injury: An Overview of Clinical Trials." *International Journal of Molecular Sciences* 21 (2):659.

Sobhan, P. K., and K. Funa. 2017. "TLX-Its Emerging Role for Neurogenesis in Health and Disease." *Mol. Neurobiol.* 54 (1):272-280. doi: 10.1007/ s12035-015-9608-1.

Tian, C., X. Wang, X. Wang, L. Wang, X. Wang, S. Wu, and Z. Wan. 2013. "Autologous bone marrow mesenchymal stem cell therapy in the subacute stage of traumatic brain injury by lumbar puncture." *Exp. Clin. Transplant.* 11 (2):176-81. doi: 10.6002/ect.2012.0053.

Tolar, J., J. O'Shaughnessy M, A. Panoskaltsis-Mortari, R. T. McElmurry, S. Bell, M. Riddle, R. S. McIvor, S. R. Yant, M. A. Kay, D. Krause, C. M. Verfaillie, and B. R. Blazar. 2006. "Host factors that impact the biodistribution and persistence of multipotent adult progenitor cells." *Blood* 107 (10):4182-8. doi: 10.1182/blood-2005-08-3289.

Van Kampen, J. M., T. Hagg, and H. A. Robertson. 2004. "Induction of neurogenesis in the adult rat subventricular zone and neostriatum following dopamine D3 receptor stimulation." *Eur. J. Neurosci.* 19 (9):2377-87. doi: 10.1111/j.0953-816X.2004.03342.x.

Vargas, K. G., J. Milic, A. Zaciragic, K. X. Wen, L. Jaspers, J. Nano, K. Dhana, W. M. Bramer, B. Kraja, E. van Beeck, M. A. Ikram, T. Muka, and O. H. Franco. 2016. "The functions of estrogen receptor beta in the female brain: A systematic review." *Maturitas* 93:41-57. doi: 10.1016/j. maturitas.2016.05.014.

Walczak, P., J. Zhang, A. A. Gilad, D. A. Kedziorek, J. Ruiz-Cabello, R. G. Young, M. F. Pittenger, P. C. van Zijl, J. Huang, and J. W. Bulte. 2008. "Dual-modality monitoring of targeted intraarterial delivery of mesenchymal stem cells after transient ischemia." *Stroke* 39 (5):1569-74. doi: 10.1161/strokeaha.107.502047.

Wang, S., H. Cheng, G. Dai, X. Wang, R. Hua, X. Liu, P. Wang, G. Chen, W. Yue, and Y. An. 2013. "Umbilical cord mesenchymal stem cell transplantation significantly improves neurological function in patients with sequelae of traumatic brain injury." *Brain Res.* 1532:76-84. doi: 10. 1016/j.brainres.2013.08.001.

Xu, P., and X. Yang. 2019. "The Efficacy and Safety of Mesenchymal Stem Cell Transplantation for Spinal Cord Injury Patients: A Meta-Analysis and Systematic Review." *Cell Transplant* 28 (1):36-46. doi: 10.1177/ 0963689718808471.

Yang, N., J. B. Zuchero, H. Ahlenius, S. Marro, Y. H. Ng, T. Vierbuchen, J. S. Hawkins, R. Geissler, B. A. Barres, and M. Wernig. 2013. "Generation of oligodendroglial cells by direct lineage conversion." *Nat. Biotechnol.* 31 (5):434-9. doi: 10.1038/nbt.2564.

Chapter 17

Rehabilitation in Peripheral Nerve Injuries Including Brachial Plexus

Jitin Bajaj[1,*], Pawan Agarwal[2], Ambuj Kumar[1], Narayan Swamy[1] and Y. R. Yadav[1]

[1]Department of Neurosurgery, Superspeciality Hospital, NSCB Medical College, Jabalpur, India

[2]Plastic Surgery Unit, Department of Surgery, NSCB Medical College, Jabalpur, India

Abstract

Peripheral nerve and brachial plexus injuries are common debilitating injuries. These require rehabilitation for a good outcome. The rehabilitation programs comprise of reducing pain, maintaining flexibility and muscle mass, muscle strengthening, enhancing functions, improving balance and gait, and preparing the patient for volitional activities. The program involves a multidisciplinary team. This chapter describes various techniques to regain the functions lost after traumatic peripheral and brachial plexus injuries.

Introduction

Peripheral nerve and brachial plexus injuries are some of the most debilitating injuries and lead to the loss of many working years. (Bergmeister et al., 2020) Traumatic lesions are generally focal in comparison to the non-traumatic ones, which are generalized or multifocal. Thus, one can have a directed plan for

---

* Corresponding Author's Email: bajaj.jitin@ gmail.com.

In: Rehabilitation in Neurotrauma
Editors: VD Sinha, Amit Chakraborty, Jitin Bajaj et al.
ISBN: 978-1-68507-787-7

surgical repair and rehabilitation after the traumatic pathology. The average loss of muscle strength after denervation is about 8% per week, reaching about 48% after six weeks. (MacDougall et al., 1980) The sarcoplasmic reticulum reduces significantly at 18 months, and muscles disintegrate at about two years. (Smania et al., 2012) A delay in surgery and rehabilitation program thus may lead to permanent complications.

Rehabilitation is vital in these injuries whether during conservative or postoperative treatment. It aims at reversing the deficit, maintenance of strength and function, prevent the complications like contractures and muscle atrophy, treat symptoms such as pain, improve quality of life, and enhances integration back into society. The rehabilitation team should also set realistic goals for better compliance. The team should be multidisciplinary with a physiotherapist, occupational therapist, dietician, etc., under the medical supervision of a neurosurgeon or plastic surgeon.

The rehabilitation programs for achieving these goals include three phases:

1. Initial phase to reduce pain, maintain flexibility of joints, and prevent muscle atrophy
2. Second phase is to build muscle strength
3. Third phase is functional and includes improving balance and preparing the patient to return to normal activities.

The Initial Phase

A) Pain reduction

It is vital to reduce pain and do sensory desensitization of the patient to increase his compliance. Neuropathic pain responds to tricyclic antidepressants (amitryptyline, nortryptyline), anticonvulsants (gabapentin, pregabalin), and serotonin reuptake inhibitors (duloxetine, venlafaxine) as first-line agents (level A). Tramadol can be considered in refractoriness. Lignocaine 5% patches are another line of pain management in refractoriness. They are effective for the cold allodynia component.(Krumova et al., 2012) Nerve blocks are an effective way to treat pain both during the initial and chronic phases. These are applied under either freehand or ultrasound guidance. Various nerve blocks for peripheral nerves include cervical plexus block and cervical paravertebral block for shoulder and upper neck; and brachial plexus block, elbow block, and wrist block for respective dermatomes. Nerve blocks are, however, short-acting and the duration depends upon the drug utilized.

B) Maintaining the muscle mass and flexibility

This has to be begun with passive muscle exercises. The therapist should initiate and maintain the range of motion (ROM) and flexibility with slow and steady stretch to place the joints in the extreme ROM for 10-30 seconds, and this is repeated 8-10 times every day. Stretching increases the formation of actin and myosin.(Goldspink 1999) Figure 1 and 2 describes the passive ROM for upper limbs.

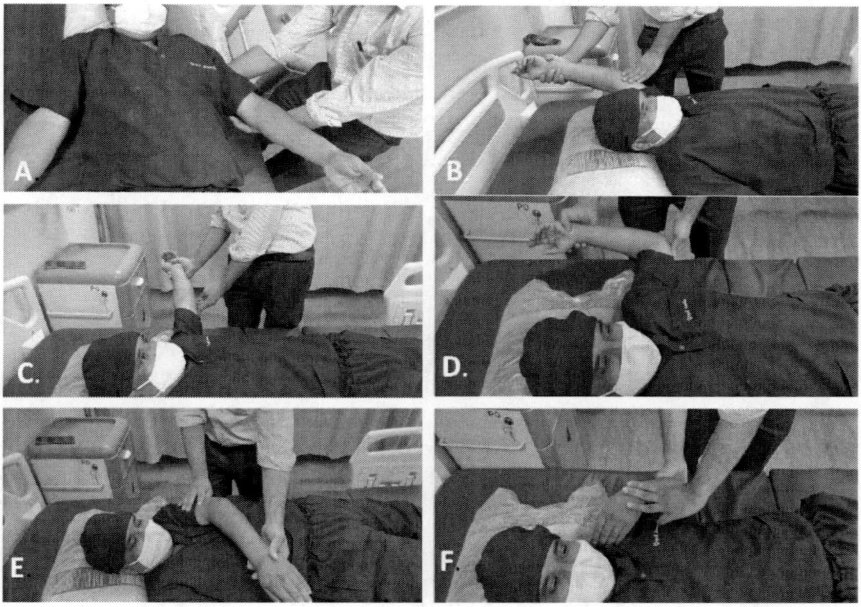

Figure 1. Passive range of motion of the shoulder and elbow. A. Scapular protraction, B. Shoulder flexion, C. Shoulder abduction, D. Shoulder external rotation, E. Shoulder horizontal adduction, F. Elbow flexion.

Firstly, we have to explain to the patient what we are doing, its purpose, and expectations. It is designed to maintain flexibility. The patient can relax and communicate in case of discomfort. Each movement requires three to five repetitions. The ROM for upper limbs begins with scapular movements. The therapist holds the patient's arm by his own elbow, and the patient's scapula by his other hand (Figure 1A). The scapular movements include protraction (Figure 1A), retraction, elevation, and depression. The shoulder movements include flexion (Figure 1B), extension, abduction (Figure 1C), adduction, and circumduction. For abduction, the thumb should point outwards, which requires a little bit of external rotation. For external rotation, the patient's elbow is flexed 90 degrees and guided back (Figure 1D). For internal rotation, the opposite is done. The horizontal adduction (Figure 1E) and abduction are done thereafter. For the elbow joint, the therapist fixes the arm with one hand, and flexes (Figure 1F), and extenses the forearm using his other hand. The flexion is done in the supination position and extension in the pronation. Similarly, supination and pronation are performed at the elbow joint. For the wrist joint, we hold the hand with a finger across the knuckles and perform flexion and extension (Figure 2A), and then radial and ulnar deviation of the wrist. Thereafter, for the fingers, the therapist performs flexion (Figure 2B), extension, and abduction (Figure 2C). The therapist can give special attention to an individual finger in case of its pathology. For the thumb, the therapist holds it and performs abduction (Figure 2D), adduction, flexion (Figure 2E), extension, and opposition. Lastly, the therapist does multi-joint movements by doing flexion of fingers in a flexed wrist and extension of fingers in an extended wrist (Figure 2F).

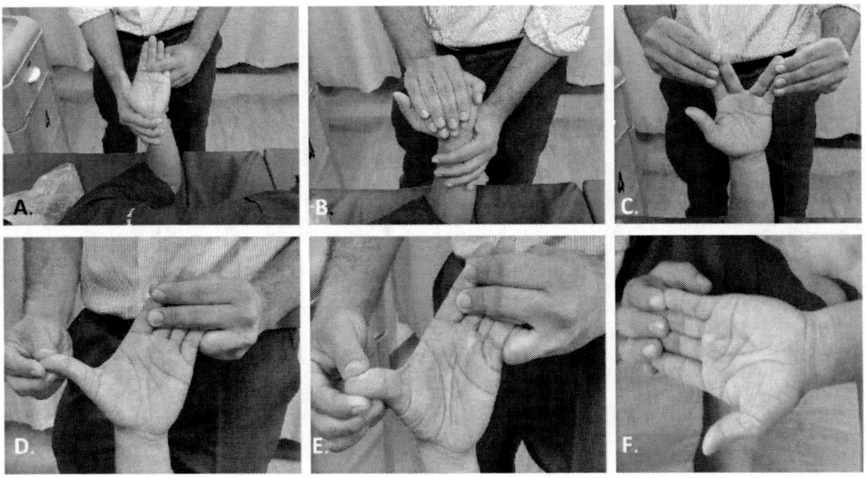

Figure 2. Passive range of motion of the wrist and fingers. A. Wrist extension, B. Finger flexion, C. Finger abduction, D. Thumb abduction, E. Thumb flexion, F. Multi-joint movement with the extension of fingers in an extended wrist.

The ROM for the lower extremity involves movements for the hip, knee, ankle, and toes. The therapist informs the patient and gives instructions to remain relaxed. Appropriate draping is performed to cover both the front and back and protect the patient's privacy. A towel/pillow is kept under the patient's knees. The hip movements include flexion (Figure 3A), extension, abduction (Figure 3B), and adduction. Holding the leg and rotating it in and out will perform the leg's internal and external rotation (Figure 3C). Gentle pressure over the leg in a flexed hip position creates knee flexion. The knee extension happens by extending the hip and bringing the leg in a lying-down position. Thereafter, the towel below the knees is removed. For the multi-joint stretch, the therapist holds the leg in an extended knee position and flexes the patient's hip. For the ankle joint, the therapist holds the leg with one hand and calcaneum with the other and moves the ankle joint in dorsiflexion (Figure 3D) and plantar flexion. The therapist's forearm supports the patient's foot. Giving extra downward pressure over the foot increases the plantar flexion. The therapist then does inversion and eversion as shown in Figures 3E being careful to stay away from the tickle area. He then performs plantar and dorsiflexion of the toes. Lastly, the knee roll is removed and gastrocnemius stretch is performed as shown in Figure 3F. As the condition allows the active movements are encouraged.

C) Neuromuscular electrical stimulation (NMES)

NMES is a proven technique to maintain muscle mass and enhance axonal regeneration.(Ahlborn, Schachner, and Irintchev 2007) It has a favorable effect on neuromuscular junction and prevents muscle atrophy. It involves stimulating a peripheral nerve to enhance the synaptic recruitment of motor units. The stimulation is given either by transcutaneous or by implanted means. The implantable wireless stimulator is a novel technique and has been shown helpful in facilitating recovery in animal models.(MacEwan et al., 2018) Generally, due to the invasive nature, the implanted electrodes are less preferred. The NMES therapy helps improve outcomes in peripheral nerve and brachial plexus injuries. Daily electrical stimulation therapy of muscle or nerve may prevent disuse atrophy and loss of muscle architecture. It also improves central plasticity. This therapy after one week of injury and using high frequency (100 Hz) has a better effect than immediate or low-frequency stimulation.(Su et al., 2018)

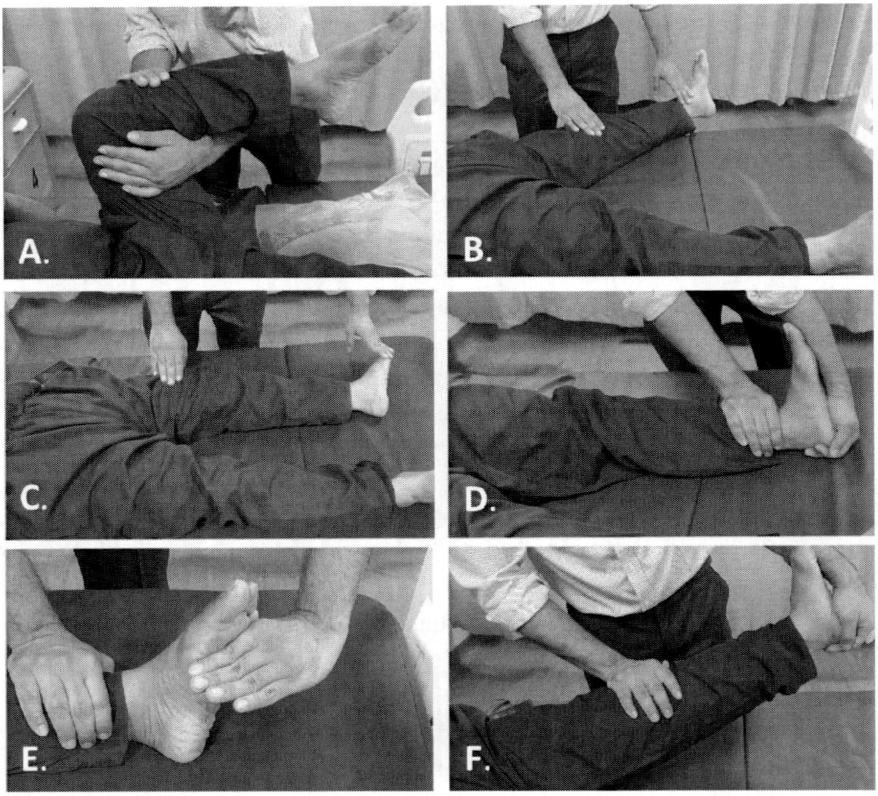

Figure 3. Passive range of motion of the lower limb. A. Hip flexion, B. Hip abduction, C. Hip external rotation, D. Ankle dorsiflexion, E. Ankle inversion, F. Gastrocnemius stretch.

D) Prevention of further injuries and deformities

Patients are told to prevent further injuries by protecting the anesthetized areas. They may wear appropriate hand gloves and footwear to avoid ulcers. Splints aid in preventing overstretching and joint contracture, however, should not provide excessive pressure, and the therapists should regularly examine for erythema and blisters. Good hygiene is also critical to prevent infections. Maintaining ROM prevents joint contractures and deformities. Muscle-strengthening exercises go hand-in-hand in a progressive manner.

Edema may develop in a dependent limb, and slings can help to prevent it. Slings can be applied both during day and night. Constrictive splints and tight casts should be avoided as these may prove detrimental and enhance edema. Intermittent pneumatic compression devices with pressure below the diastolic blood pressure are also helpful. Likewise, contractures have to be prevented. It can be done by a combination of splinting, stretching, and medications. Appropriately applied splints can also prevent overstretching of affected weak muscles, and shortening of normal antagonistic muscles.

Phase II

This phase involves muscle strengthening and reeducating the patient to perform functions. These are done through the following mechanisms.

A) Proprioceptive neuromuscular facilitation (PNF)

It is a method involving different exercises of active and passive relaxation of agonist and antagonist muscles. It improves ROM, flexibility, and neuromuscular function by stimulating the Golgi tendon organs and nerve endings. These exercises should be done 1-5 times twice a week. The stretching of the target muscle should be done slowly to prevent muscle spindle excitation and resistance. It involves the following techniques:

a) *Contract-relax*: The therapist moves the target muscle at the range of motion (Figure 4A). The patient submaximally (20-50%) contracts the affected muscle for 3-10 seconds (Figure 4B) and then relaxes. Thereafter, the therapist elongates it further (Figure 4C) for 5-10 seconds until the perceived stretch sensation diminishes.
b) *Antagonist-contract*: The therapist stretches the affected muscle to the end of range (Figure 4D). The patient contracts the antagonistic muscle for few seconds (Figure 4E). Thereafter, the patient relaxes and the therapist stretches the affected muscle further for 5-10 seconds till the end of range (Figure 4F).
c) *Contract-relax-antagonist-contract*: It is a combination of the earlier two techniques consecutively.

B) Resistance Exercises

The resistance exercises help in muscle strengthening. The exercises increase axonal growth through the neurotrophin-dependent mechanism.(Molteni et al., 2004) These can be of the following types:

a) *Isometric exercises*: This involves constant muscle length against a variable resistance. These are used when joint motion is restricted in the early phase of rehabilitation.
b) *Isotonic exercises*: This involves constant resistance against a variable length. The joints in the isotonic exercises. Three sets of 6-10 repetitions are performed to strengthen the target muscle. As the muscle adapts, additional weights are added.
c) *Isokinetic exercises*: This involves controlling the speed against resistance. The joints are mobile throughout the entire range of motion.

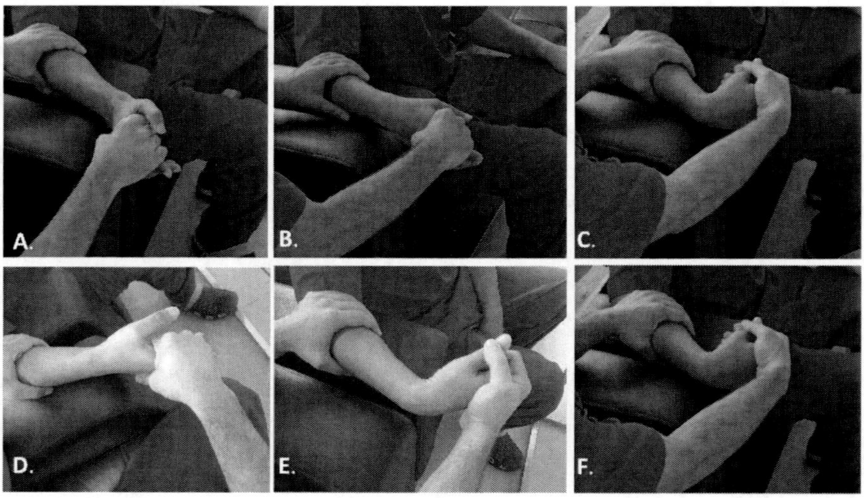

Figure 4. Contract-relax technique for weak wrist extensors (A-C). A. Target muscle at the end of the range of motion, B. Submaximal contraction by the patient, C. Target muscle movement by the therapist at the end of the range. Antagonist-contract technique for weak wrist extensors (D-E). D. The therapist has stretched the affected weak wrist extensor, E. The patient has contracted the antagonistic wrist flexors, F. The therapist has stretched the affected wrist extensors further.

It is critical to put appropriate weights for exercises to get both hypertrophy and hyperplasia of muscle fibers without any additional injury. Excessive weights may even be harmful and cause further weakness. Appropriate resistance is 30% of maximal isometric force for 12 weeks.(Aitkens et al., 1993).

A proven way of maximizing outcomes after nerve transfers has been the donor activation focussed rehabilitation approach.(Kahn and Moore 2016) It entails activating the donor nerve functions to activate and train the receptive muscles. Table 1 shows different splints and exercises for brachial plexus transfers based on this approach. Similar exercises can be made for the lower limb transfers.

Table 1. Showing splints and specific exercises for different brachial plexus nerve injuries and nerve transfers

S. No.	Nerve	Rehabilitation program
1	Suprascapular nerve (after transfer from spinal accessory nerve)	Patient/splint place the arm in partial external rotation and abduction. In the early phase, shoulder shrugging exercises and backward shoulder rolls or pulls. Later, active-assisted shoulder abduction and external rotation with active scapular retraction. Lastly, "wall slides" exercise is introduced.
2	Triceps branch to axillary nerve transfer	Initially, patient performs active extension of the forearm. Later, patient performs shoulder abduction and extension exercises in the prone position.
3	Radial Nerve	Cock-up dynamic splint, wrist joint mobilization, resistance training for wrist flexors and extensors, forearm supinator and pronator.
4	Musculocutaneous nerve (after double fascicular transfer from ulnar and median nerves)	The arm is held at 90 degrees of elbow flexion. Patient places the arm on a surface and performs co-contraction of the elbow and wrist flexor muscles, there by contracting the biceps and brachialis muscles.
5	Musculocutaneous nerve (after transfer from phrenic nerve)	Breathing exercises while doing elbow flexion.
6	Musculocutaneous nerve (after transfer from intercostal nerve)	Patient curls his trunk with forced exhalation and actively flexes his elbow.
7	Ulnar nerve (after transfer from anterior interosseus nerve)	Splint makes the metacarpophalangeal joint in slight flexion to avoid the claw position. Patient performs pinching action in pronation.

Table 1. (Continued)

S. No.	Nerve	Rehabilitation program
8	Median nerve	Splint keeps the thumb in the palmar abduction position and maintains the first space. For strengthening the patient places his hands together and forearms in a horizontal plane, and moves his arms side-to-side.
9	Median nerve (after extensor carpi radialis brevis to pronator teres nerve transfer)	Patient extends his wrist with forearm in pronation.
10	Anterior interosseus nerve (after transfer from flexor digitorum superficialis branch)	Patient wears finger-based splints to block hyperextension of distal interphalangeal joints of the index and thumb, and performs simple gripping exercises.
11	Anterior interosseus nerve (after transfer from brachialis branch of musculocutaneous nerve)	Patient performs elbow flexion in a pronated position. Splint support the wrist and positions and thumb and index finger in distal joint flexion.
12	Distal median to radial (Flexor carpi radialis branch to posterior interosseus nerve or Flexor digitorum superficialis branch to extensor carpi radialis brevis)	The splint is placed to make the wrist, thumb, and the proximal fingers in extension. The patient does finger interphalangeal joint flexion and isometric wrist flexion.
13	Anterior interosseus nerve (pronator quadratus branch) to ulnar motor nerve	Initially, a neutral wrist splint and later an anti-claw splint is helpful. Patient spreads the fingers while resisting pronation. Patient also performs active finger abduction and adduction.

C) Aerobic exercises

These exercises are helpful for both the cardiovascular and skeletal muscle systems. Low-impact moderate exercises are prescribed. Aerobic exercises help in improving psychological well-being also.

D. Splints

Splints help in preventing and treating contractures, and restoring muscle functions. An ideal splint has the properties of being lightweight, able to maintain joints in physiological position, allow for a variety of positions, adjustable, easy to clean and maintain, and inexpensive. A universal arm splint is an excellent option for brachial plexus injuries.(Sadra 1995) The addition of springs and powered devices, known as dynamic splinting, aids the affected muscle and maintains a balance with antagonist muscles thus preventing a contracture and facilitating early prehension.(Chan 2002) Dynamic splinting also helps in an established contracture to stretch out the joints and tendons. During the recovery course, dynamic splints can also replace the lost functions of a muscle. Sup-ER splint is a device, especially for birth-related brachial plexus injuries.(Verchere 2017) It is vital to remove the splints at least twice a day and check for any skin ulcerations.

E. Combined exercise program
A combined program of resistance, aerobic, and balance & gait is helpful for most patients, particularly with lower limb peripheral nerve injuries. The different exercises may be synergistic to each other and are more beneficial than individual treatments.

F. Biofeedback
This modality is helpful for patients who have difficulty in using the reinnervated muscles. The triggered electromyographic signals from the affected and antagonistic muscle are shown to the patient. It enhances motivation.(Sturma et al., 2018) Though proven efficacious for stroke patients, this modality is currently controversial for peripheral nerve injuries.(Duarte-Moreira et al., 2018)

Phase III: Function Enhancement and Return to Normal Activities

This phase is critical for the return of the patient to his routine activities and can be individualized for every patient. The therapist focuses on fine motor skills for the upper limb, and gait & balance for the lower limb.

A) *Fine motor skills*: The patient holds coins (for eg. of carrom board) and performs building towers, collecting them, and passing them. Consistent efforts yield results.
B) *Cross-education*: This involves training of the affected limb through training of the opposite normal limb. Voluntary efforts, electrical stimulation, and mental imagery are helpful for this. Both upper and lower limbs can be benefitted. Cross-education can help in rehabilitation during acute painful stages and immobilization of the

affected limb. Formal recommendations are, however, presently not present for this technique.

C) *Balance and gait*: Lower-limb peripheral nerve injuries may impair balance and gait. For functional mobility and independence, both balance and gait are vital. A therapist-supervised exercise program in combination with equipment like an oscillating powered platform increases the vestibular responsiveness and leads to improvement of balance.(Nardone et al., 2010) Muscle and balance strengthening will lead to improvement of gait. Yoga and other mind-body exercises are also helpful.

D) *Orthoses and ambulatory aids*: Assistive devices including shoe modifications, crutches, ankle-foot appliances, power wheelchairs, etc., optimize residual motor functions. Vibrating insoles improve balance by improving reaction time and improving proprioception.

E) *Functional electrical stimulation*: It is a useful technique. This technology senses the lifting of the paralyzed limb and in turn stimulates to contract the accessory muscles. For instance, stimulating the tibialis anterior muscle during the swing phase of gait can help a case of foot drop. These neuroprosthetics can be used for the upper limb, lower limb, bladder, bowel, and respiratory systems.(Peckham and Knutson 2005) These are however costly.

F) *Motor relearning*: This modality is based on strengthening task-specific functions for a patient. The therapist trains the patient in the specified task, which is then carried over for the daily activities. For the upper limb, activities like opening and closing the lid of bottles, picking and dropping objects, turning the pages, etc., are designed. The training focuses on the required task based on cognitive control. It also eliminates unwanted activity by conscious efforts. If the task is difficult to perform, then the patient may fragment it into varied components. Each exercise is repeated 5-10 times, which along with feedback is helpful. For instance, after a tibialis posterior tendon transfer for foot drop, the focus should be on (after the subsidence of pain and swelling) dorsiflexing the foot and wiggling the toes. The therapist gives appropriate feedback, and progressively, the difficulty is increased to achieve full function.

G) *Sensory reeducation*: The patient needs to be reeducated for sensations. The sensory training is done through the graded application of coarse to fine, blunt to mildly irritative substances, taking visual cues, etc. The recovery happens through cortical plasticity. Memory and attention are also involved in the training. The training begins with the return of the first sensation.(Parry and Salter 1976) The patient in a blindfolded state identifies shapes like rectangles, squares, cylinders, etc. The patient also trains for variable weights and temperature, and compares them from the normal side. Texture identification (leather, rubber, silk, etc.) is also useful. The patient then identifies common daily-life objects with their shape, weight, texture, and temperature. In a case of failure, he may open his eyes and watch the object to retrain his mind. Instruments like Semmes-Weinstein monofilaments can also be used.(Abiodun and Voola 2019) Generally, pain and temperature sensations come first followed by vibration and touch. Localization is also an important modality. The therapist labels the patient's desired area, for instance, different divisions of the volar aspect of hand in a median nerve injury, and trains for localization.(Parry and Salter 1976) In a blindfold state, the patient identifies the stimulation at variable divisions. In a case of failure, he opens his eyes and learns it.

H) *Management of chronic pain*: Pain may occur even several months after the initial injury. It may be neuropathic or as a result of chronic regional pain syndrome (CRPS). Both of these may have a sudden onset and may be dysesthetic. The CRPS also has autonomic symptoms. Similar to acute injury pain, chronic pain is also managed initially with drugs (tricyclic antidepressants, anticonvulsants, opioids, etc.) Transcutaneous electrical nerve stimulation (TENS) is another modality as an adjunct to medications. Based on Melzack and Wall's gate control theory of pain, a low-frequency TENS with intensity just above the motor threshold is helpful to inhibit the descending pain pathways and spinal gating mechanism. It selectively activates non-noxious A-beta afferents to reduce the pain afferents. Its efficacy varies from 20-65%.(Lovaglio et al., 2019) TENS is a non-invasive self-administered technique. It lacks the potential for overdose and is thus free from any major adverse effects. In refractoriness, non-pharmacological treatment like dorsal root entry zone lesions, spinal cord stimulation, or peripheral nerve stimulation may be tried. Elaboration of the surgical options is out of the scope of this chapter.

I) *Psychological management*: Many nerve injury patients develop depression, anxiety, and other psychological disorders. Appropriate management by drugs and behavior therapy is helpful for them.

J) *Bionic arm*: These are specialized artificial limbs designed for amputees. These have special sensors to detect naturally generated electromyogram signals from the remaining muscles of the limb. The signals are collected by a multichannel sensor for a different set of functions, such as fisting, spreading fingers, waving, etc. The signals are decoded through a specialized algorithm, for instance, the support vector machine algorithm, for the user's intention. Using the algorithm, the artificial arm then performs the desired set of actions. The device is 3-D printed for the patient. Activities like crude writing, holding a notebook, working with a computer mouse, holding a ball have been shown using it.(Said et al., 2020) Recently, these devices also allow sensory feedback that further improves the serviceability of the limb.(Abbasi 2020).

Conclusion

Peripheral nerve injuries require multidisciplinary management in rehabilitative care. Neurorehabilitation is required for both conservative and postoperative management. The management plan is individualized for every patient depending on the level and severity of the injury. Early conception, well designed, and the long-term program is the key to regain the lost functions.

References

Abbasi, Jennifer. 2020. "Bionic Arm With Real-Time Sensation." *JAMA* 323 (22): 2239–2239. https://doi.org/10.1001/jama.2020.8836.

Abiodun, Odeyoyin Yusuph, and Shilpa Immanuel Voola. 2019. "Effects of a New Sensory Re-Education Training Tool on Hand Sensibility, Manual Dexterity and Functional Activities of Daily Living in People with Traumatic Brachial Plexus Injury (Pilot Study)." *Health Science Journal* 13 (2). https://www.hsj.gr/abstract/effects-of-a-new-sensory-reeducation-training-tool-on-hand-sensibility-manual-dexterity-and-functional-rnactivities-of-daily-living-in-people-with-traumatic-brachial-plexus-injury-pilot-study-24353.html.

Ahlborn, Peter, Melitta Schachner, and Andrey Irintchev. 2007. "One Hour Electrical Stimulation Accelerates Functional Recovery after Femoral Nerve Repair." *Experimental Neurology* 208 (1): 137–44. https://doi.org/ 10.1016/j.expneurol. 2007.08.005.

Aitkens, S. G., M. A. McCrory, D. D. Kilmer, and E. M. Bernauer. 1993. "Moderate Resistance Exercise Program: Its Effect in Slowly Progressive Neuromuscular Disease." *Archives of Physical Medicine and Rehabilitation* 74 (7): 711–15. https://doi.org/10.1016/0003-9993 (93) 90031-5.

Bergmeister, Konstantin D., Luisa Große-Hartlage, Simeon C. Daeschler, Patrick Rhodius, Arne Böcker, Marius Beyersdorff, Axel Olaf Kern, Ulrich Kneser, and Leila Harhaus. 2020. "Acute and Long-Term Costs of 268 Peripheral Nerve Injuries in the Upper Extremity." *PLOS ONE* 15 (4): e0229530. https://doi.org/10.1371/journal.pone.0229530.

Chan, Rebecca K. Y. 2002. "Splinting for Peripheral Nerve Injury in Upper Limb." *Hand Surgery: An International Journal Devoted to Hand and Upper Limb Surgery and Related Research: Journal of the Asia-Pacific Federation of Societies for Surgery of the Hand* 7 (2): 251–59. https://doi.org/10.1142/s0218810402001229.

Duarte-Moreira, Rafael Jardim, Kamyle Villa-Flor Castro, Cleber Luz-Santos, José Vicente Pereira Martins, Katia Nunes Sá, and Abrahão Fontes Baptista. 2018. "Electromyographic Biofeedback in Motor Function Recovery After Peripheral Nerve Injury: An Integrative Review of the Literature." *Applied Psychophysiology and Biofeedback* 43 (4): 247–57. https://doi.org/10.1007/s10484-018-9403-7.

Goldspink, G. 1999. "Changes in Muscle Mass and Phenotype and the Expression of Autocrine and Systemic Growth Factors by Muscle in Response to Stretch and Overload." *Journal of Anatomy* 194 (Pt 3) (April): 323–34. https://doi.org/10.1046/j.1469-7580.1999.19430323.x.

Kahn, Lorna Canavan, and Amy M. Moore. 2016. "Donor Activation Focused Rehabilitation Approach: Maximizing Outcomes After Nerve Transfers." *Hand Clinics* 32 (2): 263–77. https://doi.org/10.1016/j.hcl.2015.12.014.

Krumova, Elena K., Martina Zeller, Andrea Westermann, and Christoph Maier. 2012. "Lidocaine Patch (5%) Produces a Selective, but Incomplete Block of Aδ and C Fibers." *Pain* 153 (2): 273–80. https://doi.org/ 10.1016/j.pain.2011.08.020.

Lovaglio, Ana Carolina, Mariano Socolovsky, Gilda Di Masi, and Gonzalo Bonilla. 2019. "Treatment of Neuropathic Pain after Peripheral Nerve and Brachial Plexus Traumatic Injury." *Neurology India* 67 (7): 32. https://doi.org/10.4103/0028-3886.250699.

MacDougall, J. D., G. C. Elder, D. G. Sale, J. R. Moroz, and J. R. Sutton. 1980. "Effects of Strength Training and Immobilization on Human Muscle Fibres." *European Journal of Applied Physiology and Occupational Physiology* 43 (1): 25–34. https://doi.org/ 10.1007/ BF00421352.

MacEwan, Matthew R., Paul Gamble, Manu Stephen, and Wilson Z. Ray. 2018. "Therapeutic Electrical Stimulation of Injured Peripheral Nerve Tissue Using Implantable Thin-Film Wireless Nerve Stimulators." *Journal of Neurosurgery* 130 (2): 486–95. https://doi.org/10.3171/ 2017.8.JNS163020.

Molteni, Raffaella, Jun-Qi Zheng, Zhe Ying, Fernando Gómez-Pinilla, and Jeffery L. Twiss. 2004. "Voluntary Exercise Increases Axonal Regeneration from Sensory Neurons." *Proceedings of the National Academy of Sciences of the United States of America* 101 (22): 8473–78. https://doi.org/10.1073/pnas.0401443101.

Nardone, Antonio, Marco Godi, Alessia Artuso, and Marco Schieppati. 2010. "Balance Rehabilitation by Moving Platform and Exercises in Patients With Neuropathy or

Vestibular Deficit." *Archives of Physical Medicine and Rehabilitation* 91 (12): 1869–77. https://doi.org/10.1016/ j.apmr. 2010.09.011.

Parry, C. B., and M. Salter. 1976. "Sensory Re-Education after Median Nerve Lesions." *The Hand* 8 (3): 250–57. https://doi.org/10.1016/0072-968x(76)90010-3.

Peckham, P. Hunter, and Jayme S. Knutson. 2005. "Functional Electrical Stimulation for Neuromuscular Applications." *Annu. Rev. Biomed. Eng.* 7: 327–60.

Sadra, Hardeep. 1995. "Universal Arm Splint for Brachial Plexus Injuries." *Canadian Journal of Occupational Therapy* 62 (4): 216–19. https://doi.org/ 10.1177/000841749506200407.

Said, Sherif, Ilyes Boulkaibet, Murtaza Sheikh, Abdullah S. Karar, Samer Alkork, and Amine Nait-ali. 2020. "Machine-Learning-Based Muscle Control of a 3D-Printed Bionic Arm." *Sensors* 20 (11): 3144. https://doi.org/10.3390/s20113144.

Smania, N., G. Berto, E. La Marchina, C. Melotti, A. Midiri, L. Roncari, A. Zenorini, et al., 2012. "Rehabilitation of Brachial Plexus Injuries in Adults and Children." *European Journal of Physical and Rehabilitation Medicine* 48 (3): 483–506.

Sturma, Agnes, Laura A. Hruby, Cosima Prahm, Johannes A. Mayer, and Oskar C. Aszmann. 2018. "Rehabilitation of Upper Extremity Nerve Injuries Using Surface EMG Biofeedback: Protocols for Clinical Application." *Frontiers in Neuroscience* 12: 906. https://doi.org/10. 3389/fnins.2018.00906.

Su, Hong-Lin, Chien-Yi Chiang, Zong-Han Lu, Fu-Chou Cheng, Chun-Jung Chen, Meei-Ling Sheu, Jason Sheehan, and Hung-Chuan Pan. 2018. "Late Administration of High-Frequency Electrical Stimulation Increases Nerve Regeneration without Aggravating Neuropathic Pain in a Nerve Crush Injury." *BMC Neuroscience* 19 (1): 37. https://doi.org/10.1186/s12868-018-0437-9.

Verchere, Cynthia. 2017. "Sup-ER Splinting: Does Early Passive Positioning in Supination and External Rotation in Children With Birth Related Brachial Plexus Injury Have Benefit?" *Clinical trial registration NCT01663428.* clinicaltrials.gov. https://clinicaltrials.gov/ct2/show/ NCT01663428.

Chapter 18

Neurorehabilitation: Orthoses and Neurostimulation

Orlin Pavlov[1,*], MD and Kalina Koleva[2], MD, PhD

[1]Department of Neurosurgery, Klinikum Fulda, University Medicine Marburg, Germany
[2]Department of Pharmacology and Toxicology, Medical University of Sofia, Sofia, Bulgaria

Abstract

The application of orthoses for neurorehabilitation has experienced tremendous development in the past years, evolving from simple ankle–foot orthoses (AFOs) and knee–ankle–foot orthoses (KAFOs) to a brain–computer interface coupled with robotic limbs. Several national societies for the treatment of strokes and other neurological diseases recommend the application of classical orthotic devices (AFO, KAFO, and hip–knee–ankle–foot orthosis). Emerging technologies have also influenced orthoses. In the group of the modern orthoses, the upper and lower robotic exoskeletons, biosignal-based interfaces for robotic tool control (EMG-based and EEG-based interfaces), have limited clinical usage due to their respective costs. Moreover, some exoskeletons (lower limbs) are too large; therefore, these exoskeletons must be installed in neurorehabilitation facilities. Apart from orthoses, neurostimulation and neuromodulation can also be used to induce recovery in sensory or motor functions, induce reduction in joint stiffness, and improve memory dysfunctions. Neurostimulation is a branch of neuromodulation that employs electromagnetic currents. Neurostimulation is divided into non-invasive and invasive stimulation. Microelectrodes (invasive stimulation) and transcranial magnetic stimulation (non-invasive

* Corresponding Author's Email: orlinpavlov88@gmx.de

In: Rehabilitation in Neurotrauma
Editors: VD Sinha, Amit Chakraborty, Jitin Bajaj et al.
ISBN: 978-1-68507-787-7

stimulation), are used to modulate nervous system responses. Neurostimulation is essential to the development of neural, hearing, artificial vision, and limbs prosthetics. Transcranial magnetic stimulation has been widely used to improve the level of paralysis in stroke patients. Orthosis, in contrast, uses the patient's capabilities, extends their range of motion, and improves the precision of motion and quality of life. Both orthoses and neurostimulation help with the complex management of patients undergoing neurorehabilitation. Only a team of experienced physicians can manage the diversity and complexity of patients requiring neurorehabilitation.

Introduction

The application of orthoses for neurorehabilitation has experienced tremendous development in the past years, evolving from simple ankle–foot orthoses (AFOs) and knee–ankle–foot orthoses (KAFOs) to a brain–computer interface coupled with robotic limbs. Orthoses play a vital role in neurorehabilitation, as they allow for faster, easier rehabilitation by facilitating standing and walking at an early stage of neurorehabilitation (Young and Moss 2019). For didactic purposes, orthoses will be divided into two groups: classical orthotic devices and high-tech orthoses.

Classical Orthotic Devices

AFOs and KAFOs are considered classical orthoses and are used in neurorehabilitation for many neurological diseases, including spinal cord injuries, multiple sclerosis, and strokes. Many neurological and neuromuscular diseases require AFOs and KFAOs at some stage. One of the factors for stable gait is knee stability. The knee instability may occur in all three anatomical planes: sagittal, coronal, and transverse (McDaid et al. 2017). Orthoses aim to stabilize, protect, and improve the function of an affected limb (Hebert 2006). AFOs provide direct control of the foot and ankle and achieve indirect control of the knee and hip joints. The simplicity of these devices explains their market availability. A recent meta-analysis of AFOs has shown that in post-stroke hemiplegic patients, AFOs led to the improvement of gait patterns and walking ability (Kim et al. 2013). The current guidelines for stroke management of several national societies, including the Heart and Stroke Foundation, the Royal College of Physicians, and the National Stroke

Foundation, recommend AFOs for individuals with foot drop to improve the everyday activities.

However, a KAFO is necessary when knee instability persists in more than one anatomical plane. The range of materials used for constructing KAFOs typically includes plastic and metal components: polypropylene for calf and thigh shells and shoe inserts, aluminum, magnesium, titanium, steel for uprights, and steel for joints (Edelstein and Bruckner 2002, McDaid et al. 2017). KAFOs can be further classified according to the type of locking mechanism into simple locked KAFOs, polycentric knee joints, and stance control knee joints, the latest of which have a microprocessor or mechanical controlled knee joint that unlocks during the swing phase of walking and locks during the stance phase, thus making walking more natural.

Hip–knee–ankle–foot orthosis (HKAFO) systems, including hip guidance orthosis (ParaWalker) and reciprocal gait orthosis systems, have been developed for individuals with higher spinal cord dysfunction. Both systems use lateral weight shift from one limb to the other as the basis for orthotic-assisted reciprocal gait (Campbell 2006). Advanced reciprocating gait orthosis and isocentric reciprocating gait orthosis are further modifications of the reciprocal gait orthosis system, with improved designs in which changing the position from sitting to standing up and vice versa is more natural. Several studies have been conducted comparing hip guidance orthosis and reciprocal gait orthosis systems, which have shown that the differences among all the contemporary orthotic options are small in terms of general gait parameters (Campbell 2006).

High-Tech Orthoses

Emerging technologies have left their footprints in orthoses as well. In the group of high-tech orthoses, the upper and lower robotic exoskeletons and the biosignal-based interface for robotic tool control (EMG-based interfaces and EEG-based interfaces) will be reviewed.

Robotic aided therapy has been shown to be more effective than conventional methods for neurorehabilitation because it provides high-intensity exercise and better movement controllability and measurement reliability (Frisoli et al. 2016). Several studies have shown the effectiveness of robot-aided therapy for the upper extremities. Upper limb exoskeletons lead to improvements in motor–task performance (Lo et al. 2010). Lower limb exoskeletons offer patients freedom from wheelchairs. As a drawback of lower limb exoskeletons, it has to be mentioned that they are heavy, expensive, and immobile, thus making them difficult to use on a daily basis. The main role of these systems is to support the patient's weight and create anatomical gait patterns (Frisoli et al. 2016). Nevertheless, they allow for more intensive locomotor training, provide objective feedback, and monitor functional improvements over time. (R. (2016))

Biosignal-based interfaces for robotic tool control systems recognize the user's intentions and provide assistance. The two main methods used in the biosignal-based interface are EEG and EMG. An EMG-based interface involves the placement of a surface EMG on the muscles undergoing neurorehabilitation. The robot observes the ongoing motion and, in triggered assistance mode, detects when the movement is incomplete and activates to complete the task. The surface EMG-controlled robot provides assistance based on the level of muscle activation. In an EEG-based interface, brain signals trigger the external devices without the movement of the extremities (Frisoli et al. 2016). There are two types of brain–computer interfaces: assistive and restorative. Assistive brain–computer interface systems help perform the activities of daily life by stimulating paralyzed muscles. In contrast, the restorative brain–computer interface system induces use-dependent neuroplasticity, which is important to neurorehabilitation. A brain–computer interface coupled with robotic hand orthosis is used to treat stroke patients with upper limb paralysis. Negrette et al. demonstrated the superiority of this method over conventional neurorehabilitation techniques (Cantillo-Negrete et al. 2021).

Neurostimulation and Neuromodulation

Neurostimulation is a branch of neuromodulation that uses electromagnetic currents. It is an essential part of neural, hearing, limbs prosthetics and artificial vision. Neurostimulation can be divided into non-invasive stimulation and invasive stimulation. In neurostimulation, microelectrodes (invasive stimulation) or non-invasive stimulation (e.g., transcranial magnetic stimulation [TMS] and transcranial electric stimulation, such as transcranial direct current stimulation and transcranial alternating current stimulation) modulate the nervous system's responses. TMS has also been widely used for stroke patients to improve their levels of paralysis.

Transcranial Magnetic Stimulation

Repetitive transcranial magnetic stimulation is used in stroke patients for prognostic, diagnostic, research, and therapeutic purposes. TMS generates subthreshold or suprathreshold currents in real life. The primary site of stimulation is the primary motor cortex. From here the impulses produce a motor response on the contralateral side, which with the help of electromyography electrodes is recorded. TMS modulates the excitability of the stimulated cortex, with its effects lasting longer than the stimulation period. The precise mechanisms by which TMS modulates the brain's action potential are complex, but they can be summarized as long-term potentiation and depression (Hoogendam, Ramakers, and Di Lazzaro 2010). The treatment of stroke patients with TMS is based on the suppression of "maladaptive plasticity" and the enhancement of adaptive plasticity (Takeuchi and Izumi 2012, Jang 2013). The International Federation of Clinical Neurophysiology recommend low-frequency TMS of the contralateral motor cortex, which is not affected by a stroke, and high-frequency TMS of the ipsilateral motor cortex. The positive effects of TMS are based on modifying local cortical excitability and improving and/or modulating the connectivity of the neuronal network (Lefaucheur et al. 2014). TMS has also been used to assess white matter tracts' connectivity via a TMS-evoked response. This response changes when the patient emerges from a vegetative to a minimally conscious state (Rosanova et al. 2012), which plays a crucial role in assessing prognosis after a traumatic brain injury (TBI).

Deep Brain Stimulation

Deep brain stimulation (DBS) has been proposed as a surgical treatment for multiple movement disorders, depression, obsessive–compulsive disorder, Tourette's syndrome, chronic pain, and hyperthermia (Koleva et al. 2020). The precise incidence of Parkinsonism after a TBI remains unknown, although it has been reported in the literature that patients with moderate–to–severe head injuries develop Parkinsonism more often than patients with mild TBIs (Abu Talh et al. 2017). Given the proven efficacy of DBS in patients with Parkinson's disease, increasing attention has been paid to patients with post-TBI Parkinsonism. This attentiveness led to one of the first case reports in the literature by Issar et al. of DBS being used to treat Parkinsonism after a TBI. The authors concluded that unilateral or bilateral stimulation of the ventral intermediate nucleus and bilateral stimulation of the globus pallidus internus are safe, effective treatment options for patients with intractable post-traumatic tremor (Issar et al. 2013).

DBS has also been used to treat consciousness disorders. Tsubokawa et al. were the first to report a case series of patients in vegetative state in which a DBS of mesencephalic reticular formation or nonspecific thalamus was performed (Tsubokawa et al. 1990). In their study, four out of eight patients emerged from vegetative states to follow commands. Other possible applications of DBS in post-TBI patients include modulation of cognitive performance and memory. For the anatomical sites for DBS for specific disorders, see Table 1.

Table 1. Post-TBI disorders treated with DBS

Disorder	**Anatomical sites for DBS**
Post-TBI tremor/Parkinsonism	Ventral intermediate nucleus and globus pallidus internus
Disorders of Consciousness (Vegetative State)	Mesencephalic reticular formation or nonspecific thalamus
Disorders of Cognition	Nucleus accumbens and anterior limb of internal capsule
Major depressive disorder	Subgenual cingulate gyrus, habenula, medial forebrain bundle, inferior thalamic peduncle, and ventral capsule/ventral striatum

Intrathecal Baclofen Administration

Neuromodulation (intrathecal baclofen administration, spinal cord stimulation, and peripheral nerve stimulation) is another important part of the complex plan for neurorehabilitation. Spasticity is yet another debilitating complication caused by a number of neurological disorders. The implantation of intrathecal baclofen pumps improves the quality of life of patients with spasticity on the Ashworth scale (Santin-Amo et al. 2019). While baclofen was introduced for the treatment of epilepsy in 1960, it was not until 1971 that it was used for the treatment of muscle spasticity. Since then, baclofen has been an FDA-approved medicament for managing spastic sequel in flexor muscle groups, clonus, and concomitant pain. The indications for the intrathecal application of baclofen are intolerable adverse effects or a failure to respond to oral therapy. Baclofen (beta-[4-chlorophenyl]-GABA) is an agonist of the beta subunit of gamma-aminobutyric acid of mono and polysynaptic neurons at the spinal cord level and brain (Albright 1996, Ghanavatian S 2021 Jan-.). The intrathecal application of baclofen begins with a screening phase. After the lumbar catheter is inserted, the patient receives a single dose of 50 mcg and is admitted to an intermediate-care unit. Monitoring after the application of intrathecal baclofen is mandatory due to its possible severe adverse effects, including sedation, confusion, and extreme muscle weakness. Neuropsychiatric disorders, including hallucinations, have also been reported.

If the screening dose results in a positive response, the patient receives an intrathecal catheter and an implantable pump. Dose adjustments can be made on a daily basis: a 10%–30% dose increase for spasticity of spinal origin and a 5%–15% dose increase for spasticity of cerebral origin (Ghanavatian S 2021 Jan-.). A dose adjustment is necessary to achieve the best possible effects using a minimal dose. Spasticity of cerebral origin usually requires a daily dose of between 90 and 703 mcg to overcome spasticity, while spasticity of spinal origin requires a slightly higher daily dose of between 300 and 800 mcg. In the author's experience, patients can even tolerate doses between 1,500 are 2,000 mcg without any adverse effects. In general practice, acute withdrawal from baclofen represents a serious caregiver problem. The most common problem, in the author's opinion, remains the pump system. Despite technological advances, pump delivery problems are common. Patients with baclofen pumps presenting with acute hallucinations or seizures must be screened for intrathecal pump insufficiency after another cause has been ruled out. There are no strict guidelines for screening for baclofen withdrawal, but in the author's experience, the following protocol has proven effective:

1. Admitting the patient to an intensive care or intermediate-care unit
2. Ruling out another possible cause for the two most common baclofen withdrawal problems: hallucinations and seizures
3. Reading the pump to search for failures
4. Taking X-rays of the pump to rule out disconnection
5. Applying 50 mcg to 100 mcg of intrathecal baclofen to reverse or improve the symptoms of withdrawal every four to six hours (most pumps have a secondary port in which the direct application of intrathecal baclofen is possible). If this dosage is ineffective, increasing it to as much as 200 mcg could be necessary, depending on the severity of the symptoms.

The acute withdrawal symptoms from intrathecal baclofen application include acute rhabdomyolysis and multi-organ system failure, severe spasticity, a hypermetabolic state with hyperpyrexia, and impaired mental status (Ghanavatian S 2021 Jan-.). This colorful clinical presentation is potentially dangerous; sometimes, even experienced physicians may have difficulty managing it.

Spinal Cord Stimulation

Since Wall and Melzack introduced the gate control theory in 1965, spinal cord stimulation (SCS) has undergone significant development. Ever since, the indications for SCS have expanded to include failed back surgery syndrome, neuropathic pain, and the reduction of opioid administration doses. According to this theory, pain control can be achieved by selectively activating large, rapidly conducting fibers (Melzack and Wall 1965).

The evolution of SCS has led to the development of several new devices and modalities for stimulation, including high-frequency technology, dorsal root ganglion stimulation, and burst stimulation (Sdrulla, Guan, and Raja 2018). SCS's precise action mechanism is based on electrical current between two epidurally placed electrodes. The generated field leads to alternation in electrical potential across membranes, depending on whether the surrounding tissue contains liquor, epidural fat, or white matter. Due to the midline position of the electrodes above the dorsal columns, the activation of the electrodes leads to the activation of the axons, which results in the orthodromic and antidromic transmission of action potentials, which, in turn, generate segmental and supraspinal effects (Sdrulla, Guan, and Raja 2018, Smits et al. 2013, Miller et al. 2016). Large axons are preferably activated due to their lower action potential threshold than smaller axons. From an anatomical perspective, the SCS preferably activates large A-beta dorsal column axons. This activation can be measured by the antidromical propagation of the action potential of the peripheral nerves as epidural action potential (Machida et al. 1985, Rudin and Eisenman 1954), as somatosensory evoked potentials, and as muscle twitches in the limbs (Halter et al. 1983, Dimitrijevic et al. 1980). The patient experiences these impulses as paresthesias. The stimulation of touch and vibration nerves "closes the gate" for ascending pain stimuli (Shealy, Mortimer, and Reswick 1967). This process can occur in simple, everyday settings. After a minor trauma, individuals unconsciously rub the trauma site to "cool down" the pain impulses.

The response to SCS therapy is divided into patient-related and indication-related factors. The most important patient-related factors are anxiety, depression, poor coping skills, somatization, general condition, and the patient's active participation in treatment (Garcia K 2021 Jan-). The ultima of neurosurgery, "The lesser the indication, the greater the complication," also applies to SCS. Careful patient selection must be undertaken prior to surgical intervention. Currently, there is Level A evidence of the efficacy of SCS for failed back surgery syndrome, peripheral ischemia, peripheral neuropathy, and angina pectoris (Kumar et al. 1998). A study by North et al. included 27 patients with failed back surgery syndrome. They were divided into two groups: those who underwent a repeat laminectomy and those who underwent SCS implantation. A total of 47% of the patients in the SCS group experienced over 50% pain relief, compared to only 12% in the repeat laminectomy group. The intake of opioids was also statistically significantly higher in the repeat laminectomy group (North et al. 2005). For patients with complex regional pain syndrome, a Level B recommendation supports the positive effects of SCS. In the author's opinion, this could also be Level A evidence, but the quality of the research in terms of selection criteria, randomizing, and bias is limited; accordingly, no Level A recommendations are yet possible.

Table 2. SCS percutaneous trial versus permanent SCS trial

Type	**SCS percutaneous trial**	**Permanent SCS trial**
Technique:	After the placement of the lead on the designated spinal level, the epidural needle is removed. The lead is adhered to the skin using skin glue, surgical sutures (the author's favorite), or surgical adhesive.	After the placement of the lead, a midline incision is made through the skin down to the supraspinous fascia. The lead is anchored with sutures and an anchoring device.
Advantages	1. Less risk of infection 2. Less pain during the trial period (only one incision) 3. Easier to handle	1. No second operation is needed 2. A more cost-effective method since the same device is used for testing and permanent stimulation. The location of the leads remains the same if SCS is permanently implanted.
Disadvantage	1. If successful, a second OR is necessary.	1. Greater risk of infection 2. More local pain after implantation 3. Longer OR time

After the evaluation period and patient selection, SCS implantation, like intrathecal baclofen application, is divided into two phases: trial and permanent. There are two types of SCS trials: percutaneous lead trials and permanent lead trials. Both have advantages and disadvantages (Table 2).

Pain treatment for patients in neurorehabilitation improves their quality of life and thus patient-related factors, such as motivation. SCS is another treatment modality that could significantly impact pain management in selected cases.

Peripheral Nerve Stimulation

Peripheral nerve stimulation (PNS) is yet another treatment modality for patients with chronic pain. As with SCS, in this setting, the leads are placed near the affected nerve, ideally parallel to the selected nerve. Common indications for PNS are median, ulnar, and radial neuropathy; occipital and pudendal neuralgias; femoral and sciatic obturator neuropathy; and brachial and lumbar plexus neuropathy. Since patients in neurorehabilitation may simultaneously suffer from different neuropathies, the most painful one should be treated with PNS first. After fulfilling the selection criteria for PNS, patients undergo a two-phase implantation: trial PNS and permanent implantation. The test phase begins with injecting a local anesthetic precisely where the needle will be placed. Under ultrasound guidance, the needle, which has an electrical stimulator on the tip, is inserted 0.5 cm–1 cm from the selected nerve. If the patient experiences uncomfortable sensations, the needle is placed too superficially. If the patient experiences muscle contractions, the needle is placed too deeply, and readjustments are necessary for optimal placement. Once the correct placement has been determined, the electrical stimulator is removed, and the lead is inserted through the needle. After the lead is placed, the needle is removed, and the lead is connected to an external stimulator. The clinical significance of PNS could dramatically change the paradigm of postoperative opioid pain management. The concept of replacing opioids with perioperative PNS could lead to a drastic reduction in opioid intake for pain management. Several studies have evaluated the feasibility and efficacy of PNS for postoperative pain management. The use of PNS in orthopedic surgery has led to a reduction in opioid intake for postoperative pain management (Ilfeld et al. 2017).

Conclusion

Both orthoses and neurostimulation are useful tools for the complex management of patients in neurorehabilitation. Only a team of experienced physicians can comprehend the diversity and complexity of neurorehabilitation patients. Pain control and management leads to an improvement in the patient's motivation and ability to participate in rehabilitation. The orthoses, on the other hand, use the patient's own capabilities, extend the range of motion, and improve the precision of the motion and the quality of life.

References

Abu Talh, Khandaker, Mohammad Sulaiman, Deepak Joshi, and Sameh Hamed. 2017. "Development of Parkinsonism symptoms immediately after severe head injury." *Neurosciences (Riyadh, Saudi Arabia)* 22 (4):308-310. doi: 10.17712/nsj.2017.4.20170240.

Albright, A. L. 1996. "Baclofen in the treatment of cerebral palsy." *J Child Neurol* 11 (2):77-83. doi: 10.1177/088307389601100202.

Campbell, James H. 2006. "Linked Hip-Knee-Ankle-Foot Orthoses Designed for Reciprocal Gait." *JPO: Journal of Prosthetics and Orthotics* 18 (7).

Cantillo-Negrete, Jessica, Ruben I. Carino-Escobar, Paul Carrillo-Mora, Marlene A. Rodriguez-Barragan, Claudia Hernandez-Arenas, Jimena Quinzaños-Fresnedo, Isauro R. Hernandez-Sanchez, Marlene A. Galicia-Alvarado, Adan Miguel-Puga, and Oscar Arias-Carrion. 2021. "Brain-Computer Interface Coupled to a Robotic Hand Orthosis for Stroke Patients' Neurorehabilitation: A Crossover Feasibility Study." *Frontiers in Human Neuroscience* 15 (293). doi: 10.3389/fnhum.2021. 656975.

Dimitrijevic, M. R., J. Faganel, P. C. Sharkey, and A. M. Sherwood. 1980. "Study of sensation and muscle twitch responses to spinal cord stimulation." *Int Rehabil Med* 2 (2):76-81. doi: 10.3109/09638288009163961.

Edelstein, Joan E, and Jan Bruckner. 2002. *Orthotics: a comprehensive clinical approach*: Slack Incorporated.

Frisoli, Antonio, Massimiliano Solazzi, Claudio Loconsole, and Michele Barsotti. 2016. "New generation emerging technologies for neurorehabilitation and motor assistance." *Acta myologica: myopathies and cardiomyopathies: official journal of the Mediterranean Society of Myology* 35 (3):141-144.

Garcia K, Wray JK, Kumar S. 2021 Jan-. "Spinal Cord Stimulation. [Updated 2021 Apr 7]. In: *StatPearls* [Internet]. Treasure Island (FL): StatPearls Publishing;." *https://www.ncbi.nlm.nih.gov/books/NBK553154/?report=classic*.

Ghanavatian S, Derian A. 2021 Jan-. "Baclofen. [Updated 2021 May 15]. In: *StatPearls* [Internet]. Treasure Island (FL): StatPearls Publishing;." doi: https://www.ncbi.nlm.nih.gov/books/NBK526037/.

Halter, J., V. Dolenc, M. R. Dimitrijevic, and P. C. Sharkey. 1983. "Neurophysiological assessment of electrode placement in the spinal cord." *Appl Neurophysiol* 46 (1-4):124-8. doi: 10.1159/000101251.

Hebert, Jackie S. 2006. "Ambulatory KAFOs: A Physiatry Perspective." *JPO: Journal of Prosthetics and Orthotics* 18 (7).

Hoogendam, J. M., G. M. Ramakers, and V. Di Lazzaro. 2010. "Physiology of repetitive transcranial magnetic stimulation of the human brain." *Brain Stimul* 3 (2):95-118. doi: 10.1016/j.brs.2009.10.005.

Ilfeld, Brian M., Christopher A. Gilmore, Stuart A. Grant, Michael P. Bolognesi, Daniel J. Del Gaizo, Amorn Wongsarnpigoon, and Joseph W. Boggs. 2017. "Ultrasound-guided percutaneous peripheral nerve stimulation for analgesia following total knee arthroplasty: a prospective feasibility study." *Journal of orthopaedic surgery and research* 12 (1):4-4. doi: 10.1186/s13018-016-0506-7.

Issar, N. M., P. Hedera, F. T. Phibbs, P. E. Konrad, and J. S. Neimat. 2013. "Treating post-traumatic tremor with deep brain stimulation: report of five cases." *Parkinsonism Relat Disord* 19 (12):1100-5. doi: 10.1016/j.parkreldis.2013.07.022.

Jang, S. H. 2013. "Motor function-related maladaptive plasticity in stroke: a review." *NeuroRehabilitation* 32 (2):311-6. doi: 10.3233/nre-130849.

Kim, Deog Young, Seung Ki Kim, Jong Bum Park, and Jin Kyu Yang. 2013. "Effects of Ankle Foot Orthosis on Post-stroke Hemiplegic Gait -A Meta-analysis." *bn* 6 (1):1-8. doi: 10.12786/bn.2013.6.1.1.

Koleva, K., O. Pavlov, R. Nikolov, and R. Behr. 2020. "Deep brain stimulation as a possible treatment of hyperthermia in patients with serotonin syndrome." *Med Hypotheses* 139:109704. doi: 10.1016/j.mehy.2020.109704.

Kumar, K., C. Toth, R. K. Nath, and P. Laing. 1998. "Epidural spinal cord stimulation for treatment of chronic pain--some predictors of success. A 15-year experience." *Surg Neurol* 50 (2):110-20; discussion 120-1. doi: 10.1016/s0090-3019(98)00012-3.

Lefaucheur, J. P., N. André-Obadia, A. Antal, S. S. Ayache, C. Baeken, D. H. Benninger, R. M. Cantello, M. Cincotta, M. de Carvalho, D. De Ridder, H. Devanne, V. Di Lazzaro, S. R. Filipović, F. C. Hummel, S. K. Jääskeläinen, V. K. Kimiskidis, G. Koch, B. Langguth, T. Nyffeler, A. Oliviero, F. Padberg, E. Poulet, S. Rossi, P. M. Rossini, J. C. Rothwell, C. Schönfeldt-Lecuona, H. R. Siebner, C. W. Slotema, C. J. Stagg, J. Valls-Sole, U. Ziemann, W. Paulus, and L. Garcia-Larrea. 2014. "Evidence-based guidelines on the therapeutic use of repetitive transcranial magnetic stimulation (rTMS)." *Clin Neurophysiol* 125 (11):2150-2206. doi: 10.1016/j.clinph. 2014.05.021.

Lo, A. C., P. D. Guarino, L. G. Richards, J. K. Haselkorn, G. F. Wittenberg, D. G. Federman, R. J. Ringer, T. H. Wagner, H. I. Krebs, B. T. Volpe, C. T. Bever, Jr., D. M. Bravata, P. W. Duncan, B. H. Corn, A. D. Maffucci, S. E. Nadeau, S. S. Conroy, J. M. Powell, G. D. Huang, and P. Peduzzi. 2010. "Robot-assisted therapy for long-term upper-limb impairment after stroke." *N Engl J Med* 362 (19):1772-83. doi: 10.1056/NEJMoa0911341.

Machida, M., S. L. Weinstein, T. Yamada, and J. Kimura. 1985. "Spinal cord monitoring. Electrophysiological measures of sensory and motor function during spinal surgery." *Spine (Phila Pa 1976)* 10 (5):407-13.

McDaid, Catriona, Debra Fayter, Alison Booth, Joanne O'Connor, Rocio Rodriguez-Lopez, Dorothy McCaughan, Roy Bowers, Cynthia P. Iglesias, Simon Lalor, Rory J. O'Connor, Margaret Phillips, and Gita Ramdharry. 2017. "Systematic review of the evidence on orthotic devices for the management of knee instability related to neuromuscular and central nervous system disorders." *BMJ open* 7 (9):e015927-e015927. doi: 10.1136/bmjopen-2017-015927.

Melzack, R., and P. D. Wall. 1965. "Pain mechanisms: a new theory." *Science* 150 (3699):971-9. doi: 10.1126/science.150.3699.971.

Miller, J. P., S. Eldabe, E. Buchser, L. M. Johanek, Y. Guan, and B. Linderoth. 2016. "Parameters of Spinal Cord Stimulation and Their Role in Electrical Charge Delivery: A Review." *Neuromodulation* 19 (4):373-84. doi: 10.1111/ner.12438.

North, R. B., D. H. Kidd, F. Farrokhi, and S. A. Piantadosi. 2005. "Spinal cord stimulation versus repeated lumbosacral spine surgery for chronic pain: a randomized, controlled trial." *Neurosurgery* 56 (1):98-106; discussion 106-7. doi: 10.1227/01.neu.0000144839.65524.e0.

Riener. R., (2016). *Technology of the Robotic Gait Orthosis Lokomat, Neurorehabilitation Technology*.

Rosanova, Mario, Olivia Gosseries, Silvia Casarotto, Mélanie Boly, Adenauer G. Casali, Marie-Aurélie Bruno, Maurizio Mariotti, Pierre Boveroux, Giulio Tononi, Steven Laureys, and Marcello Massimini. 2012. "Recovery of cortical effective connectivity and recovery of consciousness in vegetative patients." *Brain* 135 (4):1308-1320. doi: 10.1093/brain/awr340.

Rudin, D. O., and G. Eisenman. 1954. "The action potential of spinal axons in vitro." *J Gen Physiol* 37 (4):505-38. doi: 10.1085/jgp.37.4.505.

Santin-Amo, José María, Ana Flores-Justa, Paula Román-Pena, Martín Raposo-Furelos, Carla Frieiro-Dantas, Ramón Serramito García, Juan Manuel Villa, and Miguel Gelabert-González. 2019. "Baclofeno intratecal para el tratamiento de la espasticidad: revisión de los casos presentes tratados en nuestro servicio." *Neurocirugía* 30 (6):288-293. doi: https://doi.org/10.1016/j.neucir.2019.05.001.

Sdrulla, A. D., Y. Guan, and S. N. Raja. 2018. "Spinal Cord Stimulation: Clinical Efficacy and Potential Mechanisms." *Pain Pract* 18 (8):1048-1067. doi: 10.1111/ papr.12692.

Shealy, C. N., J. T. Mortimer, and J. B. Reswick. 1967. "Electrical inhibition of pain by stimulation of the dorsal columns: preliminary clinical report." *Anesth Analg* 46 (4):489-91.

Smits, H., M. van Kleef, J. Holsheimer, and E. A. Joosten. 2013. "Experimental spinal cord stimulation and neuropathic pain: mechanism of action, technical aspects, and effectiveness." *Pain Pract* 13 (2):154-68. doi: 10.1111/j.1533-2500.2012.00579.x.

Takeuchi, N., and S. Izumi. 2012. "Maladaptive plasticity for motor recovery after stroke: mechanisms and approaches." *Neural Plast* 2012:359728. doi: 10.1155/2012/359 728.

Tsubokawa, T, T Yamamoto, Y Katayama, T Hirayama, S Maejima, and T Moriya. 1990. "Deep-brain stimulation in a persistent vegetative state: follow-up results and criteria for selection of candidates." *Brain Inj* 4:315-327. doi: 10.3109/02699059009026185.

Young, Joshua, and Cameron Moss. 2019. "Orthotic care needs in a cohort of neurological rehabilitation inpatients." *Disability and Rehabilitation: Assistive Technology*:1-5. doi: 10.1080/17483107.2019.1685018.

About the Editors

Dr. V. D. Sinha
Senior Professor and Ex-Head of Department
Department of Neurosurgery
SMS. Medical College and Hospital, Jaipur, India

Dr. Amit Chakraborty
Senior Consultant and Neurosurgeon
Eternal Hospital, Jaipur, India

Dr. Jitin Bajaj
Associate Professor, Department of Neurosurgery,
Superspeciality Hospital, NSCB Medical College, Jabalpur, India
Email: bajaj.jitin@ gmail.com

Dr. Gaurav Jain
Assistant Professor, Neurosurgery,
SMS Medical College and Hospital, Jaipur, India
Email: drgauravjain9@gmail.com

Amit Agrawal
Department of Neurosurgery, All India Institute of Medical Sciences,
Bhopal, Madhya Pradesh, India
Email: dramitagrawal@gmail.com

Index

T

V